Talley & O'Connor's Clinical Examination

A guide to specialty examinations

9th edition

VOLUME TWO

Talley & O'Connor's Clinical Examination

A guide to specialty examinations

9th edition

VOLUME TWO

NICHOLAS J TALLEY

MBBS (Hons)(NSW), MD (NSW), PhD (Syd), MMedSci (Clin Epi)(Newc.), FRACP, FAFPHM, FAHMS, FRCP (Lond. & Edin.), FACP, FACG, AGAF, FAMS, FRCPI (Hon)

Distinguished Laureate Professor, University of Newcastle and Senior Staff Specialist, John Hunter Hospital, NSW, Australia; Adjunct Professor, Mayo Clinic, Rochester, MN, USA; Adjunct Professor, University of North Carolina, Chapel Hill, NC, USA; Foreign Guest Professor, Karolinska Institutet, Stockholm, Sweden

SIMON O'CONNOR

FRACP, DDU, FCSANZ

Cardiologist, The Canberra Hospital, Canberra;
Senior Clinical Lecturer, Australian National University Medical School, Canberra, ACT, Australia

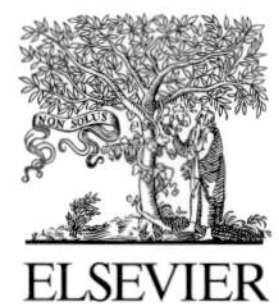

ELSEVIER

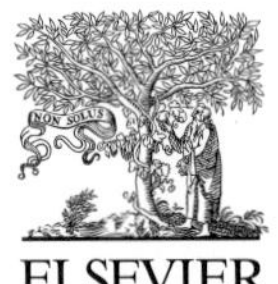

ELSEVIER

Elsevier Australia. ACN 001 002 357
(a division of Reed International Books Australia Pty Ltd)
Tower 1, 475 Victoria Avenue, Chatswood, NSW 2067

ISBN: 978-0-7295-4438-2

National Library of Australia Cataloguing-in-Publication Data

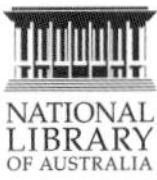

A catalogue record for this book is available from the National Library of Australia

Head of Content: Larissa Norrie
Content Project Manager: Shubham Dixit
Edited by Chris Wyard
Proofread by Melissa Faulkner
Permissions Editing and Photo Research: Priyadarshini Gnanasurian
Cover design by Georgette Hall
Typeset and Index by Aptara
Printed in Singapore

Last digit is the print number: 9 8 7 6 5 4 3 2 1

Foreword

Medicine is so broad a field, so closely interwoven with general interests, dealing as it does with all ages, sexes and classes, and yet of so personal a character in its individual appreciations, that it must be regarded as one of those great departments of work in which the cooperation of men and women is needed to fulfill all its requirements.

Dr Elizabeth Blackwell
(first woman physician in the USA)

Talley & O'Connor has long been a favourite amongst students, noted for its clarity, clear diagrams, tables and of course the 'essentials' boxes. This latest edition places clinical methods within their historical context, from the time when disease was viewed as having a single cause to our current understanding of illness as a biopsychosociocultural phenomenon. In the past 12 months we have seen both of these truths in action as we have experienced a pandemic, sparked by a single entity known as the SARS-CoV-2 virus. The virus has set off a flywheel of reactions that began with the identification of a strange new disease initiated using the tried and tested clinical methods described within these pages. While the stethoscope, thermometer and watch were close clinical companions during the realisation of the importance of the emerging problem, it was the eyes and ears of clinicians that enabled the first alarm to be raised. Ensuring that the next generation of clinicians continues to build a solid foundation grounded in the clinical method of history and examination will be made much easier by continuing access to resources such as *T&O'C*. For all those who pick up this text, may you use your eyes, your ears and your hands as described in this book, but—most importantly—may you bring your whole self to every clinical encounter and listen to the patient with an open and curious mind.

Professor Jane Gunn
FAHMS, FRACGP, PhD, MBBS, MAICD
Dean of Medicine, Dentistry and Health Science, and
Chair of Primary Care Research
The University of Melbourne,
VIC, Australia
May, 2021

Contents

Preface

Listen to your patient, he (she) is telling you the diagnosis.

Sir William Osler (1849–1918)

Diagnosticians are great medical detectives who apply rigorous methodology to uncover the truth, solve a puzzle and commence the healing process.

Nick Talley & Simon O'Connor
Clinical Examination, 2017

Clinical medicine is exciting, and clinical skills continue to form the basis of modern clinical practice in order to make an accurate diagnosis. Thirty-five years ago, encouraged by the success of our first textbook on clinical skills *Examination Medicine,* which was aimed at postgraduate physician trainees sitting their barrier specialist internal medicine examinations, we set out to write *Clinical Examination*. The textbook was written over a year while we were senior registrars at the Royal North Shore Hospital, a major teaching hospital of the University of Sydney, Australia. Our goal was simple but ambitious: to write a new type of clinical skills textbook that would speak (and appeal) to medical students in all their clinical years from first patient exposure to final examinations (and beyond), and to teach a modern, systematic and comprehensive method of history taking and examination including an approach to rigorous clinical thinking and diagnosis.

A number of innovations have aided the success of this textbook and have been employed again here. The text is carefully organised and illustrated to maximise comprehension, including chapter summaries, essential lists and useful tables. Full-colour illustrations provide a visual guide for key signs including ethnic variations so important to recognise in clinical practice. We have included amusing comments and anecdotes with the view that optimal learning must be fun. We've added historical footnotes because these can be an *aide-mémoire*, and we believe students should know medicine is ever changing but we all stand on the shoulders of those who came before us. Videos illustrate how to examine in real time.

The book has extensively evolved over multiple editions and includes all specialty areas taught in undergraduate curriculums. We are pleased that generations of students have responded so positively to each edition, and medical schools around the world have adopted the textbook in their medical degree programs. We were very proud to be awarded First Prize in the Medicine category in the 2018 British Medical Association (BMA) Medical Book Awards, and hope this brand new revised edition will be similarly well received.

Every edition including the current one has undergone rigorous peer review by experts, and we have paid careful attention to the comments and suggestions. The book has received numerous reviews in major journals and readers have sent us many suggestions, and again we have taken the opportunity to try and address all reasonable recommendations with every revision. Before embarking on each revision, we also conduct a thorough literature search to identify new key references that inform the text and, where necessary, new references are added (and old ones replaced) for further reading. A strong emphasis on evidence-based medicine continues to permeate this edition. This is because today it takes only about 3 months for existing medical knowledge to double in size, compared with about 50 years mid last century. Despite rapidly accelerating knowledge, an understanding of the diagnostic value of important symptoms and signs is essential to excellent clinical practice. There remain huge research gaps and we hope readers of this book will aspire to fill many of them in the coming years.

The SARS-CoV-2 pandemic has shaken the globe and emphasised the importance of clinical skills and expertise in frontline care. We want to acknowledge all of the expert contributors to this new edition who willingly assisted us despite the pandemic, and the excellent peer reviewers and everyone who has provided us with feedback and encouragement. Do write to the publisher with any suggestions. We also thank all our colleagues and patients who continue to educate and inspire us on a daily basis.

Nicholas J. Talley, AC
Simon O'Connor
Newcastle and Canberra, 2021

Acknowledgements

This book provides an evidence-based account of clinical skills. We are very grateful for the reviews, comments and suggestions from the many outstanding colleagues over the years who have helped us to develop and refine this book. All chapters have again been peer reviewed, a hallmark of our books, and we have taken great care to revise the material based on the detailed reviews obtained. We take responsibility for any errors or omissions.

We would like to especially acknowledge **Professor Ian Symonds**, Dean of Medicine, University of Adelaide, and **Professor Kichu Nair**, Professor of Medicine and Associate Dean Continuing Medical Professional Development, University of Newcastle, for helping produce the videos for the OSCEs.

Dr Tom Wellings, Staff Specialist in Neurology, John Hunter Hospital, provided expert input into the neurology chapters for this edition. **Dr Philip McManis** provided invaluable input into neurology for earlier editions. **Professor Alan Cooper** prepared the original dermatology chapter.

Dr A Manoharan and **Dr J Isbister** provided the original blood film photographs and the accompanying text. **Associate Professor L Schreiber** provided the original section on soft-tissue rheumatology. We have revised and updated all of these sections again.

We thank **Professor Alex Ford** (Leeds Teaching Hospitals Trust, UK) and his team for their systematic review of the evidence supporting (or refuting) key clinical signs that has been retained.

Professor Brian Kelly, Dean of Medicine at the University of Newcastle, provided valuable comments on the psychiatry chapter. **Professor Phillip Boyce** provided the original psychiatry chapter.

Thank you to **Dr Malcolm Thomson** who provided a number of the X-rays and scans for this title. Others have been provided by the Medical Imaging Department at the Canberra Hospital X-ray Library.

We would like to thank **Associate Professor Lindsay Rowe**, Staff Specialist Radiologist at the John Hunter Hospital, for preparing the text and images within the gastrointestinal system section retained from the last edition.

We would like to acknowledge and thank **Glenn McCulloch** for the photographs he supplied for this title. We would also like to acknowledge Coleman **Productions** and the **Hunter Medical Research Institute** who provided with photographic assistance.

The authors thank **Dr Michael Potter, Dr. Yamini Yadav** and **Dr Stephen Brienesse** for their assistance. The authors and publishers also wish to thank **Jasmine Wark**, BBiomedSc, DipLang for her expert editorial support.

Elsevier Australia and the authors extend their appreciation to the following reviewers for their comments and insights on the entire manuscript:

REVIEWERS

Carlos El-Haddad, MBBS, PhD candidate, FRACP, Conjoint Lecturer, School of Medicine, Western Sydney University, Campbelltown, NSW, Australia

Randall Faull, MBBS, PhD, FRACP, FRCP, Royal Adelaide Hospital, Adelaide, SA, Australia

Stephen Fuller, MBBS, PhD, FRACP, FRCPA, The University of Sydney Nepean Clinical School, Faculty of Medicine and Health, The University of Sydney, NSW, Australia

Wayne Harris, MBBS, MRCP(UK), FRACP, Department of Paediatrics and Child Health, University of Queensland, Brisbane; Ipswich Hospital, West Moreton Health District, Ipswich, QLD, Australia

Andrew Korda, MBBS, AMMA, FRCOG, FRANZCOG, Conjoint Professor of Obstetrics and Gynaecology, Western Sydney University, Sydney, NSW, Australia

Kypros Kyprianou, MBBS, FRACP, Department of General Paediatrics, Monash Children's Hospital, Clayton, VIC, Australia

Sue Lynn Lau, MBBS, Grad Dip Med Stat, PhD, FRACP, Western Sydney University, University of Sydney, Western Sydney Local Health District, NSW, Australia

Jennifer Martin, MBBS, MA, PhD, Chair of Clinical Pharmacology, School of Medicine and Public Health, The University of Newcastle, NSW, Australia

Peter Pockney, BSc, MBBS, DM, FRCS (Gen Surg), FRACS, Conjoint Snr Lecturer Surgery, NHMRC Centre of Research Excellence in Digestive Health, University of Newcastle, NSW, Australia

David Simmons, MBBS, MD (Cantab), MA (Hons Cantab), FRACP, FRCP, Western Sydney University, South Western Sydney Local Health District, NSW, Australia

Saxon D Smith, MBChB, GAICD, MHL, PhD, FAMA, IFAAD, FACD, The Dermatology and Skin Cancer Centre, St Leonards, NSW, Australia; Sydney Adventist Hospital, Wahroonga, NSW, Australia

Joerg Mattes, MBBS, MD, PhD, FRACP, Professor and Chair of Paediatrics & Child Health; Director Priority Research Centre GrowUpWell; BMedSc/MD Joint Medical Program Convenor HMRI, University of Newcastle, Newcastle, NSW, Australia; Senior Staff Specialist, Department of Paediatric Respiratory & Sleep Medicine, John Hunter Children's Hospital, Australia

Bryony Ross, BBiomedSc, MBBS, FRACP, FRCPA, Consultant Haematologist and Haematopathologist, Children's Hospital at Westmead; Conjoint Lecturer at the University of Newcastle, NSW, Australia

Ian Symonds, BMBS, MMedSci, MD, FRCOG, FRANZCOG, Dean of Medicine, Professor of Obstetrics & Gynaecology, International Medical University, Malaysia; University of Adelaide, SA, Australia

CONTRIBUTORS

Wendy Carseldine, MBBS, BSc(Hons), FRANZCOG, DDU, MPH, CMFM, Consultant Obstetrician and Gynaecologist, Maternal Fetal Medicine Subspecialist, John Hunter Hospital, NSW, Australia

Clinical methods: an historical perspective

The best physician is the one who is able to differentiate the possible and the impossible.

Herophilus of Alexandria (335–280BC)

Since classical Greek times interrogation of the patient has been considered most important because disease was, and still is, viewed in terms of the discomfort it causes. However, the current emphasis on the use of history taking and physical examination for diagnosis developed only in the 19th century. Although the terms 'symptoms and signs' have been part of the medical vocabulary since the revival of classical medicine, until relatively recently they were used synonymously. During the 19th century, the distinction between *symptoms* (subjective complaints, which the clinician learns from the patient's account of his or her feelings) and *signs* (objective morbid changes detectable by the clinician) evolved. Until the 19th century, diagnosis was empirical and based on the classical Greek belief that all disease had a single cause: an imbalance of the four humours (yellow bile, black bile, blood and phlegm). Indeed the Royal College of Physicians, founded in London in 1518, believed that clinical experience without classical learning was useless, and physicians who were College members were fined if they ascribed to any other view. At the time of Hippocrates (460?–375BC), observation (inspection) and feeling (palpation) had a place in the examination of patients. The ancient Greeks, for example, noticed that patients with jaundice often had an enlarged liver that was firm and irregular. Shaking a patient and listening for a fluid splash was also recognised by the Greeks. Herophilus of Alexandria (335–280BC) described a method of taking the pulse in the 4th century BC. However, it was Galen of Pergamum (AD130–200) who established the pulse as one of the major physical signs, and it continued to have this important role up to the 18th century, with minute variations being recorded. These variations were erroneously considered to indicate changes in the body's harmony. William Harvey's (1578–1657) studies of the human circulation, published in 1628, had little effect on the general understanding of the value of the pulse as a sign. Sanctorius (1561–1636) was the first to time the pulse using a clock, while John Floyer (1649–1734) invented the pulse watch in 1707 and made regular observations of the pulse rate. Abnormalities in heart rate were described in diabetes mellitus in 1776 and in thyrotoxicosis in 1786. Fever was studied by Hippocrates and was originally regarded as an entity rather than a sign of disease. The thermoscope was devised by Sanctorius in 1625. In association with Gabriel Fahrenheit (1686–1736), Hermann Boerhaave (1668–1738) introduced the thermometer as a research instrument and this was produced commercially in the middle of the 18th century. In the 13th century Johannes Actuarius (d. 1283) used a graduated glass to examine the urine. In Harvey's time a specimen of urine was sometimes looked at (inspected) and even tasted, and was considered to reveal secrets about the body. Harvey recorded that sugar diabetes (mellitus) and dropsy (oedema) could be diagnosed in this way. The detection of protein in the urine, which Frederik Dekkers (1644–1720) first described in 1673, was ignored until Richard Bright (1789–1858) demonstrated its importance in renal disease. Although Celsus described and valued measurements such as weighing and measuring a patient in the 1st century AD, these methods became widely used only in the 20th century. A renaissance in clinical methods began with the concept of Battista Morgagni (1682–1771) that disease was not generalised but rather arose in organs, a conclusion published in 1761. Leopold Auenbrugger invented chest tapping (percussion) to detect disease in the same year. Van Swieten, his teacher, in fact used percussion to detect ascites. The technique was forgotten for nearly half a century until Jean Corvisart (1755–1821) translated Auenbrugger's work in 1808.

The next big step occurred with René Laënnec (1781–1826), a student of Corvisart. He invented the stethoscope in 1816 (at first merely a roll of stiff paper) as an aid to diagnosing heart and lung disease by listening (auscultation). This revolutionised chest examination, partly because it made the chest accessible in patients too modest to allow a direct application of the examiner's ear to the chest wall, as well as allowing accurate clinicopathological correlations. William Stokes (1804–78) published the first treatise in English on the use of the stethoscope in 1825. Josef Skoda's (1805–81) investigations of the value of these clinical methods led to their widespread and enthusiastic adoption after he published his results in 1839. These advances helped lead to a change in the practice of medicine. Bedside teaching was first introduced in the Renaissance by Montanus (1498–1552) in Padua in 1543. In the 17th century, physicians based their opinion on a history provided by an apothecary (assistant) and rarely saw the patients themselves. Thomas Sydenham (1624–89) began to practise more modern bedside medicine, basing his treatment on experience and not theory, but it was not until a century later that the scientific method brought a systematic approach to clinical diagnosis.

This change began in the hospitals of Paris after the French Revolution, with recognition of the work of Morgagni, Corvisart, Laënnec and others. Influenced by the philosophy of the Enlightenment, which suggested that a rational approach to all problems was possible, the Paris Clinical School combined physical examination with autopsy as the basis of clinical medicine. The methods of this school were first applied abroad in Dublin, where Robert Graves (1796–1853) and William Stokes worked. Later, at Guy's Hospital in London, the famous trio of Richard Bright, Thomas Addison (1793–1860) and Thomas Hodgkin (1798–1866) made their important contributions. In 1869 Samuel Wilks (1824–1911) wrote on the nail changes in disease and the signs he described remain important. Carl Wunderlich's (1815–77) work changed the concept of temperature from a disease in itself to a symptom of disease. Spectacular advances in physiology, pathology, pharmacology and the discovery of microbiology in the latter half of the 19th century led to the development of the new 'clinical and laboratory medicine', which is the rapidly advancing medicine of the present day. The modern systematic approach to diagnosis, with which this book deals, is still, however, based on taking the history and examining the patient by looking (inspecting), feeling (palpating), tapping (percussing) and listening (auscultating).

Suggested reading

Bordage G. Where are the history and the physical? *Can Med Assoc J* 1995; 152:1595–1598.

McDonald C. Medical heuristics: the silent adjudicators of clinical practice. *Ann Intern Med* 1996; 124:56–62.

Reiser SJ. The clinical record in medicine. Part I: Learning from cases. *Ann Intern Med* 1991; 114:902–907.

The Hippocratic oath

I swear by Apollo the physician, and Aesculapius, and Hygieia, and Panacea, and all the gods and goddesses that, according to my ability and judgment, I will keep this Oath and this stipulation: To reckon him who taught me this Art equally dear to me as my parents, to share my substance with him and relieve his necessities if required; to look upon his offspring in the same footing as my own brother, and to teach them this Art, if they shall wish to learn it, without fee or stipulation, and that by precept, lecture, and every other mode of instruction, I will impart a knowledge of the Art to my own sons and those of my teachers, and to disciples bound by a stipulation and oath according to the law of medicine, but to none others. I will follow that system of regimen which, according to my ability and judgment, I consider for the benefit of my patients, and abstain from whatever is deleterious and mischievous. I will give no deadly medicine to any if asked, nor suggest any such counsel; and in like manner I will not give a woman a pessary to produce abortion. With purity and with holiness I will pass my life and practise my Art. I will not cut persons laboring under the stone, but will leave this to be done by men who are practitioners of this work. Into whatever houses I enter I will go into them for the benefit of the sick and will abstain from every voluntary act of mischief and corruption; and further from the seduction of females or males, of freemen and slaves. Whatever, in connection with my professional practice, or not in connection with it, I may see or hear in the lives of men which ought not to be spoken of abroad I will not divulge, as reckoning that all such should be kept secret. While I continue to keep this Oath unviolated may it be granted to me to enjoy life and the practice of the Art, respected by all men, in all times! But should I trespass and violate this Oath, may the reverse be my lot!

Hippocrates, born on the Island of Cos (c.460–357 BC) is agreed by everyone to be the father of medicine. He is said to have lived to the age of 109. Many of the statements in this ancient oath remain relevant today, while others, such as euthanasia and abortion, remain controversial. The seduction of slaves, however, is less of a problem.

SECTION 10

Paediatric and neonatal history and examination

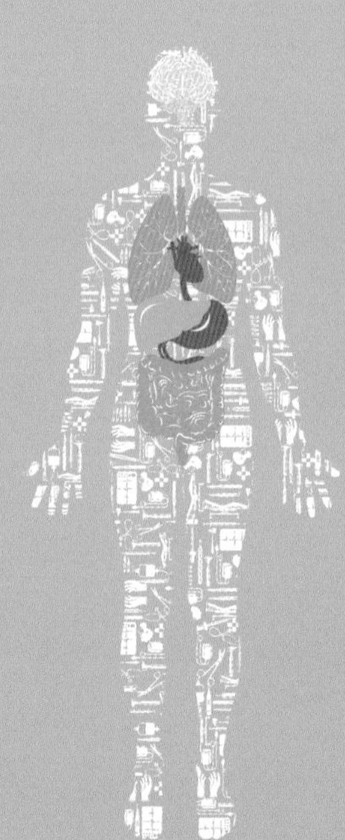

CHAPTER 37

The paediatric history and examination

Joerg Mattes and Bryony Ross

Medicine cannot exist without observation of the patient. HIPPOCRATES (460?–357BC)

PRINCIPLES OF PAEDIATRIC HISTORY TAKING AND EXAMINATION

Children are not simply little adults: the history taking and physical examination of these little people needs to be tailored to their specific needs. Like the neonatal examination (and often more so) physical examination in childhood is opportunistic: trying slavishly to follow a set sequence will almost always end in frustration and tears for the clinician, the parents and, most importantly, the child. Much of the paediatric examination is, however, identical or very similar to that of the adult. To avoid unnecessary repetition, this chapter focuses mainly on where the paediatric examination differs from that of the adult examination.

In contrast to the neonatal examination, there is no consensus regarding the timing and regularity of the paediatric examination. Many clinicians use the immunisation schedule as a convenient routine for the evaluation of children in their care. The American Academy of Paediatrics suggests that every school-aged child should have a complete physical examination and health evaluation every 1–2 years.[1]

The principal aims of well-child examination in school-aged children (kindergarten to early adolescence) are:[2]

- promoting health
- detecting disease
- counselling to prevent injury and future health problems.

It is generally accepted that children should have a physical examination every time they present to a clinician. These examinations should not be restricted to the part of the body considered to be the basis of the presenting complaint. The purpose and scope of the examination needs to be explained to the parents and child (particularly to adolescents) and should take into account their level of understanding. If any part of the examination will be physically or psychologically uncomfortable, the parents and child should be informed in advance.[3]

PAEDIATRIC HISTORY TAKING

The paediatric history is somewhat unique in medicine in that in most cases it is given by someone other than the patient—this is usually one or both parents. Children and teenagers, however, have much to say—their input in the history is extremely useful. It is important to involve children in this process, but their level of maturity should be taken into account. If the child is old enough to understand, it is best to direct simple questions to the child but in many cases to expect that the parent will answer or even repeat the question to the child, almost as an interpreter. In many cases it may be preferable to interview adolescents without their parents at some point (see section 'Adolescent history and examination' later in the chapter). Reassuring the adolescent at the start of the consultation that matters discussed will be kept confidential is a must.[4] Equally important, however, is also explaining to the adolescent when this confidentiality *may* be broken. (See 'Screening of development and social interactions' below and Table 37.19 on p 708.)

History-taking sequence

1. Review the history of the presenting chief complaints under the following headings using the mnemonic **SIC**:
   S ymptoms [severity, frequency, triggers, treatments]
   I nvestigations
   C omplications.
2. Then address any other concerns raised by the patient or the parents.
3. Perform a systems review, which is useful to cover any information that may have been omitted. It is often easiest for this to be remembered as a 'top-to-toe' checklist of questions to ask the carer (and the child as appropriate, according to the developmental stage) or young person (see Text box 37.1).
4. Next collect the antenatal and birth history (see Ch 38).
5. Ask about medications (including dose, frequency and adherence), relevant environmental exposures (e.g. tobacco smoke).
6. Ask whether immunisations are up to date (see https://www.health.gov.au/sites/default/files/national-immunisation-program-schedule-portrait.pdf for the current Australian vaccination schedule).
7. Find out whether there are any known drug allergies. Ask about other allergies and / or intolerances. Ask specifically about food allergies, asthma, eczema and hay fever.
   Ask whether there is a family history of inherited diseases. Are the child's parents related (consanguinity)?
8. Have there been unexplained premature deaths in the family?
9. Explore the psychosocial history by asking questions using the mnemonic **BEST CARE**:
   BEhavioural history: this should cover any unusual behaviours (such as frequent temper tantrums), sleep disturbances or phobias, and toileting problems (such as encopresis[a] and bed wetting).
   Screening of development and social interactions: a quick developmental surveillance in the school-aged child should cover school performance, vision, hearing, speech, gross- and fine-motor function, and social interaction. A more structured screening can be of particular importance in adolescents (HEEADSSS assessment). Ideally, this should be performed without the parents present and, again, concepts around confidentiality should be explained and respected (see Table 37.19 on p 709).
   Typical day: asking the parents to describe a typical day can give an idea of their living conditions and social history. Also check the child's habits regarding physical activity, food and diet, sleep, dental care practices and safety (e.g. use of bike helmets, seatbelts).
   Coping with hospitalisation and/or disease: explore how well the parents understand the current situation and their expectations for the future.
   Access to healthcare: find out whether the family lives in a remote area, or has transport available.
   Relationships: discuss how members of the family get on with each other, extended family support and any alternative care arrangements. Is the child in foster care? Who are the primary carers? Does the child spend time between family members?
   Effect of illness on the child and family: find out how limitations in physical, cognitive, emotional, and social functioning and the dependence on services impact on the child, siblings and parents. This is particularly important in children and teenagers with chronic medical and / or neurodevelopmental conditions (e.g. cerebral palsy, autism, Down syndrome).
10. Conclude the history by ensuring that you and the family have a shared understanding of what the main issues are. Ask the family whether there are any other concerns or issues that haven't been covered so far.

[a] Faecal incontinence of psychological cause.

The top-to-toe checklist

System	Sample questions
Head	Does your child have headaches? Has your child ever hurt his or her head?
Eyes	Does your child have blurred vision or double vision?
Ears	Have your child's ears been sore? Has your child ever had an ear infection or muck coming out of the ears?
Nose	Does your child have problems with a bleeding nose? Does anything other than snot ever come out of your child's nose? (Discharge) Does your child snore loudly?
Mouth and throat	Has your child ever had trouble swallowing food or drinks? Does your child brush their teeth after eating?
Neck	Have you ever noticed any lumps in your child's neck? If so, were they sore? Stable in size on growing? (Lymphadenopathy) Does your child have trouble keeping their neck straight? (Torticollis)
Chest	Does your child get more short of breath than his or her friends when playing sport? Does your child get wheezy? Does your child have problems with a cough? Does your child cough anything up?
Abdomen	Does your child often vomit or get pains in the tummy? Has your child had problems with runny poo when going to the toilet? Does your child sometimes find it difficult to do a poo?
Genitourinary	Does your child have pain when passing urine? Has there ever been blood in your child's urine? *For girls:* Have you ever noticed any discharge from your vagina? At what age did your periods begin? Tell me about your periods: are they painful? Do they occur regularly? Is there much blood? Are you sexually active?
Endocrine	Has your child been drinking more water lately? Does your child need to urinate at night? Has your child had more or less energy lately?
Neurological	Has your child had problems with dizziness? Tell me what it feels like. Has your child ever had a fit? Have you noticed weakness in your child's arms or legs?
Skin	Has your child had any rashes on the skin? Are they itchy? Does your child get many bruises?

TEXT BOX 37.1

GENERAL PHYSICAL EXAMINATION

(For a general summary see Text box 37.2.)

Preparing for the examination

Before you start the physical examination, roll up your sleeves to above the elbow. Clean your hands and forearms with ethanol-based hand disinfectant or soap and water before and after contact with children, before and after any procedure or exposure to bodily fluids and after touching the child's surroundings. Hand hygiene is crucial for the prevention of cross-infection and nosocomial infections.[b] It is generally advised that you do not sit on the patient's bed when you see the child as a hospital inpatient. However, a child-friendly approach may sometimes necessitate that this rule be broken. One must wear examination gloves and other personal protective equipment (PPE) when indicated so as to avoid cross-infection. Note that donning and

[b] This means an infection acquired when a person is under medical care—usually in hospital.

The paediatric history and examination: a suggested method

1. **Preparation**
   a. Wash your hands.
   b. Wear personal protective equipment (PPE) if indicated.
2. **Measurements**
   a. Document the child's weight, height and head circumference and plot on the appropriate growth chart.
   b. Calculate body mass index (BMI) in the older child.
   c. Look for disproportional growth.
   d. Measure vital parameters (blood pressure, pulse and respiratory rate, temperature).
3. **General inspection**
   Observe the child, either sitting in the parent's lap or playing to assess the child's state of wellbeing, asymmetry of movement, abnormal posturing and spontaneous movements.
4. **Upper and lower limbs**
   a. Examine limbs individually and then compare for size disparity and deformities, swelling, tenderness, flexibility and range of movement.
   b. Inspect nails and palms.
5. **Back**
   Inspect spine for neural tube defects, scoliosis and lumbar hyperlordosis.
6. **Skin**
   Look out for petechiae, bruising, rash, lesions and masses.
7. **Head**
   a. Inspect hair.
   b. Palpate for craniosynostosis, bony and soft-tissue masses.
8. **Neck**
   a. Feel for nodes and masses.
   b. Palpate the thyroid gland.
   c. Check range of active movement.
9. **Face and dysmorphology**
   a. Note face shape and symmetry.
   b. Carefully inspect eyes, nose, mandible, mouth and lips for dysmorphic features.
   c. Look out for cleft lip and palate and check size of tongue.
   d. Note abnormal ear size and shape or unusual folding.
10. **Neurological system**
    a. Examine cranial nerves.
    b. Perform 180° examination in infants and small children.
    c. Examine gait.
    d. Determine tone, power, reflexes, coordination and sensation at all four extremities.
11. **Developmental assessment**
    Assess vision, hearing, fine-motor and gross-motor skills, social interaction and language.
12. **Lymphatic system**
    Assess for lymphadenopathy, large spleen and tonsils.
13. **Respiratory and cardiac systems**
    a. Inspect chest for deformity and scars and signs of respiratory distress.
    b. Auscultate for stridor, wheeze and crackles.
    c. Percuss for dullness or hyperresonance.
    d. Check capillary refill.
    e. Palpate pulses of all four limbs and localise the apex heartbeat.
    f. Auscultate the heart sounds.
14. **Abdominal system**
    a. Inspect for distension, epigastric peristalsis, masses and scars.
    b. Auscultate for bowel sounds and bruits.
    c. Palpate for masses, tenderness and organomegaly.
    d. Percuss for ascites and to measure organ size.
15. **Genitourinary system**
    a. Inspect skin for lesions and location of the urethral meatus.
    b. Palpate the scrotum for both testes, hernias and abnormal masses.
    c. Visualise the labia, clitoris, urethral meatus and vaginal introitus.
    d. Inspect the anus.
    e. Tanner staging.
16. **Ear, nose and throat (last, but not least)**
    a. Inspect ears for size, shape and position, and malformations.
    b. Perform otoscopy.
    c. Examine the mouth for stomatitis, ulcers, pallor and cyanosis.
    d. Visualise the oropharynx and palatine tonsils.

TEXT BOX 37.2

doffing PPE safely is a skill that needs to be learnt (http://cec.health.nsw.gov.au/keep-patients-safe/COVID-19/personal-protective-equipment). Otherwise, there is a high risk to inadvertently self-contaminate eyes, face, hands and clothes. Clean your examination tools (e.g. stethoscope) thoroughly with appropriate antimicrobial agents before and after use as recommended by the manufacturer.

Moving a settled, happy child from the parent's lap to start an examination may cause significant distress. This can make an already potentially challenging examination all the more difficult! Feel free to begin the examination where the child is most comfortable. **Engaging the child with play, and establishing rapport, is a key first step.** In an ideal situation, the child should be examined undressed to his or her underwear, but this is commonly not possible for small children and may cause significant distress to the adolescent patient. It is preferable for the parents to undress the young child when this is necessary.

Always consider examining adolescents fully clothed, and ask them to undress only if necessary for particular parts of the examination (e.g. the skin). Sometimes getting the older child to change in private into a hospital-type gown may help. Parents should be present for the examination of a child. Always offer to have a chaperone present for physical examination of an adolescent if the child does not want the parents present or they are absent.[3]

Examination

Observation

Much information can be gathered by observing the young child, either sitting in the parent's lap or playing on the floor. Assess the child's state of wellbeing (does the child look sick or well, under- or overnourished? How active is he or she?). Note any asymmetry of movement or abnormal posturing, and evaluate the child's skin colour and breathing pattern. Observe the way the child interacts with the parents and with other people.

Take time to allow the child to become acquainted and comfortable with you. As mentioned, much of the examination can be performed with the child in the parent's lap—usually the place where the child is likely to feel the most safe. Be prepared to play with, be silly with and interact with the child in a friendly, calm and quiet manner wherever possible. Some age-appropriate toys (well cleaned between patients) can be very helpful; when all else fails, using a bubble wand to blow a few well-timed bubbles should soothe and win over even the most upset child. Never forget to warm your hands before touching a child.

Whereas the young child may be most comfortable on the parent's lap, slightly older children usually sit happily on an examination table or bed with the examiner to one side and the parents to the other side. Approach the child in a friendly, gentle, patient way. Asking the child to show you his or her hands and praising the child for doing so often builds some trust, which allows you to start with some non-frightening palpation (e.g. brachial pulses) and gentle manoeuvres (e.g. turning the hands and inspecting the palms) before proceeding to the head-to-toe examination. Lastly, if in the hospital setting, much can be gained by a quick glance and visual exploration of the room, especially for children and teenagers with chronic medical conditions or prolonged hospital stays.

Measurements

In addition to documenting the child's **weight**, **height** and **head circumference** at the well-child examinations, it is prudent to check and document these measurements every time the child presents for review. These measurements are crucially important for the detection of serious pathologies and the monitoring of growth and development. Plot the results on the appropriate growth charts: it is generally standard practice to use gender-specific, height-for-age, weight-for-age and head-circumference charts (see Fig. 37.1). There are special growth charts for children with certain syndromic diagnoses (e.g. Down syndrome).

For children who do not walk, recumbent length is measured rather than height. A sitting height can also be useful in some situations (see below). It is best to use a stable, accurate, fixed measuring device wherever possible.

For an accurate weight to be determined, children should be undressed (underwear for older children; nappy for infants). The nappy weight needs to be considered when calculating the accurate weight. Also do not forget to remove the child's shoes and socks.

A method for measuring an accurate head circumference is outlined in Chapter 38. It may be important to measure the head circumference of both parents if benign familial macrocephaly is suspected. Head shape and craniosynostosis are explained later in this chapter.

Body mass index (BMI; see Ch 3) and waist circumference are used less in children than in adults, but can be useful tools, particularly in adolescents. BMI and growth velocity centile charts are available from the World Health Organization and should be used wherever possible. Recent studies suggest that **waist circumference** may be more useful than BMI for the assessment of Indigenous children.[5]

Other anthropometric measurements that may be useful, particularly in children who are at risk of growth failure (e.g. children with feeding difficulties, chronic illness or social difficulties), include mid-upper arm circumference and skinfold measurements, although these are rarely performed in routine practice.

Mid-upper arm circumference: first remove any clothing that may be covering the child's arm. Estimate the midpoint of the arm and use a tape measure to determine the circumference. This is usually easier with the arm lying flat against the patient's side and with the tape neither too tight nor too loose. A measurement of less than 11 centimetres in a child over 6 months old usually indicates malnutrition.[6]

Skinfold measurements: these are usually taken from the triceps and subscapular region. Using a skinfold calliper, measure the thickness of a fold of skin and underlying subcutaneous tissue (*not* muscle; see Fig. 37.2). Skinfold measurements can be compared with population averages.

Tall and short stature

Once a child's height (or length) is accurately measured and plotted, three further considerations need to take place: (1) is the child tall or short (above or below the upper / lower centiles for age and sex), (2) what is the trend or trajectory over time, and (3) what are the biological parents' heights?

The mid-parental height can be determined to give an idea of the child's growth potential:

For males:
$\frac{\text{(mother's height in cm + father's height in cm)} + 13\text{ cm}}{2}$
For females:
$\frac{\text{(mother's height in cm + father's height in cm)} - 13\text{ cm}}{2}$

The child would be expected to grow to within 2 standard deviations, or approximately 9 centimetres, of the number obtained from this equation.

When performing routine measurements in children, look for disproportionate growth and be aware of the extra measurements that can be taken (e.g. **upper and lower segment lengths**) if this is suspected. This is particularly important if there are concerns that the child may have short stature (e.g. caused by a chondrodysplastic disorder). For example, a child with achrondroplasia may have a normal sitting height, but have a marked reduction in standing height. Generally, at birth the normal upper-to-lower segment ratio is 1.7 : 1 and by the age of 10 the segments should be equal (and remain so into adulthood).[7]

Measurement of upper and lower segment lengths: the lower segment is measured from the symphysis pubis to the floor in the standing child; to calculate the upper segment, subtract the lower segment length from the total height.

In most children with short stature the cause is hereditary short stature, so parental height should always be taken into account. As with other growth parameters, if a child's height was previously within a healthy range and is now crossing height centiles *downwards* this is usually more cause for concern than a child who has followed the same, albeit lower, centile.

A wide range of diagnoses are associated with short stature, including nutritional deficiencies (see below), chromosomal abnormalities (such as Down or Turner syndrome), skeletal dysplasias (such as achondroplasia), metabolic disorders (e.g. Hunter or Hurler syndrome), endocrinopathies (such as hypothyroidism, Cushing syndrome or primary pituitary disease) and iatrogenic causes (such as craniospinal irradiation in childhood for malignancy).

Pathological tall stature is less common, but causes include Klinefelter syndrome, Marfan syndrome, gigantism, thyrotoxicosis and Beckwith–Wiedemann syndrome.

Vital signs

These (blood pressure, pulse and respiratory rates, temperature) should be measured at each presentation, particularly if the child is unwell.

Text continued on p 655

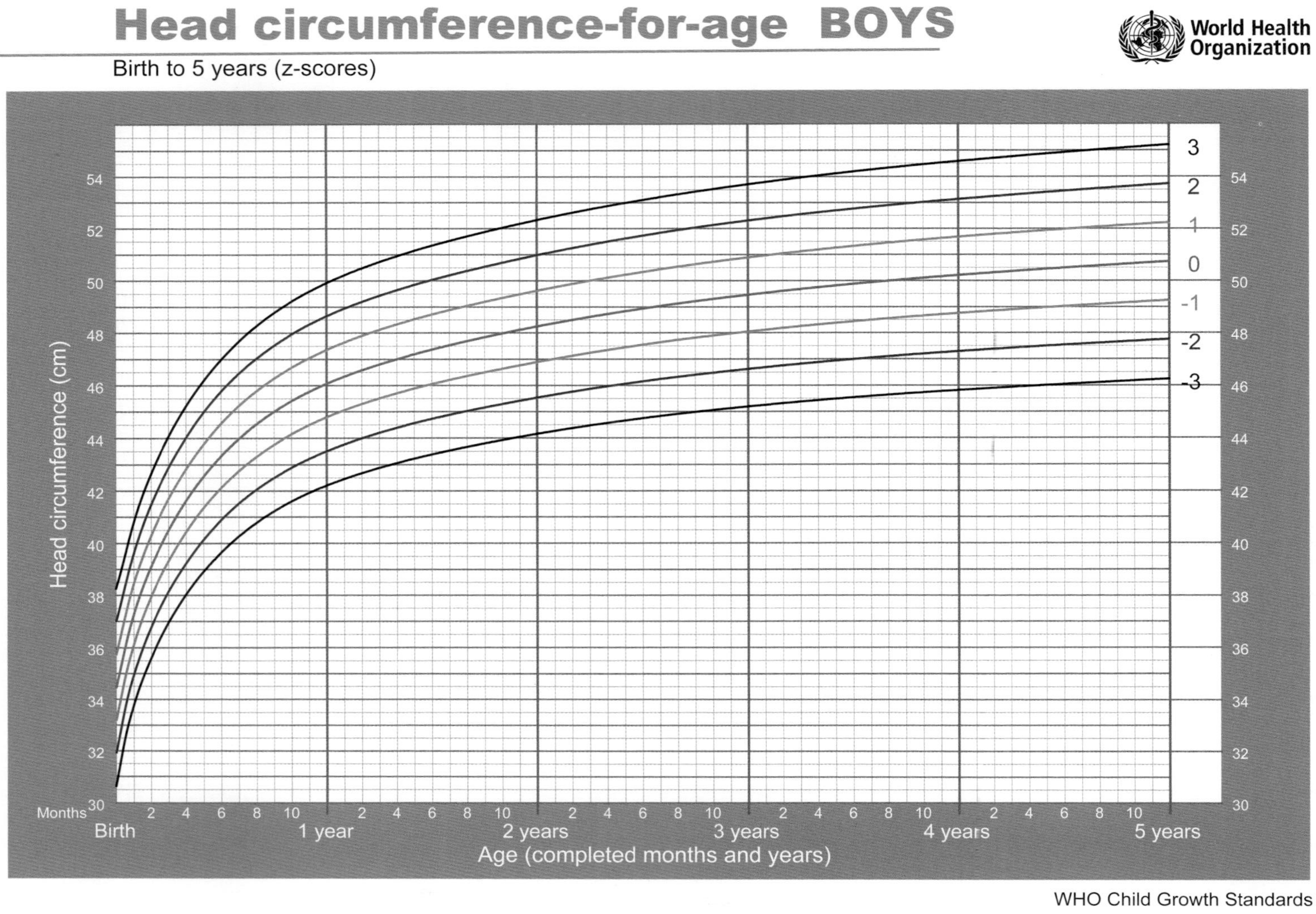

Head circumference-for-age BOYS

Birth to 5 years (z-scores)

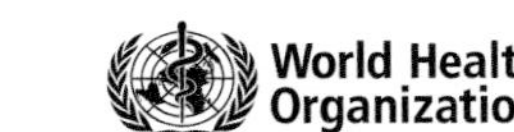

Growth charts from birth to 5 years

(Reprinted from World Health Organization Child Growth Standard Charts, https://www.who.int/tools/child-growth-standards/standards/.)

FIGURE 37.1

Continued

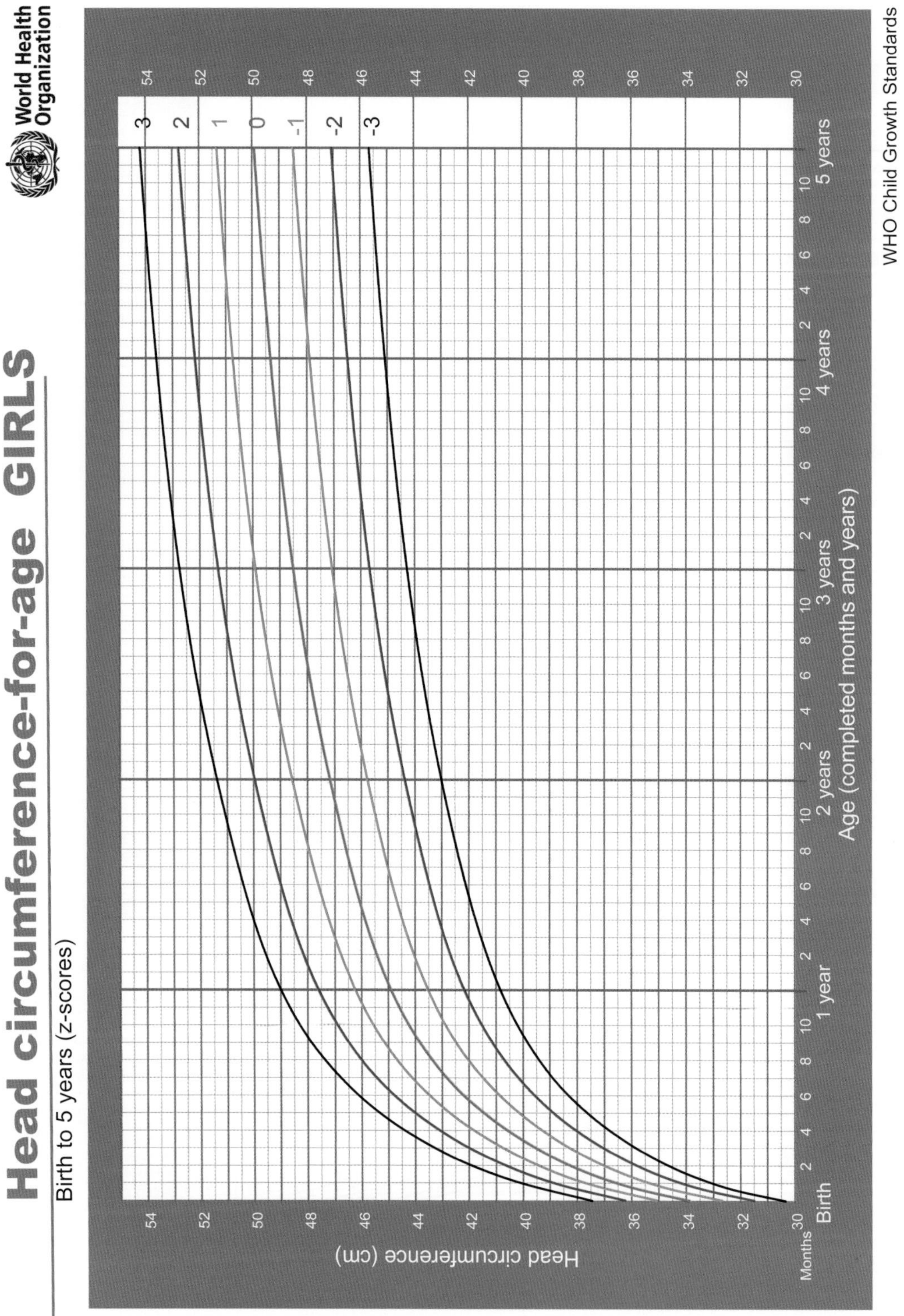

Head circumference-for-age GIRLS

Birth to 5 years (z-scores)

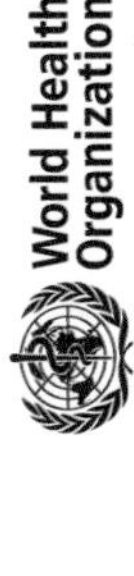

Head circumference (cm)

54
52
50
48
46
44
42
40
38
36
34
32
30

3
2
1
0
-1
-2
-3

Months
Birth 2 4 6 8 10
1 year 2 4 6 8 10
2 years 2 4 6 8 10
3 years 2 4 6 8 10
4 years 2 4 6 8 10
5 years

Age (completed months and years)

WHO Child Growth Standards

FIGURE 37.1, cont'd

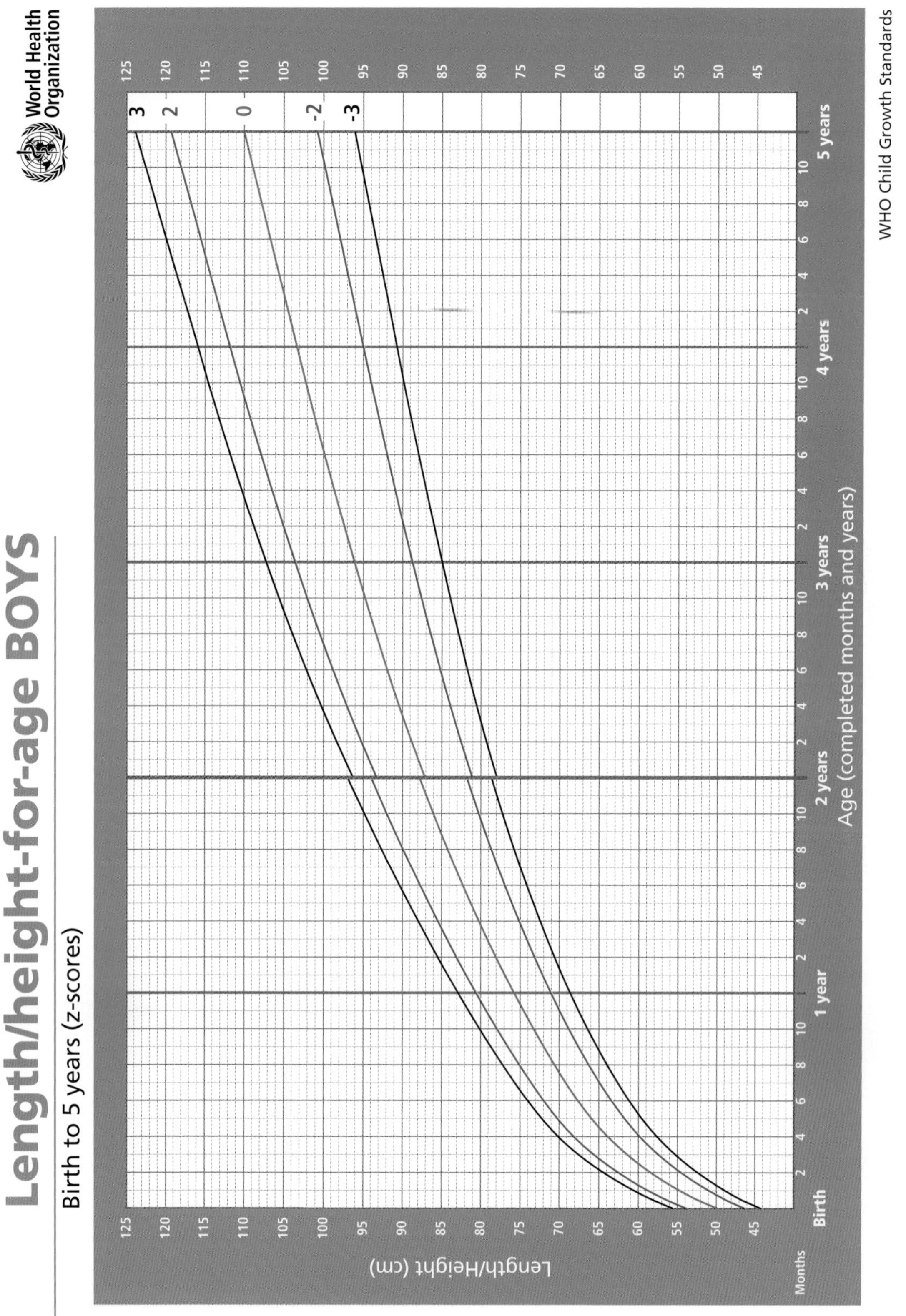

Length/height-for-age BOYS

Birth to 5 years (z-scores)

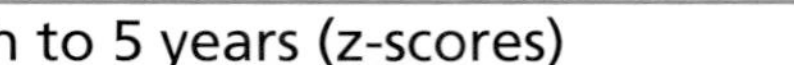

FIGURE 37.1, cont'd

Continued

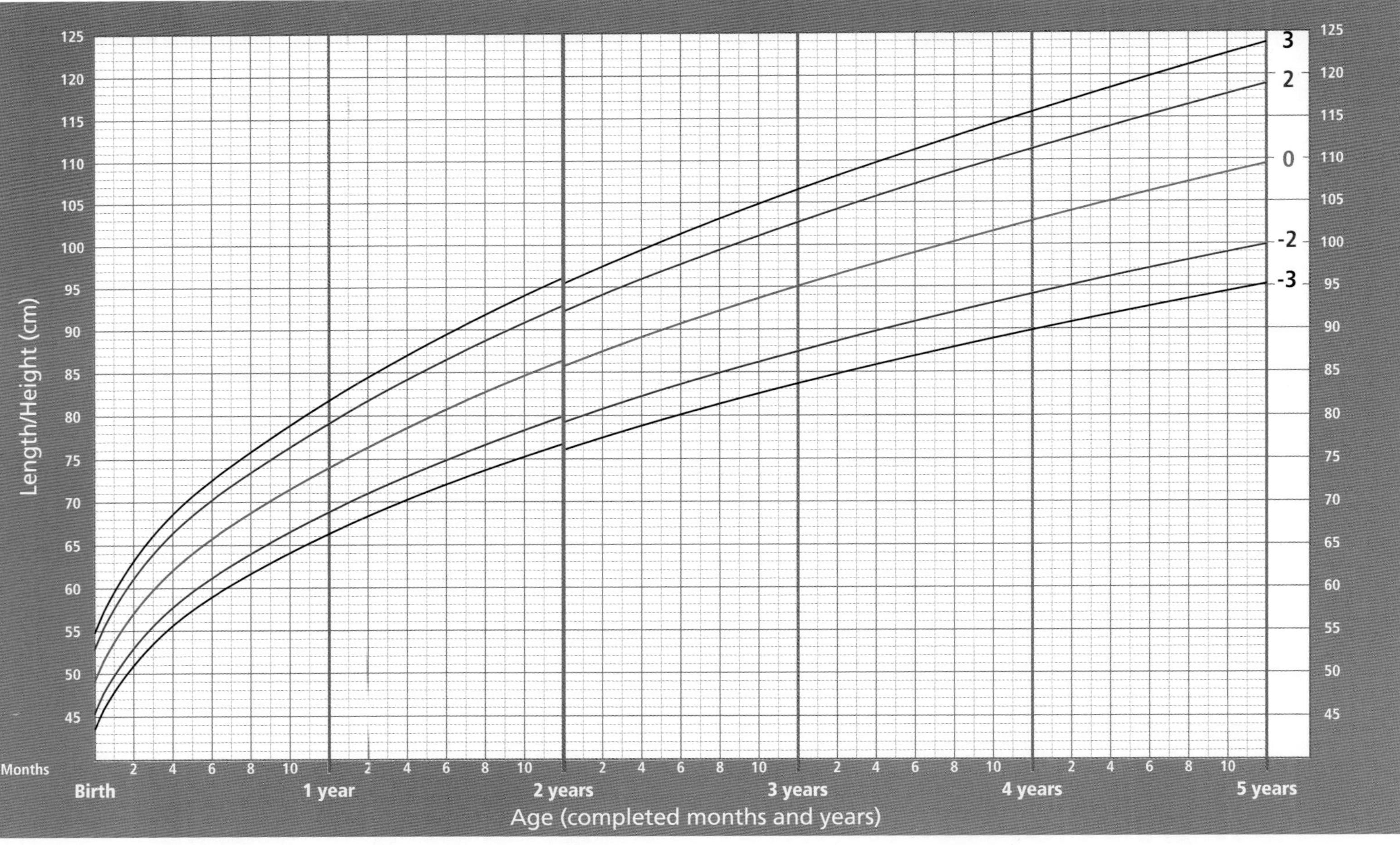

FIGURE 37.1, cont'd

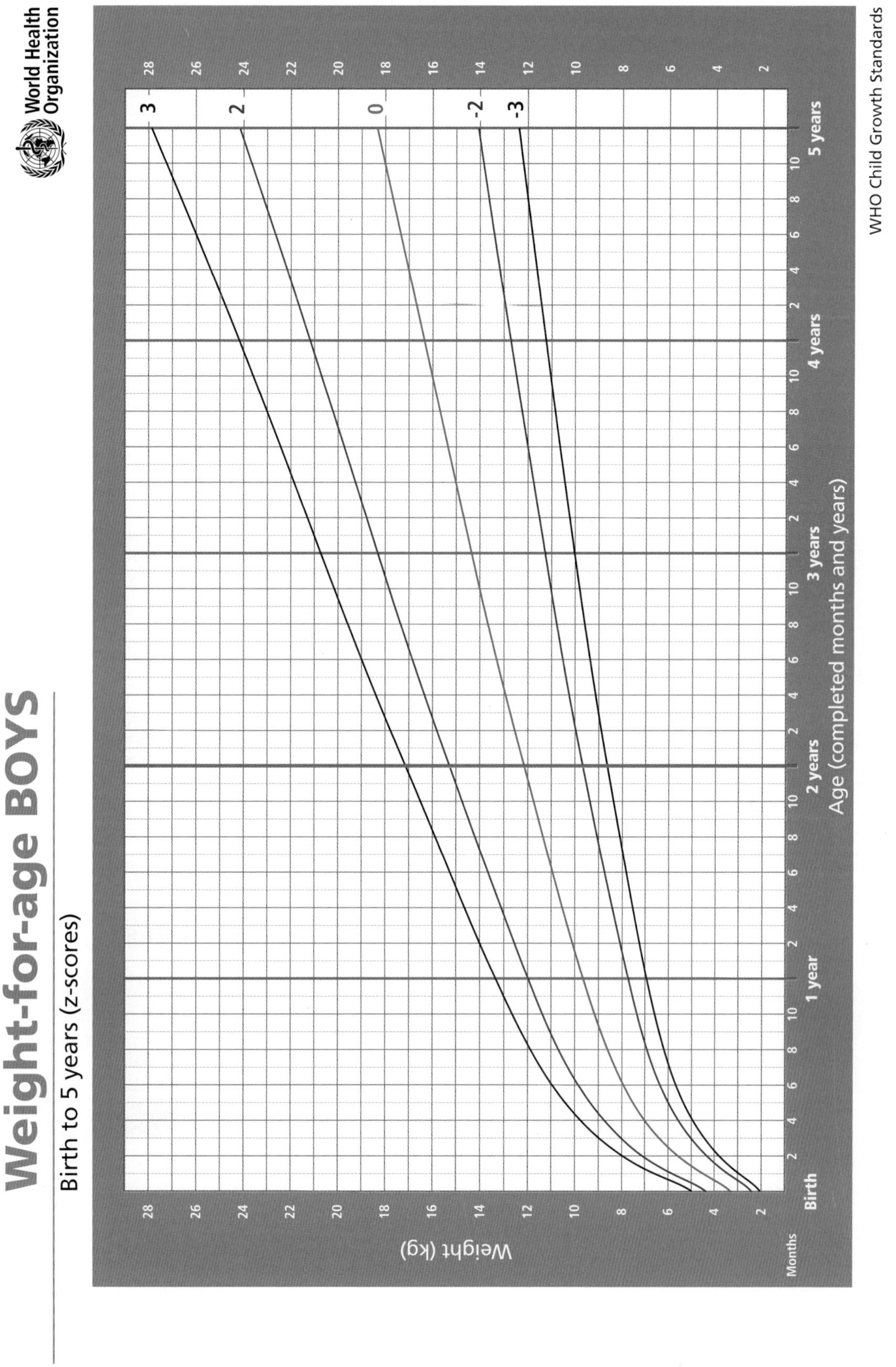

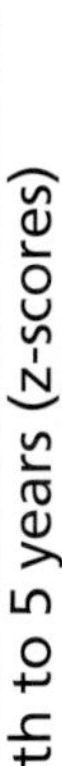

FIGURE 37.1, cont'd

Continued

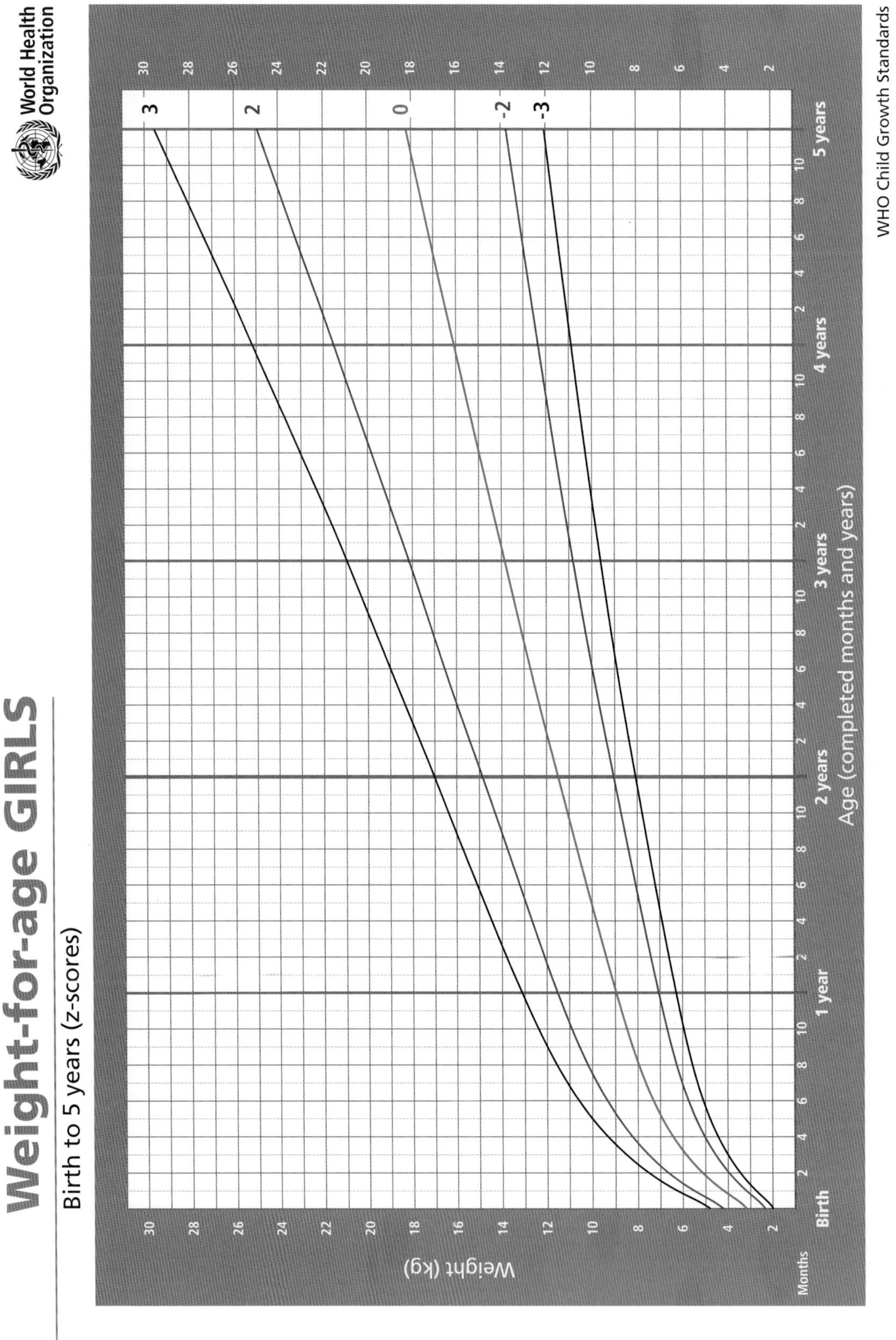
Weight-for-age GIRLS
Birth to 5 years (z-scores)
World Health Organization
Weight (kg)
30 28 26 24 22 20 18 16 14 12 10 8 6 4 2
3
2
0
-2
-3
Months
Birth 2 4 6 8 10 1 year 2 4 6 8 10 2 years 2 4 6 8 10 3 years 2 4 6 8 10 4 years 2 4 6 8 10 5 years
Age (completed months and years)
WHO Child Growth Standards

FIGURE 37.1, cont'd

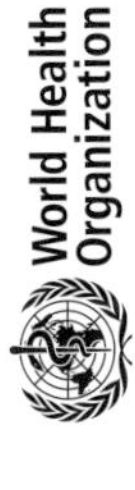

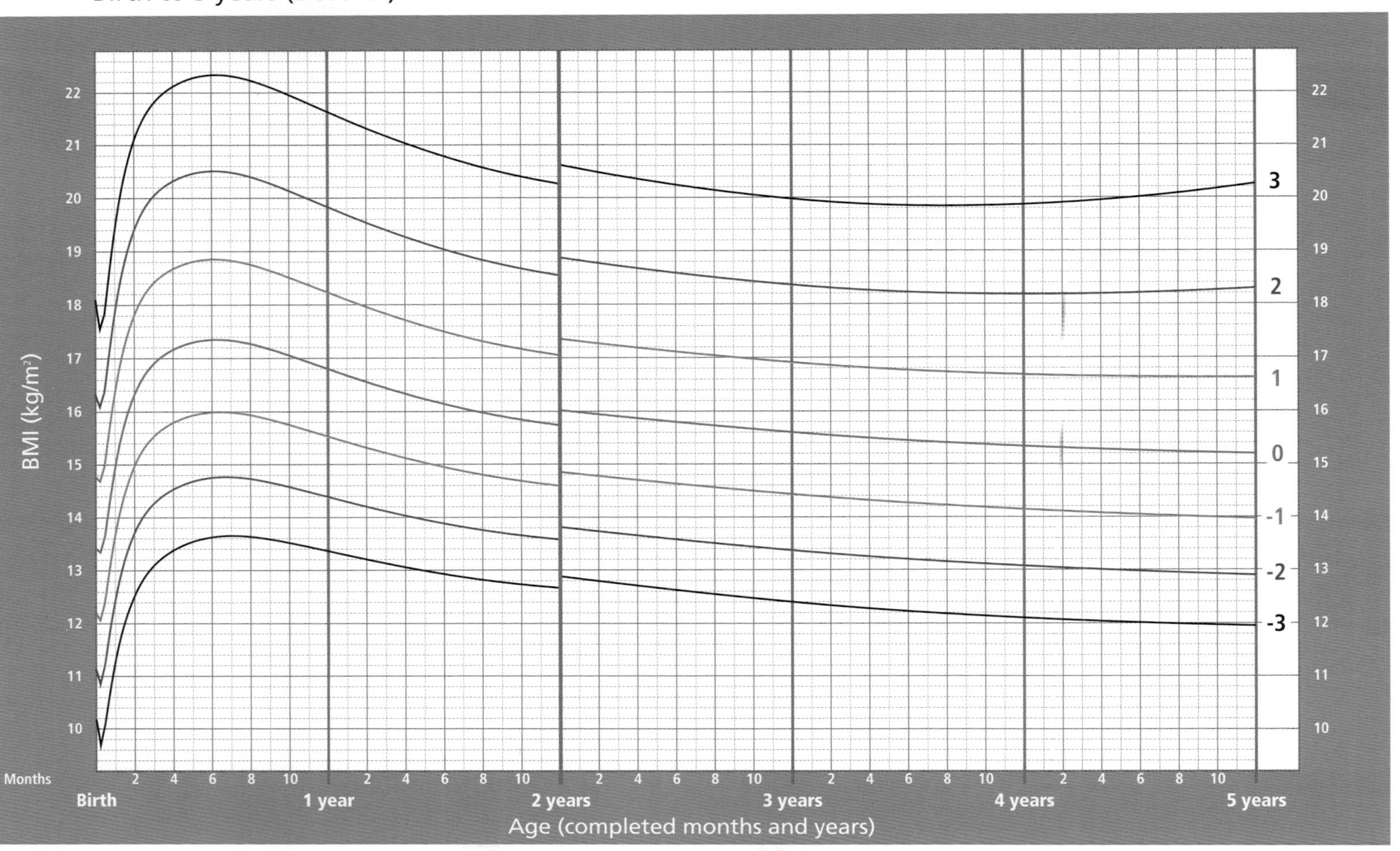

FIGURE 37.1, cont'd

Continued

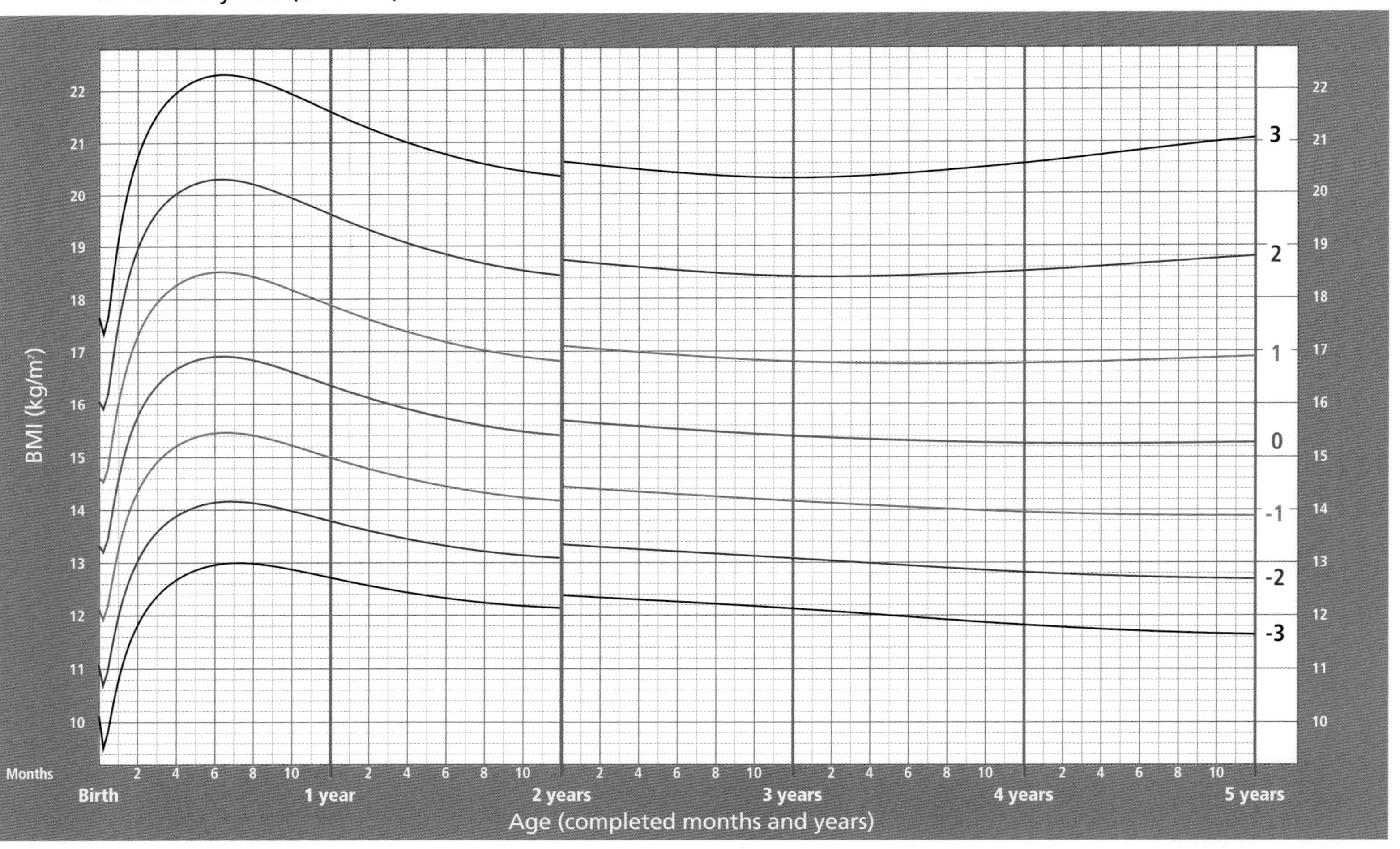

FIGURE 37.1, cont'd

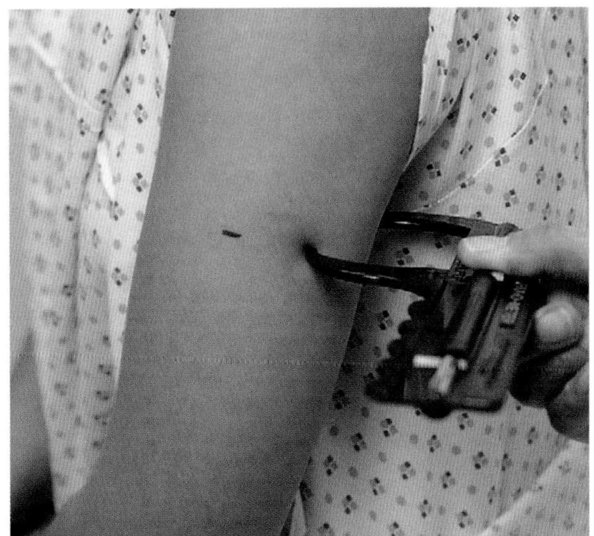

Measuring the triceps skinfold

(From Wilson SF, Giddens JF. *Health assessment for nursing practice*, 4th edn. St Louis, MO: Mosby, 2009.)

FIGURE 37.2

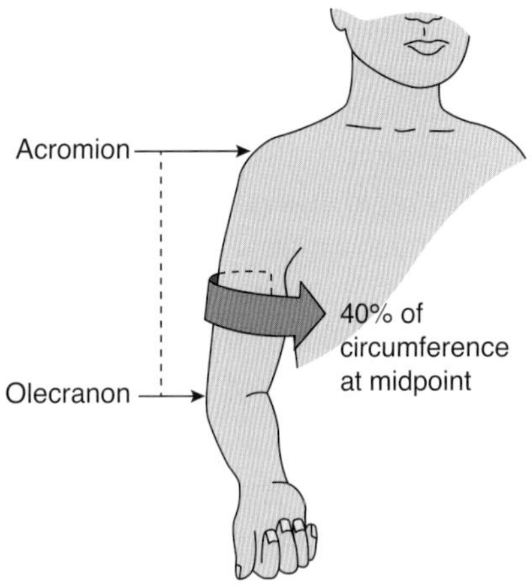

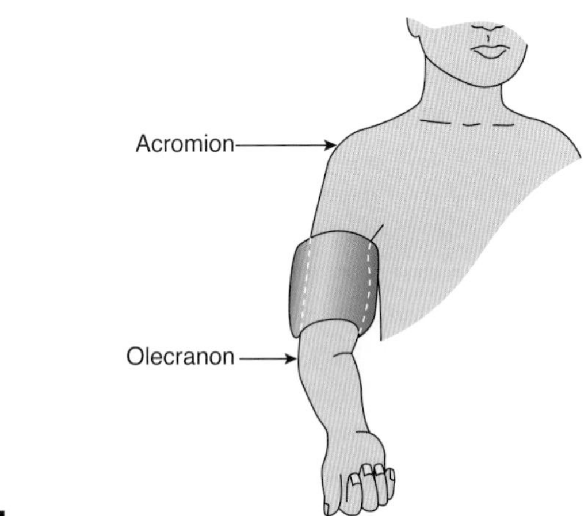

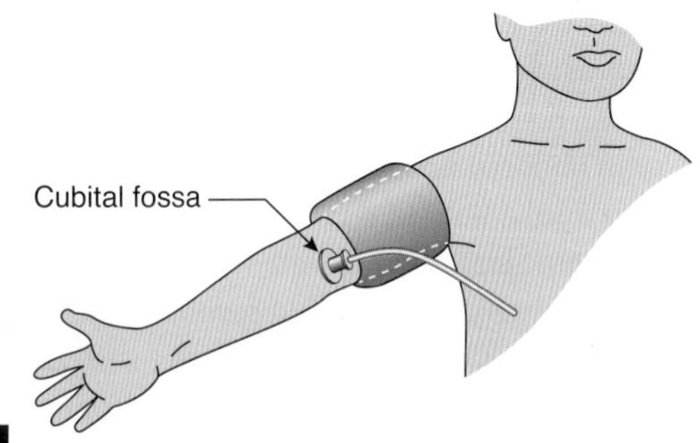

(a, b) Determining the proper cuff size. (c) Measuring the blood pressure

(From Hockenberry MJ, Wilson D. *Wong's essentials of pediatric nursing*, 8th edn. St Louis, MO: Mosby, 2009.)

FIGURE 37.3

Blood pressure

The American Academy of Pediatrics recommends routine blood pressure measurements for children from the age of 3 years.[8] The blood pressure cuff should be appropriate for the child's size (the width of the cuff bladder should equal 40% of the mid-upper arm circumference; see Fig. 37.3(a) and (b)).[9] It is best measured after the child has been sitting quietly for 5 minutes, although this is seldom possible in practice. An automatic sphygmomanometer is often used for screening, but auscultation is more precise. Listen with the diaphragm of the stethoscope over the brachial artery pulse, proximal and medial to the cubital fossa (see Fig. 37.3(c)). Systolic pressure is indicated by the appearance of the first Korotkoff sound and diastolic by the fifth Korotkoff sound (the cessation of all sound) (pp 94, 690).

Hypertension is not common in children and is usually indicative of an underlying disease, such as renal disease or cardiovascular disease. However, primary hypertension is increasingly seen in morbidly obese children and adolescents.[10] One should compare a patient's systolic and diastolic measurements with population data tables—that are age, sex and sometimes height matched—in order to diagnose hypertension accurately.[11]

Hypotension is also uncommon in children, but it warrants rapid evaluation to exclude hypovolaemia or sepsis, which can lead to shock (circulatory failure; see Table 37.1). Remember, hypotension is a *late sign* in critically ill children with other signs often present prior to hypotension (e.g. tachycardia, pallor, mottled skin).

Pulse and respiratory rates

In childhood, a **wide pulse pressure** may be seen in patients with patent ductus arteriosus, aortic regurgitation and hyperthyroidism. The most common causes of a **narrow pulse pressure** are subaortic and aortic valve stenosis. Again, it is better to count the pulse than to use an automated system, and the pulse is usually easily palpated in most children, so there are no excuses. Many clinicians find the brachial or femoral pulses easier to feel in infants and small children, although the radial or carotid pulse can also be used. It is particularly hard to feel a carotid pulse in infants and small children as they have a proportionally large head and a small, short neck.

The **heart rate** changes with age. Figure 37.4 shows the range of resting heart rates for children of different ages. In a resuscitation situation, pulselessness is indicative of either arrested or abnormal electroactivity (e.g. ventricular fibrillation) of the heart. Electroactivity is assessed using ECG monitoring.

Accurate **respiratory rate** determination can also be tricky in children and ideally should be taken when the child is awake but at rest (see Fig. 37.5). By far the most common cause of an elevated respiratory rate in children is respiratory disease, but severe infection and cardiac, neuromuscular, central nervous system and metabolic disorders should be considered. Toxins and raised intracranial pressure can depress the respiratory rate.

Pulse oximetry is becoming more and more common in the routine assessment of children (and almost universal as part of the neonatal examination—see Ch 38) and this allows for a simple, non-invasive and reasonably accurate estimation of arterial oxygen saturation.[11] Normal oxygen saturation (S_aO_2) values in paediatrics have not been established and are known to vary with altitude, but it is generally accepted that in healthy children (at sea level) the normal range for S_aO_2 is 97–100%.[12]

Blood pressure values requiring further evaluation, according to age and sex

	Male		Female	
	Systolic (mmHg)	Diastolic (mmHg)	Systolic (mmHg)	Diastolic (mmHg)
3	100	59	100	61
4	102	62	101	64
5	104	65	103	66
6	105	68	104	68
7	106	70	106	69
8	107	71	108	71
9	109	72	110	72
10	111	73	112	73
11	113	74	114	74
12	115	74	116	75
13	117	75	117	76
14	120	75	119	77
15	120	76	120	78
16	120	78	120	78
17	120	80	120	78
18	120	80	120	80

(Kaelber DC, Pickett F. Simple table to identify children and adolescents needing further evaluation of blood pressure. *Pediatrics* 2009; 123:e972e4. With permission of the American Academy of Pediatrics.)

TABLE 37.1

Temperature

There is considerable debate about the best method for checking the temperature in infants and children. It is important to remember that there can be a significant difference in each recording with different thermometers.[13] It used to be common practice to measure children's temperatures in the rectum, but this experience can be frightening for small children and may be psychologically harmful for older children.[14] Taking the temperature in the axilla is a reasonable alternative but **tympanic thermometry** is now commonly used. It is easy and quick to take the temperature from the ear and the reading is closely correlated with core

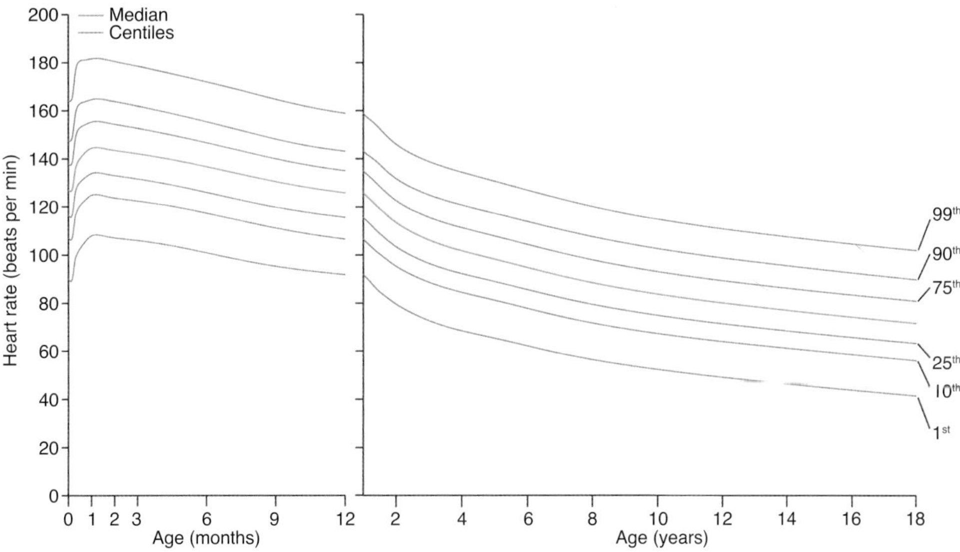

Heart rate and age

(From Fleming S, Thompson M, Stevens R et al. Normal ranges of heart rate and respiratory rate in children from birth to 18 years of age: a systematic review of observational studies. *Lancet* 2011; 377(9770):1011–1018, with permission.)

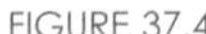

FIGURE 37.4

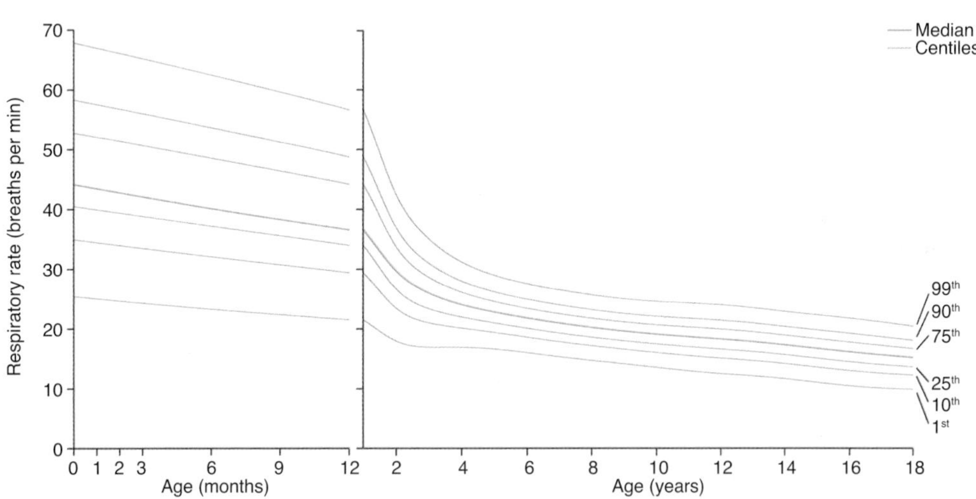

Respiratory rate and age

(From Fleming S, Thompson M, Stevens R et al. Normal ranges of heart rate and respiratory rate in children from birth to 18 years of age: a systematic review of observational studies. *Lancet* 2011; 377(9770):1011–1018, with permission.)

FIGURE 37.5

Normal temperatures at different sites

Body site	Type of thermometer	Normal range, mean (°C)	Elevated body temperature or fever (°C)
Axilla	Hg in glass, electronic	34.7–37.3, 36.4	37.4
Sublingual	Hg in glass, electronic	35.5–37.5, 36.6	37.6
Rectal	Hg in glass, electronic	36.6–37.9, 37.0	38.0
Ear	Infrared emission	35.7–37.5, 36.6	37.6

(Chamberlain JM, Terndrup TE. New light on ear thermometer readings. *Contemp Pediatr* 1994; 11(3):66–76.)

TABLE 37.2

body temperature (see Table 37.2 for normal values). Mercury thermometers should be avoided, and an oral temperature should be considered only in children who are capable of understanding the procedure (from about 6 years of age).

Specific physical examinations

Upper and lower limbs (legs and arms)

When examining the upper and lower limbs, remember to examine the limbs individually and then to compare both limbs, particularly when checking for size disparity (e.g. hemihyperplasia). Ask the child whether he or she is sore anywhere before beginning the examination. Examine the upper limbs and hands:

Look (inspect)

On the dorsal surface of the hands, examine the skin, joints and nails before turning the hands over to examine the palms, taking particular care to check the palmar creases. Examine the nails for any abnormalities (e.g. pitted nails in psoriasis, fungal infection) and the interdigital webbing for any lesions (e.g. scabies).

Feel (palpate)

Note any areas of increased heat (particularly over joints), tenderness (e.g. dermatomyositis) or swelling. A hot, swollen joint with limited and/or painful movement could signify septic arthritis, juvenile arthritis or rheumatic fever (the latter especially in the Indigenous child population).

Move and measure

Gently move the wrist and finger joints through their respective ranges of motion, looking for flexibility, asymmetry and any unusual positions. Thus if there appears to be restriction of movement in any joint, make a note of the degree of movement possible.

If there is a suggestion of hypermobility, consider calculating the Beighton score in children >6 years:

1. One point if while standing forwards bending the patient can place his or her palms on the ground with legs straight
2. One point for each elbow that bends backwards
3. One point for each knee that bends backwards
4. One point for each thumb that touches the forearm when bent backwards
5. One point for each little finger that bends backwards beyond 90° (see Fig. 37.6).

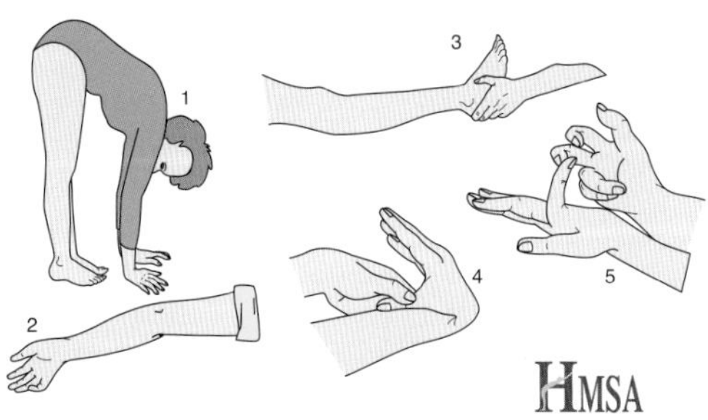

Calculating the Beighton score

((c) Hypermobility Syndromes Association, http://hypermobility.org/hypermobility-disorders-an-update-for-clinicians.)

FIGURE 37.6

This score can be used to formulate whether the child has **benign joint hypermobility syndrome (BJHS)** or needs further investigation for other conditions associated with joint hypermobility (e.g. Marfan syndrome, Ehlers–Danlos syndrome). Please see https://www.hypermobility.org/hypermobility-disorders-an-update-for-clinicians for more information.

Examine the lower limbs and feet in a similar manner:

Look (inspect)

Examine the proximal upper and lower limbs for asymmetry and deformity.

Feel (palpate)

Note muscle bulk (atrophy, hypertrophy), swelling, heat and tenderness.

Move and measure

Measure tone, strength, flexibility and range of movement.

Look for any bony or joint deformities, masses or dysmorphic features. Examine the knees. Deformities of the feet and knee are quite common. See Chapter 38 to review common deformities of the foot. The main deformities seen at the knee are genu varum (bow legs) (see Fig. 37.7) and genu valgum (knock-knees), both of which *may be normal at certain ages* (i.e. physiologically normal or normal, non-pathological, anatomical variation) and usually correct spontaneously (see Fig. 37.7(c)). Unilateral deformity, however, is less likely to be physiological and requires investigation.

Genu varum (bow legs; see Fig. 37.7)

Genu varum is common in normal children under the age of 2 years.

Ask the child to stand with the feet together and measure the **intercondylar** distance.

Pathological causes include rickets, skeletal dysplasias or Blout's disease (unilateral closure of the proximal medial tibial growth plate).

Genu valgum (knock-knees; see Fig. 37.8)

Genu valgum is common in normal young children (usually between the ages of 3 and 7 years).

Ask the child to stand and compare the limb lengths, then measure the **intermalleolar** distance.

If this condition is persistent beyond the age of 7 or increasing deformity is seen before this age, underlying causes should be sought (again, rickets and skeletal dysplasia are the usual cause).

Adolescent genu valgum is an idiopathic disorder seen after the age of 8 years.

Look for **toeing in (metatarsus varus**; see Fig. 37.9), which is physiological in the young child (aged 2 to 5 years), but may require correction in the older child,

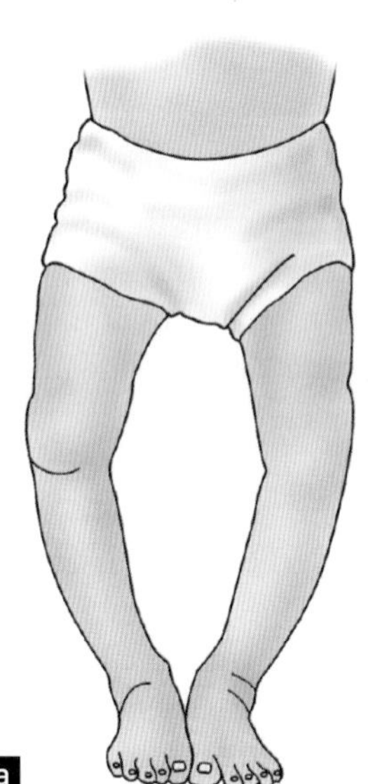

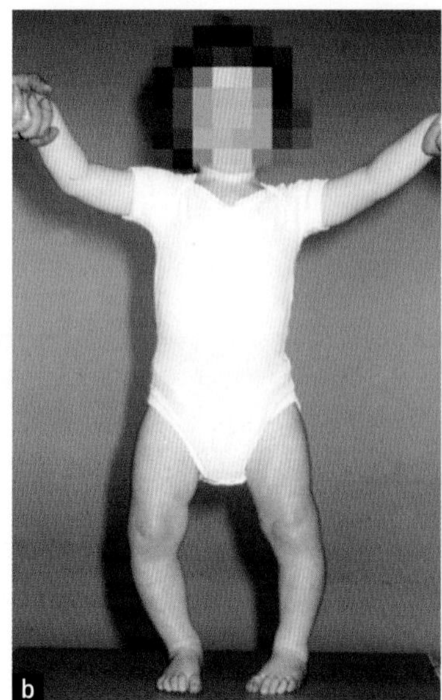

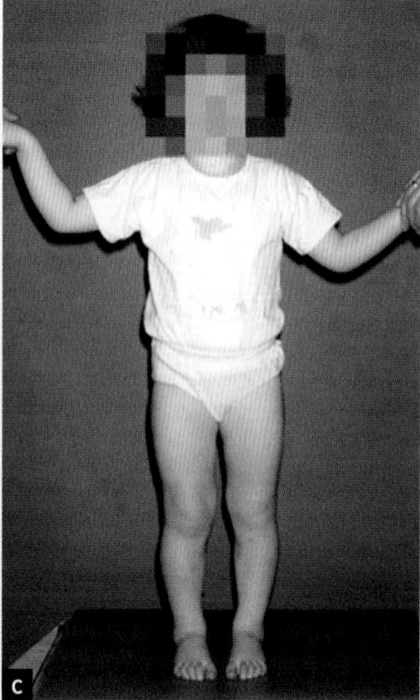

(a, b) Genu varum; (c) shows the same toddler in (b), with the deformity corrected

((a) and (b) from Scoles P. *Pediatric orthopedics in clinical practice*. Chicago: Year Book Medical Publishers, 1982, p 84; (c) from Macnicol MF. *Orthopaedics and trauma* 2010; 24(5):369–380.)

FIGURE 37.7

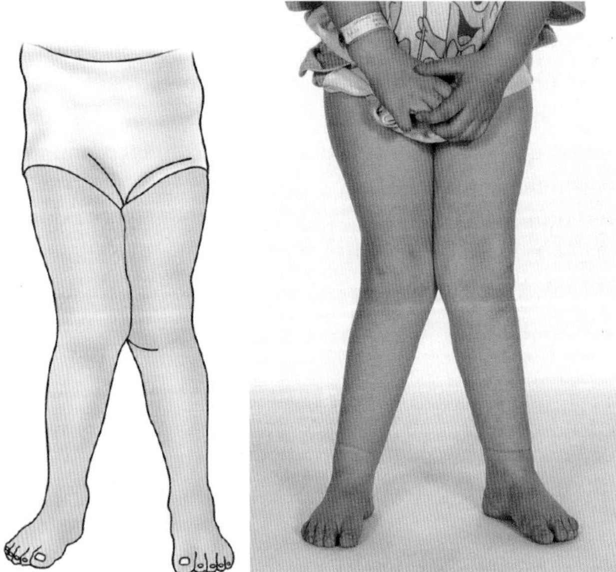

Genu valgum

(From Macnicol MF. *Orthopaed Trauma* 2010; 24(5):369–380.)

FIGURE 37.8

and **toeing out** (**metatarsus valgus**), which may require surgical correction as it *does not* self-correct with time.[15]

If there is limitation of **movement**, consider whether this is due to pain, weakness, contractures or spasticity.

It is also useful to **measure** for **limb length** discrepancies, although a small discrepancy (up to 2 centimetres) is common once patients have reached adulthood. There are two measurements traditionally used for this purpose:

1. *The true leg length:* measure from the anterior superior iliac spine to the medial malleolus.
2. *The apparent leg length:* measure from the pubic symphysis to the medial malleolus.

Clinically, it is more reliable to assess the posterior iliac crest level while the child stands with the knees and hips extended and to use blocks placed under the foot until the pelvis is level (then measure the height of the block; see Fig. 37.10).

Limb length discrepancies (true leg length discrepancy >2 cm) can be seen in hemihypertrophy syndromes such as Beckwith–Wiedemann syndrome.

Back

When examining the back, ensure that the entire length of the spine is uncovered. Examine the child standing, with the feet together and the arms at the sides. Look for obvious **neural tube defects** (meningocele and meningomyelocele; see Fig. 38.7) and any asymmetry, skin lesions or masses. Check whether the shoulders, scapulae and pelvic rims are symmetrical. Have the child bend over to touch the toes to assess the level of the pelvis. Palpate along the vertebral column, which should form a straight line from the base of the neck to the gluteal cleft, looking for tenderness or any defects in the bony spine (**spina bifida occulta**).

Lumbar hyperlordosis is sometimes seen in children between the ages of 8 and 10 years. It is usually physiological and resolves spontaneously.[16] Structural

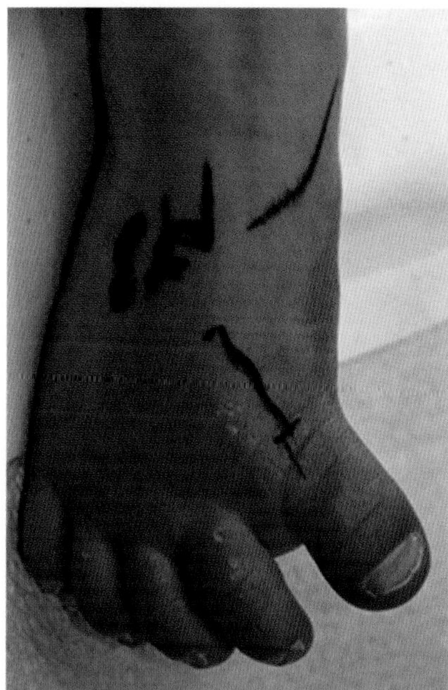

In-toeing

(From Harris E. The intoeing child: etiology, prognosis, and current treatment options. *Clin Podiatr Med Surg* 2013; 30(4):531–565.)

FIGURE 37.9

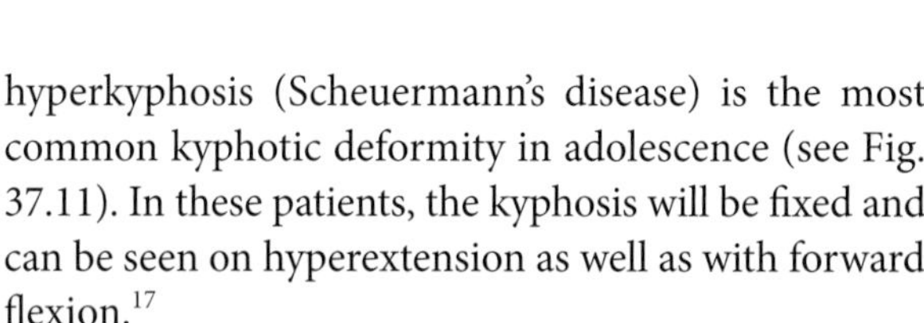

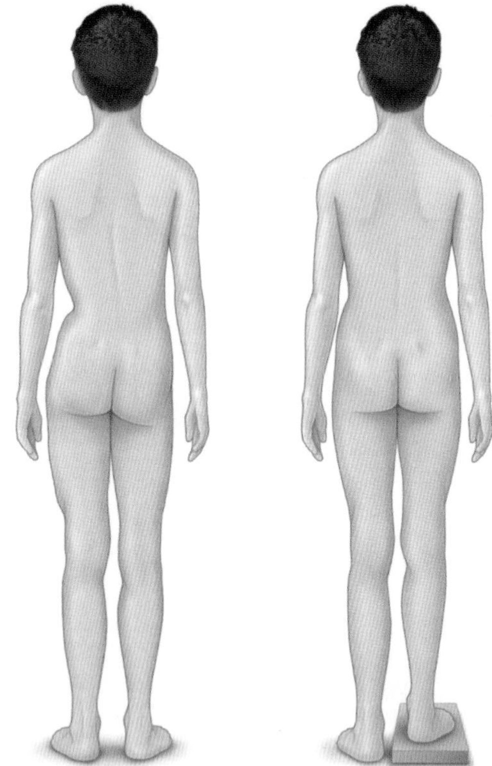

Leg length discrepancy

(From Herring JA. *Tachdjian's pediatric orthopaedics*. Philadelphia: Saunders, 2008, Ch 24, pp 1191–1271.)

FIGURE 37.10

hyperkyphosis (Scheuermann's disease) is the most common kyphotic deformity in adolescence (see Fig. 37.11). In these patients, the kyphosis will be fixed and can be seen on hyperextension as well as with forward flexion.[17]

Scoliosis (lateral curvature of the spine; see Fig. 37.12) is by far the most common spinal abnormality seen in children and adolescents. Always consider a functional scoliosis caused by leg length discrepancy—this will correct as the child bends forwards. Early-onset scoliosis occurs before the age of 5 years and is more likely to progress as the child ages and to lead to cardiovascular problems.[16] This form of scoliosis is also more likely to be associated with an underlying pathology. Thus, associated anomalies should be sought (e.g. intraspinal, cardiovascular, urogenital). Late-onset (older than 5 years of age) scoliosis is much more common and much more likely to be idiopathic. Finish the back examination by inspecting the buttocks. Flattened buttocks and shortening of the gluteal cleft may be seen in sacral agenesis. Check for sacral dimples, hair tufts and skin lesions (these are other potential signs of spina bifida occulta—see Ch 38).

An excellent resource of information for the musculoskeletal examination of children is pGALS—paediatric Gait Arms Legs and Spine, by Foster and Jandial.[18]

Skin

Look at the skin for:

- colour (pallor, plethora, jaundice, carotinaemia)
- any lesions (location, colour, raised or flat, diffuse or localised)
- haemorrhages (ecchymoses, petechiae, purpura)

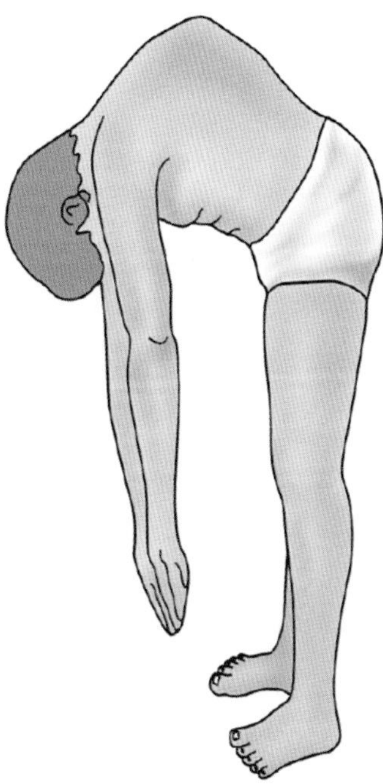

Thoracic kyphosis. Note the sharp break in the contour of a child with kyphosis

(From Behrman RE. *Nelson textbook of pediatrics*, 14th edn. Philadelphia: Saunders, 1992.)

FIGURE 37.11

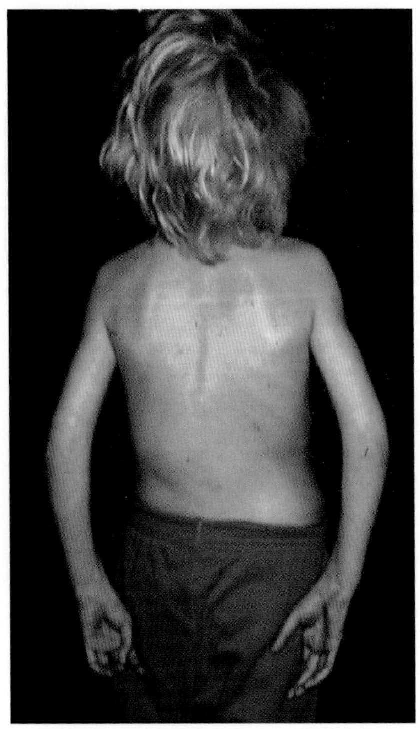

Right thoracic idiopathic scoliosis

(From Graham JM. *Smith's recognizable patterns of human deformation.* Philadelphia: Elsevier, 2007, Ch 20, pp 107–110.)

FIGURE 37.12

- peripheral stigmata of systemic disease (e.g. spider naevi in liver disease, telangiectasia in ataxia-telangiectasia).

Skin lesions can be referred to as either primary (first change to occur in the skin because of disease; see Table 37.3) or secondary (caused by external factors that may evolve from primary lesions; see Table 37.4).

Many benign skin lesions are commonly seen in childhood (e.g. warts, epidermal cysts) and may require no specific treatment. Bruising in babies is an unexpected finding and requires further investigation (e.g. coagulopathy, non-accidental injury). Although below-knee bruising in cruising[c] children is more common, this should prompt concerns if the bruises are located in *atypical* areas such as the buttocks, hands and trunk and a plausible mechanism is not identified. (See later in the chapter regarding examination for suspected child abuse.)

[c] Cruising is where an infant, prior to walking independently, uses furniture or other sturdy objects to hold onto and walk, often sideways.

Palpate the skin to feel for areas of rough, dry skin. Eczema typically presents on the face in an infant, the extensor surfaces in a young child and the flexor surfaces in an older child. Examine the groin, particularly if the child is still in nappies (nappy rash or napkin dermatitis).

Look for vascular lesions (ask the parents about 'birthmarks'), which, although relatively common, may be of clinical significance. Infantile **haemangiomas** are benign vascular tumours (see Fig. 37.13) that have a period of growth (proliferation) but eventually (over 90%) self-resolve (involute) spontaneously by the time the child is 9 years old. Thus, they do not require treatment unless they are extensive, increase in size or are in a problematic area (e.g. perioral, periorbital, anogenital, laryngeal).[19] These lesions need to be differentiated from vascular malformations, which neither *proliferate* nor *involute* (see Table 37.5).

The presence of cervicofacial or more than five cutaneous haemangiomas may indicate the presence

Primary skin lesions	
Macules	Small, flat areas of change in skin colour <1 cm (e.g. freckles)
Patches	Larger, flat areas of colour change (e.g. port-wine stain)
Papules	Elevated lesions <1 cm (e.g. molluscum contagiosum)
Plaques	Raised lesions >1 cm; the surface area is greater than the elevation (e.g. psoriasis)
Nodules	Circumscribed, elevated lesions displaying both depth and elevation; larger than pustules (e.g. capillary haemangioma)
Vesicles	Small, raised cavities containing fluid (<1 cm) (e.g. chicken pox)
Bullae	Larger (>1 cm) fluid-filled lesions (e.g. bullous impetigo)
Pustules	Similar to vesicles, but filled with pus (e.g. pustular psoriasis)
Wheal	Raised lesions that are transient and caused by dilation of local blood vessels (e.g. urticaria)
Comedones	Plugs of clumped keratin and sebum in a hair follicle (e.g. acne)
Burrows	Linear tunnels made by mites in the epidermis (e.g. scabies)
Telangiectasia	Dilated (permanently) superficial blood vessels in the skin

(Modified from Goldbloom RB. *Pediatric clinical skills*. Philadelphia: Saunders, 2010.)

TABLE 37.3

Secondary skin lesions	
Scaling	Accumulation of desquamating skin cells (e.g. ichthyosis)
Crusts	Accumulations of dried exudates or transudate (e.g. infected eczema)
Excoriations	Linear breaks in the skin (e.g. scratches seen in scabies)
Fissures	Linear cracks in the skin (e.g. cracked heels)
Erosions	Circumscribed loss of the superficial layer
Ulcer	Circumscribed loss of tissue that extends into the dermis to subcutaneous tissue or even deeper
Atrophy	Thinning of the skin layers (e.g. postradiation skin changes)
Scars	Fibrous tissue repairs of skin that has been damaged below the level of the epidermis

(Modified from Goldbloom RB. *Pediatric clinical skills*. Philadelphia: Saunders, 2010.)

TABLE 37.4

of airway or visceral haemangiomas. The infantile vascular lesions associated with **Sturge–Weber syndrome** and **Klippel–Trenaunay syndrome** are detailed in Chapter 38, but remember that these vascular lesions grow in proportion to the child and often require treatment.

Malignant skin lesions (squamous cell carcinomas, basal cell carcinomas, melanomas) are very uncommon in children, but should be considered in adolescents. Also note any hypopigmented lesions (see Fig. 37.14), which can be benign (previous scarring, vitiligo) or may indicate an underlying disorder such as **tuberous sclerosis (TS)**. Note the number of lesions in particular, because most children with one to three hypopigmented macules will *not* be at risk of TS.[19] Facial angiofibromas (see Fig. 37.15) are classic skin lesions seen in patients with TS, but these are not usually seen prior to puberty. Check also for forehead plaques, shagreen patches (see Fig. 37.16), ungual fibromas and gingival fibromas in these children.

Café-au-lait spots (see Fig. 37.17) are very common in the general population (found in up to 15%), but six or more spots rarely occur in a patient without **neurofibromatosis type 1** (NF1; see Fig. 37.18); and conversely, patients with NF1 rarely have fewer than six café-au-lait spots.[20] Always remember to check for axillary freckling in patients with suspected NF1 (see Fig. 37.19), as this is usually present after 5 years of age.

Head

Examine the **hair**. Look for areas of alopecia. It is common for babies to have a 'bald spot' from lying in one position. Look for the oily, flaky scalp of 'cradle cap' (seborrhoeic dermatitis). Other causes of dry, flaky scalp include atopic dermatitis or tinea capitis. Some rare genetic disorders have clues in the hair: 'kinky hair' (twisted, fragile hair) can be seen in Menkes disease, or discoloration (e.g. a single white forelock) can be found in Waardenburg's syndrome.

Measure the **head circumference**. If this is not within the normal range, also measure the head

Haemangioma of the cheek.

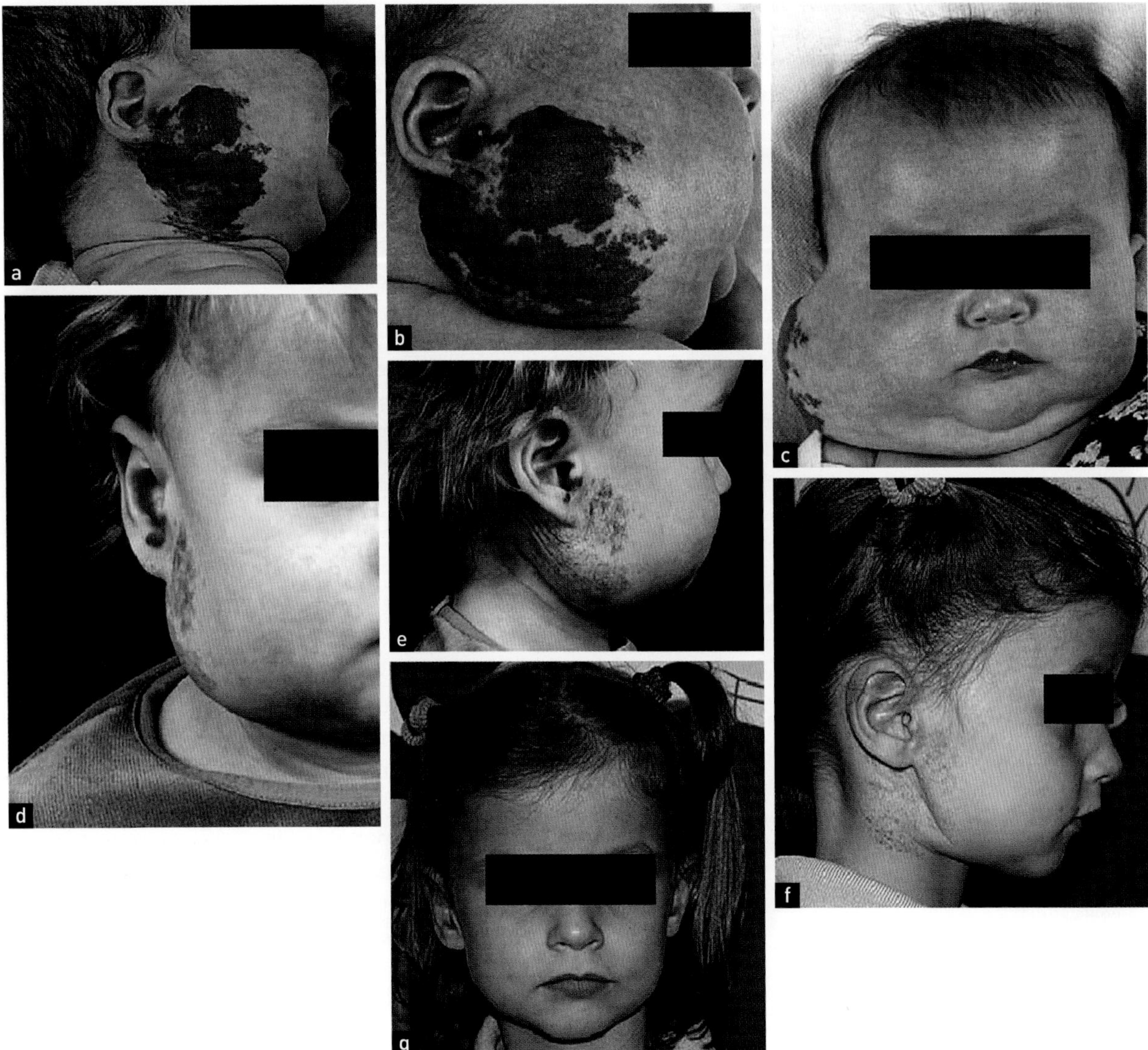

(a) Initial presentation at 2 weeks; (b, c) in proliferative phase at 2 months; (d, e) in involuting phase at 18 months; (f, g) in involuted phase at 6 years. Steroid treatment was used in infancy and surgery has been avoided

(From Leon-Villapalos J. Understanding vascular anomalies: a common language for doctors. *Surgery* 2012; 30(8):427–434, with permission.)

FIGURE 37.13

circumference of the parents and any siblings. Use a non-stretching tape to measure around the head at the widest point.

A small head (**microcephaly**) generally means a small brain. Causes can be familial or genetic. Secondary causes include congenital infection, hypoxic–ischaemic encephalopathy and fetal alcohol syndrome. Many paediatric syndromes such as Down syndrome, Rett syndrome and Edward syndrome are also associated with microcephaly.

A large head (**macrocephaly**) does not always mean a large brain. It may be the result of an enlarged brain (megalencephaly), but can also be due to fluid accumulation within the skull (hydrocephalus),

Haemangiomas and vascular malformations

Childhood haemangiomas	Vascular malformations
Development in first to fourth week of life, growth in the first 12 months	Established at birth, often later manifestation
Obligate regression phase	No tendency to regression, increasing ectasia more common while lacking true progression
Usually not completely compressible	Often compressible, differences in circumference and length, temperature differences
Histology: proliferation of endothelial cells, increase in number of mast cells	Histology: ectatic vessels, occluded vessels, variable vessel wall thickness or disturbed vessel wall architecture
High blood flow	Usually low blood flow, high in arteriovenous fistulae
Muscle and skeletal involvement rare	Muscle and skeletal involvement frequent

(Hohenleutner U, Landthaler M, Hamm H, Sebastian G. Hemangiomas of infancy and childhood. *J Dtsch Dermatol Ges* 2007; 5(4):334–338. ©John Wiley & Sons.)

TABLE 37.5

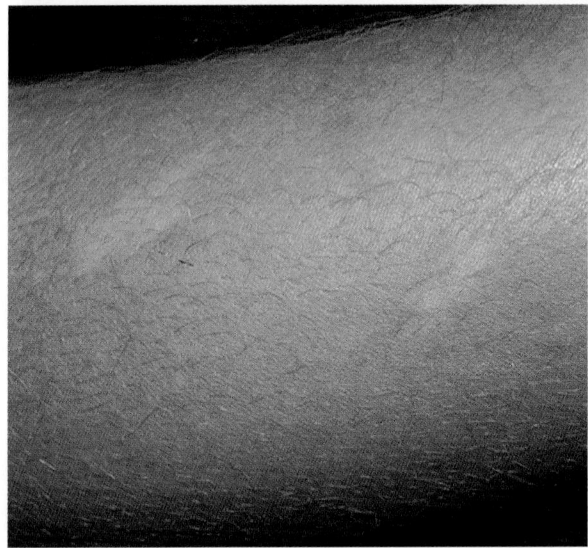

Hypopigmented lesion in tuberous sclerosis (TS)

(From Winn R. *Youmans neurological surgery*, 6th edn. Philadelphia: Saunders, 2011.)

FIGURE 37.14

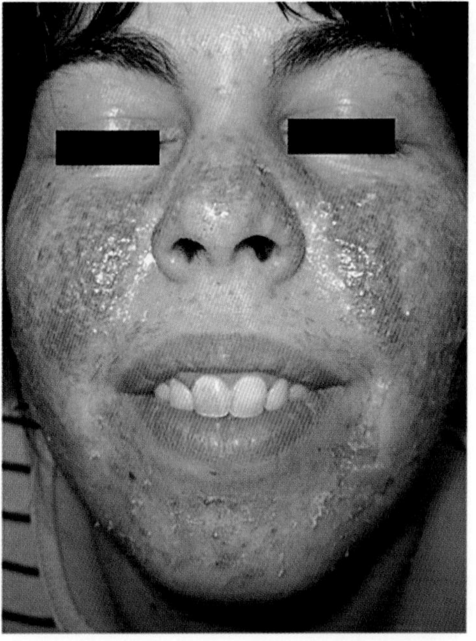

Clinical image of the lesions before the start of treatment. Multiple facial angiofibromas predominantly affecting the cheeks in tuberous sclerosis, with a prominent erythematous base

(From Valerón-Almazán P. Topical rapamycin solution to treat multiple facial angiofibromas in a patient with tuberous sclerosis. *Dermatology* (Actas Dermo-Sifiliográficas, English edn) 2010; 103(2):165–167. Copyright ©2010 Elsevier España, S.L. and AEDV.)

FIGURE 37.15

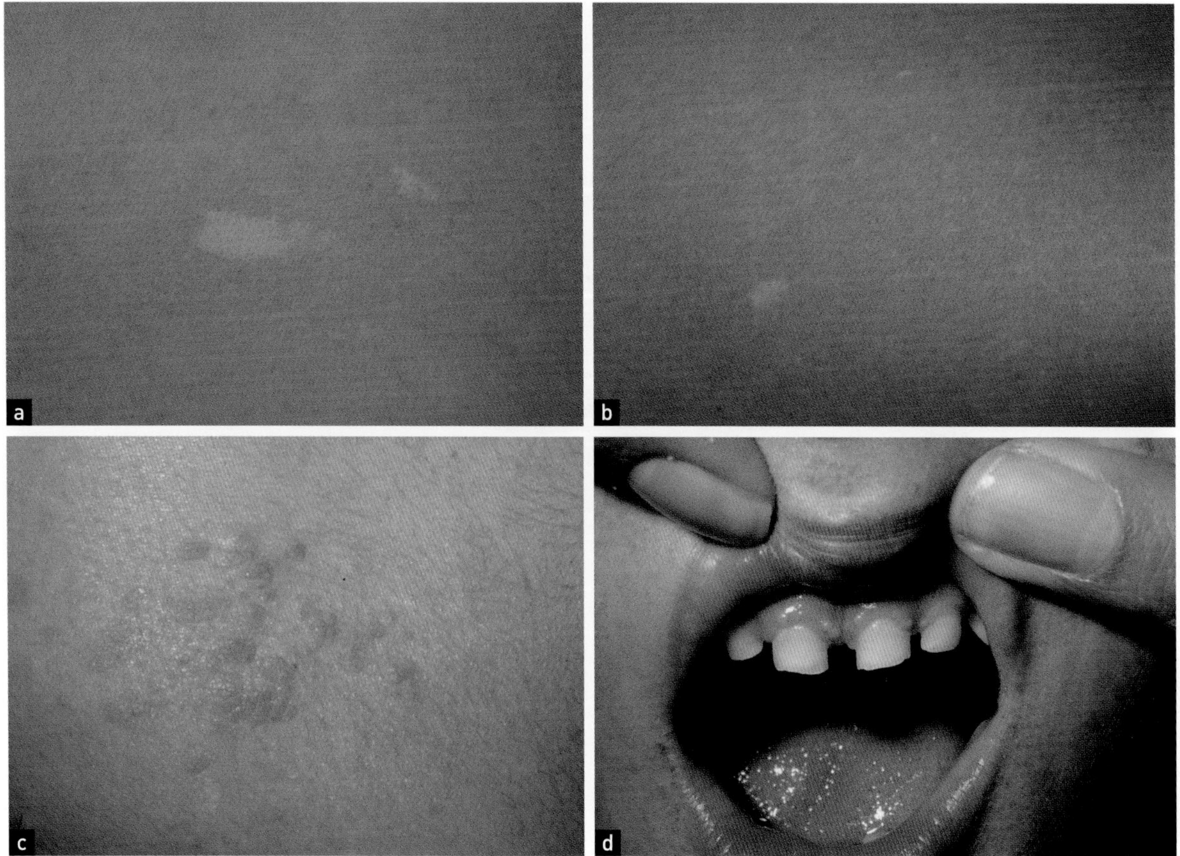

(a) Ashleaf macules are often present at birth or noted early in infancy. (b) Confetti hypopigmentation typically becomes more common over time. (c) Shagreen patch: large shagreen patches may be congenital, whereas smaller ones typically develop over time. (d) Gingival fibromas are a less common feature, but occasionally develop in young children with tuberous sclerosis

(From Morrell DS, Burkhart CN, Siegel D. In Eichenfield L, Eichenfield L, Frieden I, eds. *Neonatal dermatology*, 2nd edn. Philadelphia: Saunders, 2008, Ch 26, pp 477–501.)

FIGURE 37.16

porencephaly[d] or enlargement of the skull itself due to rickets, thalassaemia or osteogenesis imperfecta. Macrocephaly may be familial, secondary to metabolic disorders like Tay–Sachs disease, mucopolysaccharidoses (e.g. Hunter or Hurler syndrome), or syndromic (e.g. as a result of Sotos syndrome or neurofibromatosis).

If hydrocephalus is suspected in an infant or a small child, check for a bulging fontanel while the child is seated, prominent scalp veins and 'sun-setting' eyes (this failure of upward gaze means the child will have proportionally more conjunctiva visible *above* the iris than below). Smaller children are much more tolerant of increased intracranial pressure (and therefore may present late with massive hydrocephalus) than older children, who have fused cranial sutures.

Head shape should also be assessed (see Fig. 37.20). The most commonly seen head shape abnormality is positional plagiocephaly (an asymmetrical, flattened deformity of the skull secondary to positioning). Occipital plagiocephaly has been increasingly seen as parents have been encouraged to place their infants

[d] A developmental abnormality whereby one of the lateral ventricles communicates with the surface of the brain.

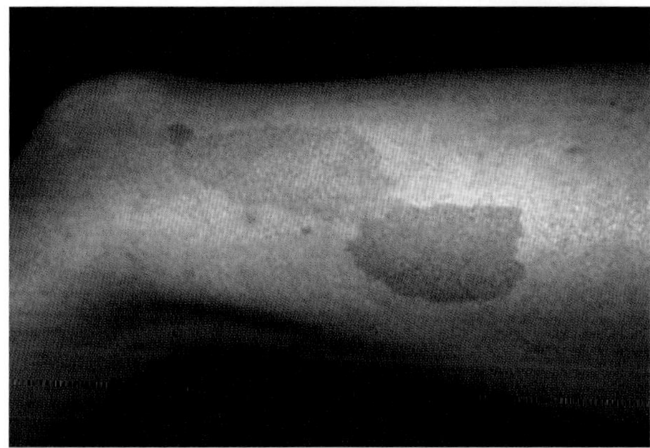

Café-au-lait macules on the thigh of a child

(From Boyd KP, Korf BR, Bruce R et al. Neurofibromatosis type 1. *J Am Acad Dermatol* 2009; 61(1):1–14.)

FIGURE 37.17

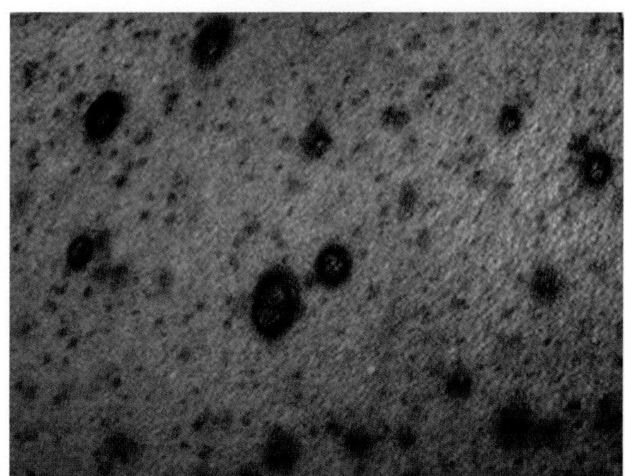

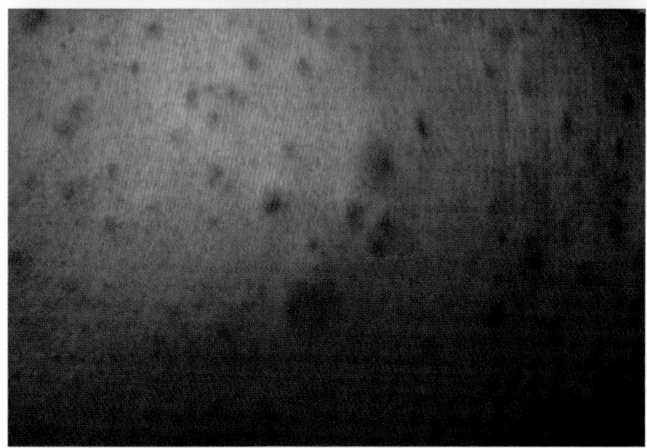

Cutaneous neurofibromas

(From Boyd KP, Korf BR, Bruce R et al. Neurofibromatosis type 1. *J Am Acad Dermatol* 2009; 61(1):1–14.)

FIGURE 37.18

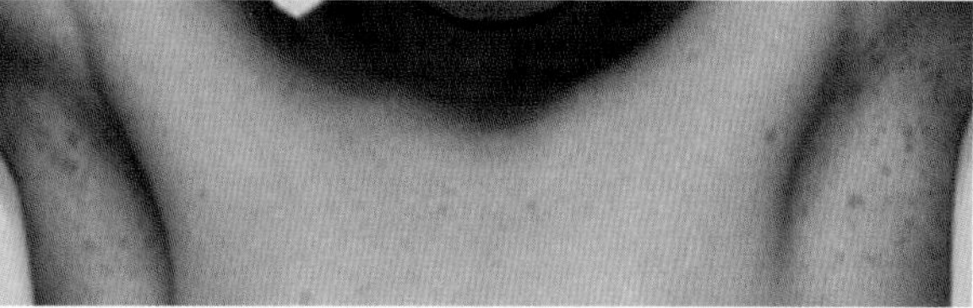

Bilateral axillary freckling

(From Boyd KP, Korf BR, Bruce R et al. Neurofibromatosis type 1. *J Am Acad Dermatol* 2009; 61(1):1–14.)

FIGURE 37.19

on their backs to sleep to decrease the risk of sudden infant death syndrome (SIDS).

Craniosynostosis (the premature fusion of the cranial sutures) is much less common and may occur as an isolated event or as part of a recognised syndrome (e.g. Crouzon or Apert syndrome).[21] The most common single suture synostosis involves the sagittal suture, but may also be seen at the coronal, metopic and lambdoid sutures. As these abnormalities may be associated with complications that affect the sensory, respiratory and neurological systems, it is important that they are recognised early and referred for treatment.[22]

Palpate over the skull for bony lumps (e.g. exostoses) and soft-tissue lumps (e.g. haemangiomas or cysts). Palpate the fontanels if still open (see Ch 38).

Examine the neck. As well as palpating for lymph nodes (see later in this chapter), look for cervical masses such as cystic hygromas, thyroglossal cysts or epidermoid cysts, which present with painless, soft or semifirm swellings. **Thyroglossal cysts** are most commonly localised in the midline at or below the level of the hyoid bone and move upwards when the tongue is protruded.[23] Epidermoid cysts are found on the floor of the mouth and superior to the hyoid bone.

Look for a **webbed neck**, which suggests Turner syndrome (see Fig. 37.21) or Noonan's syndrome; if found, look for decreased lateral rotation, which is seen in both syndromes. A **short neck** may be seen in several syndromes (e.g. Hurler syndrome and Klippel–Feil syndrome) as well as in congenital hypothyroidism.

Finally, palpate for the **thyroid gland**. This lies on either side of the trachea, below the thyroid cartilage, and is best felt by standing behind the patient and placing your hands gently on either side of the patient's

Diagnostic features of craniosynostosis.

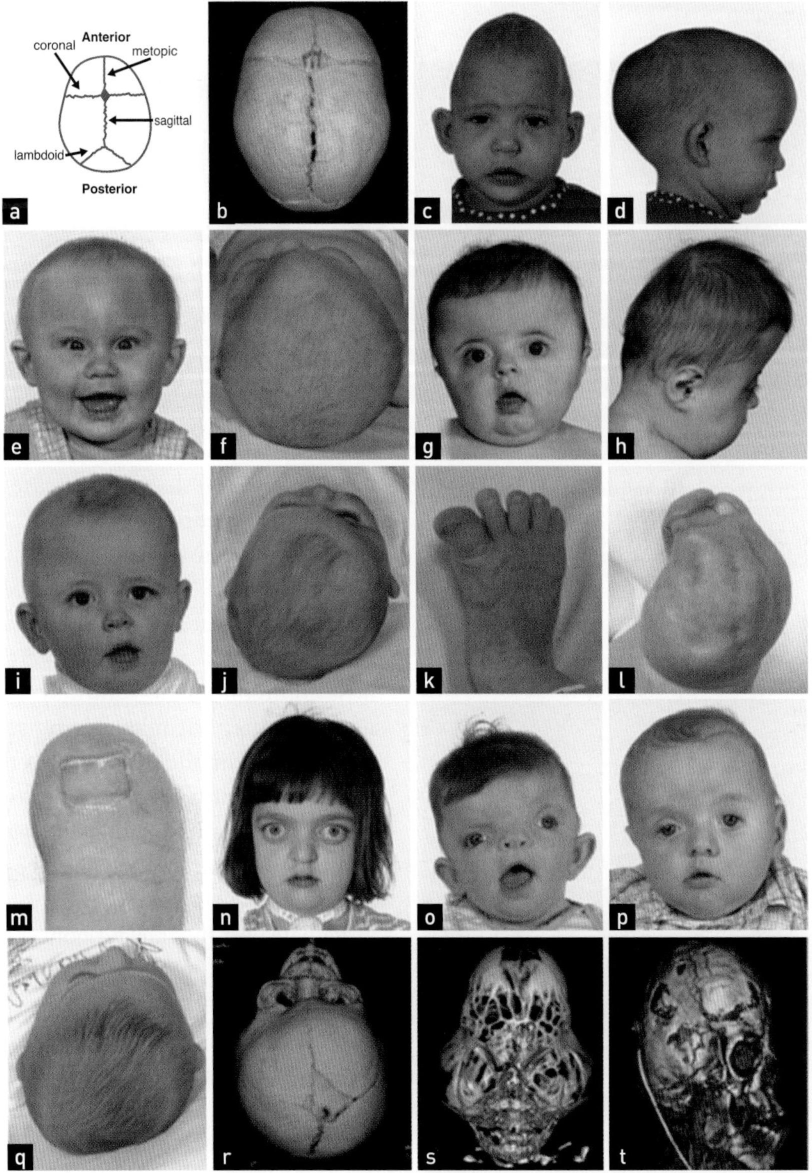

(a) Schematic diagram showing positions of the major cranial sutures. (b) CT scan (vertex view of skull) showing major sutures; anterior is at top. (c, d) Sagittal synostosis: note the long, narrow head. (e, f) Metopic synostosis: note hypotelorism and the triangular profile of the forehead. (g, h) Bicoronal synostosis: broad, flattened head. (i, j) Right unicoronal synostosis: note the flattened brow and anterior position of the ear on the affected side, deviation of the nasal tip and prominent brow on the unaffected side. Congenital anomalies of the feet or hands characteristic of (k) Pfeiffer syndrome, (l) Apert syndrome and (m) craniofrontonasal syndrome. (n) Crouzonoid facial appearance. (o) Severe hypertelorism, grooved nasal tip and left unicoronal synostosis in craniofrontonasal syndrome. (p) Ptosis and left unicoronal synostosis in Saethre–Chotzen syndrome. (q) Positional plagiocephaly: prominence on the right anteriorly and the left posteriorly, with right ear anterior and parallelogram shape to the skull. (r) CT reconstruction showing left unicoronal synostosis. (s) CT reconstruction showing clover-leaf skull. (t) CT venogram showing abnormal venous drainage in multisuture syndromic craniosynostosis

FIGURE 37.20

neck. Ask the patient to swallow and the thyroid will move upwards. This is really only possible in the older cooperative child, however; it can be very difficult to examine the neck of an infant owing to the relative size of the head compared with the neck. Also, not surprisingly, small children usually will not tolerate an examiner standing behind them putting their hands around their neck! Try to examine the thyroid with the patient sitting and facing you if that approach is more likely to be successful.

Ear, nose and throat

It is particularly important to be proficient in the ear, nose and throat (ENT) examination as infections in these organs are some of the most common presentations for children. **This is a key skill in the paediatric examination.**

Inspect the size, shape and position of the ears. Check for malformations and any preauricular tags or pits, which can be associated with hearing loss but are usually benign. **Palpate** over the tragus and pinna, which may be tender if the child has otitis externa, and over the mastoid behind the ear if mastoiditis is suspected. Mastoiditis, if present, may also push the pinna of the ear forwards, giving the child a lop-sided appearance. Infection and inflammation of the skin of the ears and the ear canal (e.g. eczema, bacterial or fungal otitis externa) are quite common. Children are also predisposed to middle ear infections. A hyperaemic (red), inflamed, bulging tympanic membrane, with loss of the light reflex (see Ch 32, Fig. 42.16), may signify **acute otitis media (AOM)** (also called otitis media with effusion—OME; see Ch 42). While genetic, infectious, immunological and environmental factors all play a role in this predisposition, the shape of the eustachian tube itself, which is shorter and less angled in children (see Fig. 37.22), means that it is easier for organisms to migrate from the nasopharynx to the middle ear and more difficult for the middle ear to drain.[22]

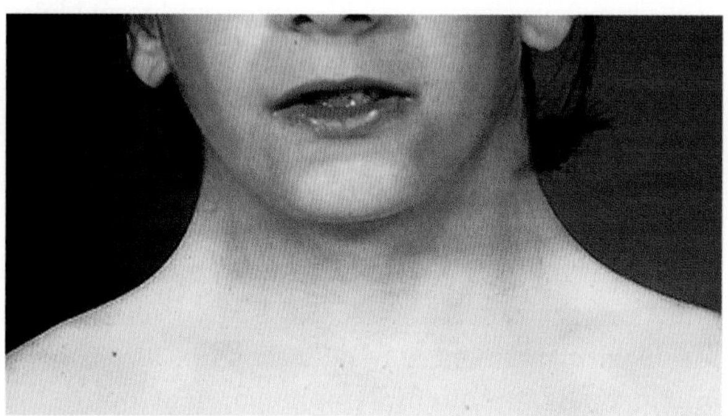

Webbed neck in Turner syndrome

(From Bouloux PM. Self-assessment picture tests. *Medicine*, vol 1. St Louis, MO: Mosby, 1996; Goljan EF. *Rapid review laboratory testing in clinical medicine.* St Louis, MO: Mosby, 2008.)

FIGURE 37.21

Although **otoscopy** should not hurt unless it is done incorrectly, it can be quite upsetting for younger children and is best performed while they are seated on their parent's lap—**and at the end of the examination.** If necessary, have the parent lock the child's lower limbs securely between their thighs (or even wrap a leg across the child's legs) and use his or her arms to embrace the child warmly, holding them tight against their chest, whilst simultaneously holding down the child's arms and head.

Ensure that you hold the otoscope with part of your hand touching the child's head so that it can move with any movements of their head to prevent injuring the tympanic membrane (see Fig. 37.23). Tips for otoscopes come in various sizes; use one that fits comfortably in the ear canal but also allows visualisation of the drum. Generally, to visualise the ear canal and eardrum adequately, gently pull the pinna downwards if the child is under the age of 2 years, and upwards and backwards if older than 2 years.[7] Take note of the ear canal as the otoscope enters the ear. Look for swelling and erythema. Bear in mind that earwax can build up in the canal and make visualisation of the tympanic membrane difficult or even impossible.

Finally, examine the eardrum itself (see Figs 37.24 and 37.25). Normally, this is a pale-pink colour, although previous infections and perforations can cause scarring. If the eustachian tube is blocked, the drum may be under negative pressure and may be retracted away from you. Retraction is also seen in chronic otitis media with effusion. If there is pus behind the drum, as in acute otitis media, it can take on a red or yellow colour and may be bulging.

Examine the shape and position of the **nose**, and look for signs of inflammation and rhinorrhoea. Palpate over the bony and cartilaginous surfaces of the nose feeling for lumps, pain and swelling. Look inside the nose. If there is pain, look for lesions or ulcers. Look

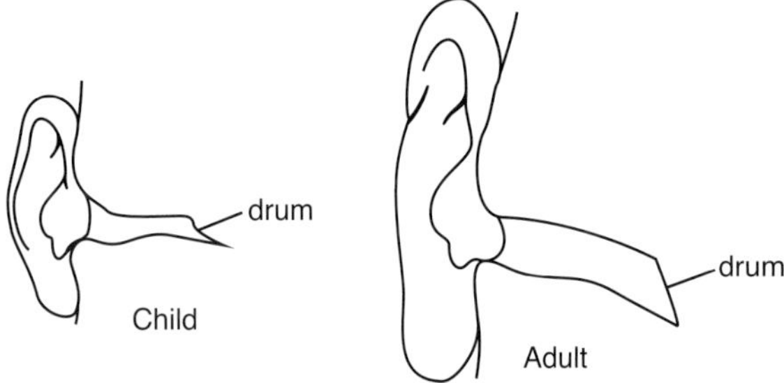

Comparison of the eustachian tubes in children and adults

(From Hockenberry MJ, Wilson D. *Wong's nursing care of infants and children*, 9th edn. St Louis, MO: Mosby, 2011.)

FIGURE 37.22

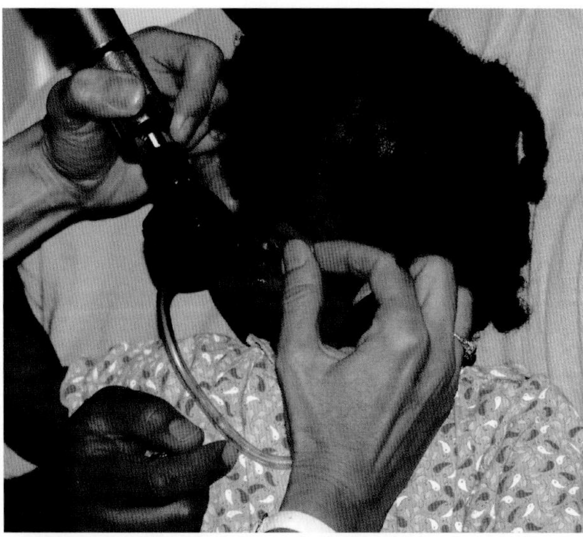

Positioning of examiner's hands for otoscopic examination. Note that the little finger of the hand holding the otoscope is braced against the child's head. (The examiner is left-handed.) The first two fingers of the other hand retract the pinna, while the remaining fingers are wrapped around the bulb of the insufflator, prepared to squeeze the bulb if the examination warrants

(From Swartz MH. *Textbook of physical diagnosis: history and examination*, 6th edn. Philadelphia: Saunders, 2009.)

FIGURE 37.23

for blood and the site of haemorrhage (often a large vessel is seen in 'Little's area' in children with recurrent epistaxis—see Ch 42). An inflamed mucosa suggests allergy, while the presence of polyps suggests cystic fibrosis. Look for a foreign body (e.g. beads, food—or pretty much anything!). In a general paediatrics setting, an otoscope can be used for this, and if a more detailed examination is required then referral to an ENT surgeon is necessary for nasal endoscopy.

Examination of the **mouth** and **throat** is fundamental in paediatrics and is one of the most common examinations in everyday practice. Again, the best place for this examination is with the child sitting in the parent's lap. It is usually best to position the child facing forwards with one of the parent's arms across the child's arms and the other hand on the child's forehead, preventing the child's head from moving. Initially, look at the lips and mouth. Check for lesions such as ulcers or angular stomatitis. Look for pallor or cyanosis and for any anatomical defects such as a cleft lip. Ask the child to show you the teeth. Note the position and signs of dental decay, which remains the most common chronic disease in children. In a cooperative (or older) child, examine the sublingual space (under the tongue), looking particularly for where the lingual frenulum attaches to the tongue. If possible, examine the buccal mucosa and look for the opening of the salivary ducts.

To visualise the **oropharynx**, a tongue depressor is often needed to move the tongue down and out of the way, and parental cooperation can be critical at this stage. Check the hard and soft palates, looking in particular for defects, including midline cleft palate defects. Inspect the uvula: a bifid uvula may be a sign of a submucous cleft along with a thin translucent bluish or white strip of lining (mucosa). If seen, palpate the hard palate looking for a defect or notch at the base of the uvula.

The palatine tonsils are commonly enlarged in children and are generally easily visualised after about 9 months of age. Look for erythema and exudate if infection is suspected (see Fig. 37.26). Unilateral tonsillar enlargement may indicate a tonsillar abscess or, much less commonly, lymphoma. Also look at the pharynx itself for erythema and exudate.

Face and dysmorphology

The goal is to determine whether the size, shape and position of a physical feature is a normal variant versus a minor or major anomaly, which can be quite challenging

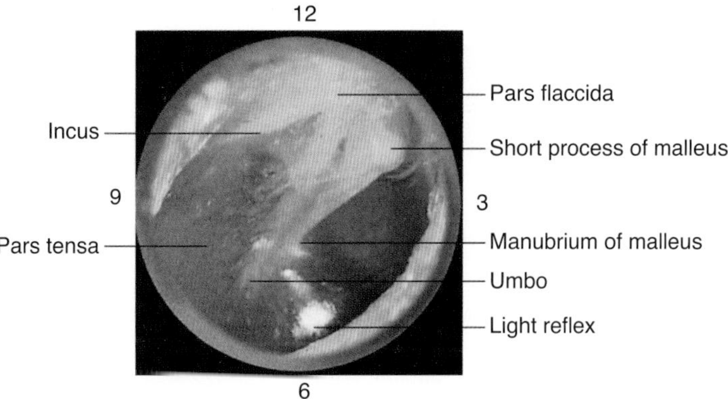

Tympanic membrane landmarks

(From Seidel HM, Ball JW, Dains JE et al. *Mosby's guide to physical examination*, 7th edn. St Louis, MO: Mosby, 2011.)

FIGURE 37.24

Acute otitis media.

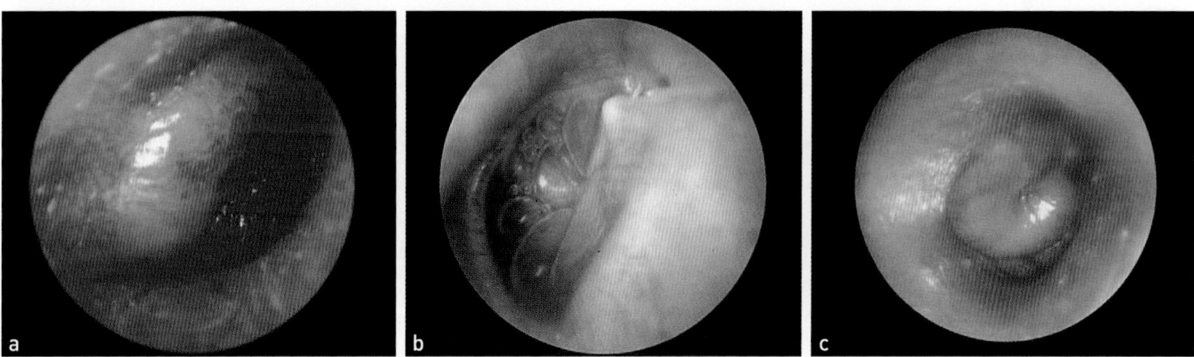

(a) This is the textbook picture: an erythematous, opaque, bulging tympanic membrane. The light reflex is reduced, and the landmarks are partially obscured. Mobility is markedly reduced. (b) In this acutely febrile child who complained of otalgia, the presence of both air and fluid formed bubbles separated by greyish-yellow menisci. Even though the drum was not injected, this finding, combined with fever and otalgia, is consistent with acute infection. (c) In this child the tympanic membrane was injected at the periphery, and a yellow purulent effusion caused the inferior portion to bulge outwards. Mobility was markedly reduced

((a) From Hawke M, Yellon RF. *Zitelli and Davis' atlas of pediatric physical diagnosis*, 6th edn. Philadelphia: Saunders, 2012.)

FIGURE 37.25

on occasions. **An empathic approach is clearly needed**, as the parents are often the first to realise their child 'looks different'. The list below is not exhaustive but outlines some common facial dysmorphisms that suggest particular diagnoses. Importantly the *entire clinical picture* needs to be taken into account as single, isolated facial anomalies may be more likely to be normal anatomical variation *without* a syndromic diagnosis.

Careful examination of the **face** (in association with other features) may reveal the presence of a syndromic or genetic abnormality (see Tables 37.6 and 37.7).[24]

Pharyngotonsillitis.

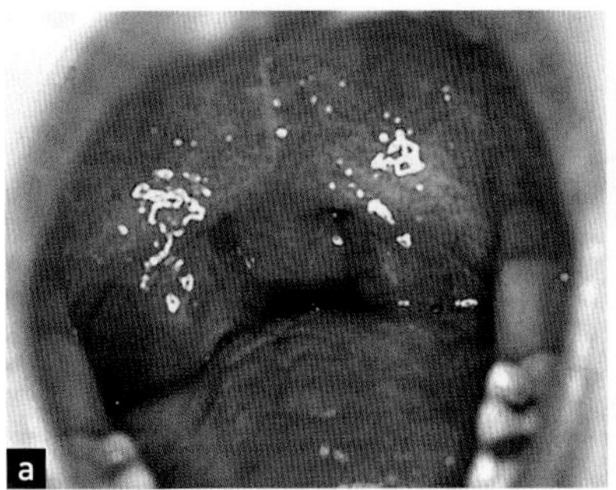
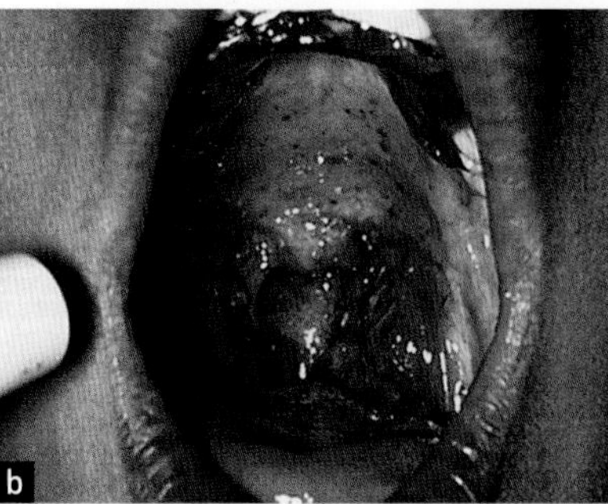
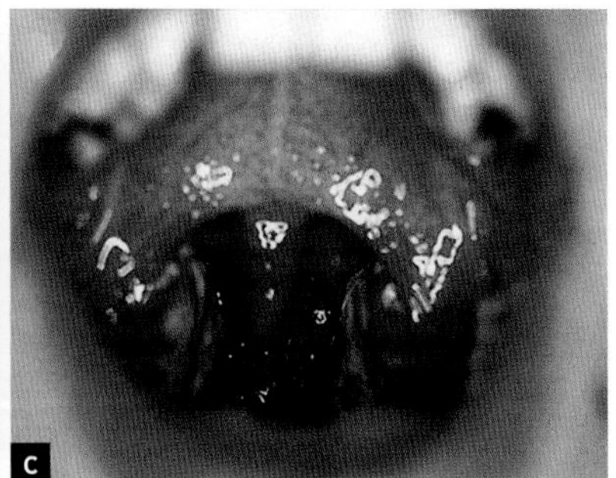

This common syndrome has several causative pathogens and a wide spectrum of severity. (a) The diffuse tonsillar and pharyngeal erythema seen here is a non-specific finding that can be produced by a variety of pathogens. (b) This intense erythema, seen in association with acute tonsillar enlargement and palatal petechiae, is highly suggestive of group A *Streptococcus* β-haemolytic infection, although other pathogens can produce these findings. (c) This picture of exudative tonsillitis is most commonly seen with either group A streptococcal or Epstein–Barr virus infection

(From Yellon RF, McBride TP, Davis HW. Otolaryngology. In: Zitelli BJ, Davis HW (eds). *Atlas of pediatric physical diagnosis*, 4th edn. St Louis, MO: Mosby, 2002, p 852.)

FIGURE 37.26

Note the general shape of the face (e.g. broad or round). Look for asymmetry (e.g. CHARGE syndrome, Goldenhar syndrome), coarse features (e.g. metabolic disorders such as mucopolysaccharidoses), midface hypoplasia (e.g. fetal alcohol syndrome) and expression (e.g. the expressionless facies of congenital myotonic dystrophy).

Look at the shape of the **forehead**: is it prominent, broad, short or bossed? Is the hairline high or low? Look at the prominence of the supraorbital ridges and the eyebrows and note the bushy and singular eyebrows (synophrys) of Cornelia de Lange syndrome.

Examine the **eyes**. Look for coloboma (defects in which tissue is missing from various parts of the structure of the eye). These may be seen in the eyelids, iris, lens and macula and even in the optic nerve (e.g. CHARGE syndrome). Look at the colour of the sclerae, which are bluish in osteogenesis imperfecta, and the iris, which appears bicoloured (heterochromic) in Waardenburg syndrome. Look for hypertelorism (widely spaced eyes)[e,f] (e.g. Apert syndrome) and, if suspected, measure the inner and outer canthal distances. Hypotelorism (closely spaced eyes) is a strong indicator for abnormal brain development.[24] Examine the eyelids looking for ptosis (e.g. Noonan syndrome), and check for ectropion (whereby the eyelids appear everted, as in Kabuki syndrome) or entropion (whereby the eyelids are turned inwards, as in DiGeorge syndrome). Look for the presence of epicanthal folds and note whether the palpebral fissures slant upwards as in Down syndrome or downwards as in Treacher Collins syndrome.

Look at the shape and size of the **nose**, particularly for a flat nasal bridge, which is common in many syndromes. The philtrum may be long, as in Cornelia de Lange syndrome, or smooth, as in fetal alcohol syndrome. Assess the mandible for micrognathia (small jaw) and prognathia (forward position of mandible relative to maxilla). Micrognathia, glossoptosis (tongue further back in mouth), and cleft palate occur in Pierre Robin sequence. Note the size of the mouth, which may be enlarged in Angelman syndrome, and the size of the lips, which may be thin, as in the thin upper lip of fetal alcohol syndrome. Look for a cleft of the lip or palate and check for the high-arched palate of Marfan syndrome.

[e] This is one of numerous parts of the paediatric examination that it is recommended should be left until the end.

[f] This means an abnormally large separation of parts of the body. It is most often used to mean abnormal separation of the eye sockets caused by enlargement of the sphenoid bone.

Select syndromes with dysmorphic features

Condition	Selected distinctive features
1p36 deletion syndrome	Deep-set eyes, straight eyebrows, flat midface
17q21.31 microdeletion syndrome	Long face, narrow palpebral fissures, bulbous nasal tip, large low-set ears
22q deletion syndrome	Short palpebral fissures, broad midnose, long tapered fingers
9q22.3 microdeletion syndrome	Large size, macrocephaly, small mouth, thin upper lip
9q34 microdeletion syndrome	Long eyebrows with synophrys, upturned nose, short philtrum, low-set ears
Angelman syndrome	Large mouth, prominent jaw
ATRX	Hypertelorism, short philtrum, macrostomia, everted lower lip
Cardiofaciocutaneous syndrome	Sparse coarse hair, high forehead, relative macrocephaly, hyperkeratotic macules
CHARGE syndrome	Dysplastic ears, which are often asymmetrical; unilateral facial palsy
Coffin–Lowry syndrome	Full lips, with the upper lip being rounded with minimal vermilion peaks; 'puffy' tapered fingers
Cornelia de Lange syndrome	Synophrys with arched eyebrows, ill-defined alae, thin lips with downturned mouth
Costello syndrome	'Coarse' appearance, sparse curly hair, deep palmar creases
Fetal alcohol syndrome	Short palpebral fissures, flat philtrum, relatively thin upper lip
Kabuki syndrome	Long palpebral fissures, prominent ears, fetal finger pads
Mowat–Wilson syndrome	Deeply set eyes, round nasal tip, uplifted earlobes
Noonan syndrome	Hypertelorism, deeply grooved philtrum
Prader–Willi syndrome	Narrow forehead, 'upslanting' palpebral fissures, small hands and feet
Smith–Magenis syndrome	Short philtrum with upturned upper lip, flat midface
Sotos syndrome	Macrocephaly, high forehead, 'downslanting' palpebral fissures
Williams syndrome	Periorbital puffiness, anteverted nares, full lips

ATRX= alpha-thalassemia syndrome, X-linked.

(Toriello HV. Role of the dysmorphologic evaluation in the child with developmental delay. *Pediatr Clin North Am* 2008; 55(5):1085–1098.)

TABLE 37.6

Look for macroglossia suggestive of Down syndrome or Beckwith–Wiedemann syndrome.

The **ears** may be large, as in fragile X syndrome, or small, as in Down syndrome. Check whether the ears are abnormal in shape or position. Inspect the pinna for unusual folding and the earlobes for size and creases (e.g. Beckwith–Wiedemann syndrome) and for preauricular pits and tags (may be normal anatomical variation; may or may not be associated with hearing issues).

An excellent online source of information on diagnosis, genetic testing, management and genetic counselling of patients and families can be found at GeneReviews™ (www.ncbi.nlm.nih.gov/books/NBK1116), a peer-reviewed and regularly updated site. Another useful site is Genetics Home Reference (http://ghr.nlm.nih.gov).

Neurological examination

Much of the neurological examination in older children is essentially identical to that in an adult. Examining the upper and lower limbs for tone, power, deep tendon reflexes, coordination and sensation and examining the gait are unchanged, as are the cerebellar examination, much of the cranial nerve (CN) examination and the ophthalmological examination (see Chs 32–34 for a detailed explanation of these examinations). In infants and younger children, keen observation and interactive play can reveal much with respect to their developing neurological system.

Select metabolic conditions with dysmorphic features

Condition	Dysmorphic features
Arginino succinic aciduria	Alopecia, brittle hair
Congenital disorders of glycosylation	Lipodystrophy, high nasal bridge, prominent jaw, inverted nipples
D-2-hydroxy glutaric aciduria	Macrocephaly, epicanthal folds, coarse facial features, single transverse palmar crease
Glutaric aciduria type I	Prenatal- or postnatal-onset macrocephaly, facial grimacing
Glutaric aciduria type II	High forehead, depressed nasal bridge, short nose, single transverse palmar crease
GM_1 gangliosidosis	Coarse facial features, expressionless face, hirsutism on forehead, long philtrum
Homocystinuria	Tall and thin, depigmented hair
I-cell disease	Similar to mucopolysaccharidosis but earlier onset
Kearns–Sayre syndrome	Progressive ptosis, short stature
Menkes syndrome	Depigmented, kinky or brittle hair; abnormal eyebrow hair
Methylmalonic acidaemia	High forehead, broad nasal bridge, epicanthal folds, long smooth philtrum, triangular mouth
Mucolipidosis III	Hirsutism, synophrys, coarse facial features
Mucopolysaccharidosis	Macrocephaly, coarse facial features, frontal bossing, prominent eyes, depressed nasal bridge, thick lips
Multiple carboxylase deficiency	Alopecia, sparse eyebrows and eyelashes
Multiple sulfatase deficiency	Postnatal microcephaly, coarse facial features, prominent eyes
Propionic acidaemia	Frontal bossing, depressed nasal bridge, epicanthal folds, open mouth with downturned corners
Pyruvate dehydrogenase deficiency	Frontal bossing, short nose, long philtrum, thin upper lip
Smith–Lemli–Opitz syndrome	High forehead, ptosis, epicanthal folds, short nose, micrognathia, syndactyly of toes 2–3
Zellweger syndrome	High forehead, large fontanels, abnormal ears, broad nasal bridge, hypoplastic supraorbital ridges

(Toriello HV. Role of the dysmorphologic evaluation in the child with developmental delay. *Pediatr Clin North America* 2008; 55(5):1085–1098.)

TABLE 37.7

Cranial nerves

CN I (olfactory nerve)

In infants: not generally able to be tested.

In older children: ask the child to close the eyes and identify a common scent (e.g. vanilla).

CN II (optic nerve)

Always remember to examine each eye individually.

In infants:

Perform fundoscopy.

Perform the swinging torch test (this tests CN II [afferent] and CN III [efferent]).

- Use a torch to shine a light onto the pupil, then move the light to the other pupil and look closely for a change in pupillary diameter.
- A defect in CN II (afferent pupillary defect) will result in less constriction of both pupils when light is shone into the affected eye; subsequently shining the light into the normal eye will result in the pupils constricting even further.

Visual fields: cannot be tested reliably.

Visual acuity: cannot be tested reliably.

In older children:

Perform fundoscopy.

Perform the swinging torch test (as above).

Visual fields:

- Have an assistant (often the parent) distract the child while you bring a toy (traditionally red in colour) from behind them into the visual field.
- The child should notice the toy and respond as soon as the toy is perpendicular to the outer canthus of the eye.
- For an older child, ask him or her to cover up one eye with the hand and focus on your nose and tell you how many fingers he or she can see being held up into each of the four visual quadrants (identical to the examination in an adult).

Visual acuity:

- For smaller children, offer small interesting objects for them to pick up (raisins or hundreds-and-thousands are particularly well received) but ensure they do not put them into their mouth and choke on it—as a bonus, this also tests fine-motor function.
- For older children, use an age-appropriate vision chart (see Fig. 37.27).

CN III, IV and VI (oculomotor, trochlear and abducens)

These three cranial nerves are examined together as they all innervate muscles of the face: the superior oblique by CN IV, the lateral rectus by CN VI and the medial rectus, superior rectus, inferior rectus and inferior oblique by CN III.

For infants:

Look for ptosis (CN III) and, if seen, look for a constricted pupil on the affected side (e.g. Horner syndrome).

Looking at the infant front-on, move your head from left to right and watch him or her fix and follow your face. Alternatively, use a picture of a face for the infant's eyes to follow, held about arm's length from the infant.

For older children:

Use a finger puppet or toy for the child to focus on and move this through the lateral, medial, upper and lower visual fields. Observe the eye movements.

In school-aged children, it is often useful to use a torch, so that you can observe the light reflection centred on both pupils.

If there is any diplopia, ask where the two images are most widely separated.

The false image (the outer image) can be determined by having the child close each eye. This can also help determine which muscle is paretic.

CN V (trigeminal)

For infants:

Observe the infant feeding and palpate over the masseter muscles as he or she sucks.

For older children:

Observe and palpate the masseter muscles while the child clenches the teeth together.

Test sensation in the ophthalmic, maxillary and mandibular divisions of the trigeminal nerve as you would in an adult.

The jaw jerk *can* be elicited by placing your thumb over the child's chin while the mouth is slightly open. Tap on your thumb with a tendon hammer and the mouth should close. An upper motor neurone lesion is suggested by a brisk mouth closure. It is really only in older children that this reflex can be elicited, as most children will not let you come anywhere near their faces with the hammer.

CN VII (facial)

For infants:

Observing the child's face during the examination is usually sufficient.

Look for drooling out of the weak side of the mouth. Subtle changes are more pronounced when the infant is crying or laughing.

For older children:

Ask the child to smile, raise the eyebrows, close the eyes and show the teeth.

Ask the child to blow on a toy or finger puppet.

The corneal reflex (CN V afferent and CN VII efferent) is rarely tested in children, but if there is serious concern, it is best to perform this by gently blowing on the eye. Use your hand to protect the other eye during the procedure.

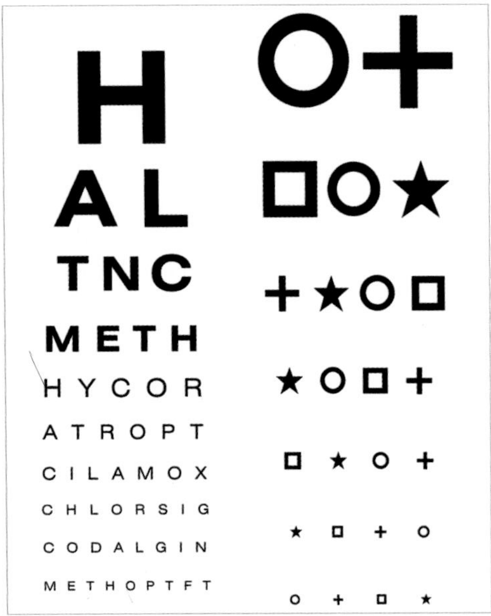

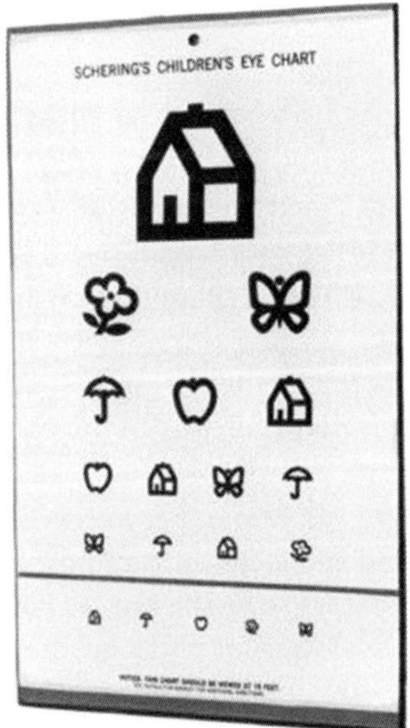

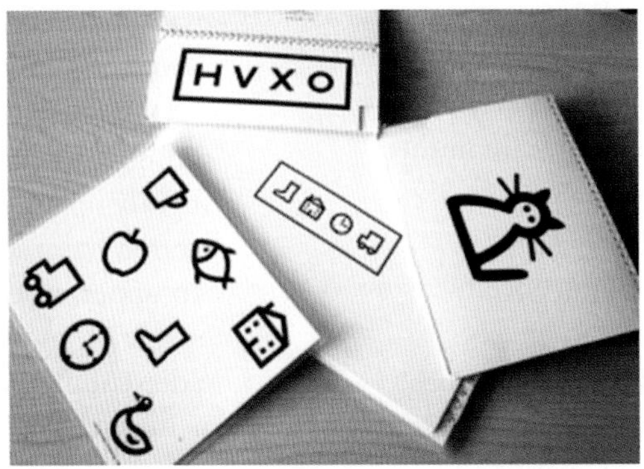

Age-appropriate visual acuity charts

(Snellen visual acuity chart, *Clinical Neurology: A Primer*, Figure 4.2, 2010, Elsevier Australia; Picture visual acuity chart, *Ophthalmic Assistant*, The Ninth Edition, Fig. 8.4, 2013, Elsevier Inc; Visual acuity charts designed for use with children, *Clinical Procedures in Primary Eye Care*, Fourth Edition, Figure. 3.2, 2014, Elsevier Limited.)

FIGURE 37.27

CN VIII (cochlear and vestibular)

For infants: generally, if there is serious concern, formal audiometry should be arranged.

For older children: test as you would for an adult, including Weber's and Rinne's tests if appropriate (see Ch 32).

CN IX and X (glossopharyngeal and vagus)

For infants:

Observe the palate if (when) the child cries at any stage during the examination.

Listen for b, d and k sounds when the child is speaking, as children with defective palate movement often have difficulty producing these sounds.

For older children:

In practice, this is usually limited to asking the child to open up and say 'Ah!' and observing palate movements.

Again, listen for b, d and k sounds when the child is speaking.

It is not recommended to test routinely for the gag reflex in children unless there is a history suggestive of swallowing difficulties or palate dysfunction. Be aware that children with a sensitive gag reflex may well vomit during this procedure.

CN XI (spinal accessory)

For infants:

Lay the infant supine on an examination table, with your arm underneath the shoulders providing support. Push gently on the head laterally and the infant should resist this movement.

Palpate the sternocleidomastoid muscles bilaterally.

For older children: as in the adult, have the child push against your hand with his or her mandible, and while you palpate the contralateral sternocleidomastoid muscle.

CN XII (hypoglossal)

For infants: examination in this age group is fairly limited—assess for tongue fasciculation and movement of the tongue if possible during the examination.

For older children: ask the child to poke the tongue out at you and to imitate you as you move your tongue from side to side (most children love this).

Motor and cerebellar examination

The majority of the motor and cerebellar examination in smaller children is best performed using a combination of observation and play. Have the child reach overhead to grasp a toy and then manipulate small objects (blocks, balls, etc.). This gives you an indication of proximal and distal strength in the upper limbs. If things are going particularly well, you can perform the **wheelbarrow test**: have the child begin on his or her hands and knees, then lift and hold the child's legs under your arms while the child 'walks' forwards on the hands. For older children, test power in the upper and lower limbs as you would in an adult.

Watch the child walk and climb stairs, or jump and hop; for the smaller child, note the infant's ability to bear weight while standing supported. These all give a good indication of strength in the lower limbs. In fact, the **gait examination** is probably the quickest and easiest test of gross-motor function in children. Where appropriate, perform a gait examination for older children as you would in the adult.

Ask the child to lie on the floor (supine) and to stand up as quickly as possible: a child with proximal weakness may roll onto the abdomen and 'climb up' his or her legs using the strength in the upper limbs (Gower's sign; see Fig. 37.28). This is usually seen in Duchenne's muscular dystrophy, but also may be seen in children with other myopathies and dystrophies (e.g. spinal muscular atrophy, Becker's muscular dystrophy or steroid myopathy).

Examining **tone** in children is of particular significance. The clinical presentation prompting examination includes the 'floppy' infant, the child with abnormal gait or the child with delayed motor milestones. In these children, inherited neuromuscular disorders must always be considered, although numerous other conditions (e.g. infectious, autoimmune, vascular) can have a similar presentation. Features from the history and examination can guide diagnosis; for example, normal-looking muscle bulk (or even pseudohypertrophy, particularly of the calves) coupled with decreased muscle tone and strength may indicate Duchenne's or Becker's muscular dystrophy.

If weakness is found during the physical examination, an attempt should be made to differentiate between an upper motor neurone (UMN) lesion, which usually presents with hypertonia, hyperreflexia, clonus, spasticity and a positive Babinski's sign (after the age of 1 year), and a lower motor neurone (LMN) lesion, where the child has hypotonia and hyporeflexia.[20] For infants, this differentiation is described as 'floppy weak' (an infant with a disorder of the LMN, e.g. spinal muscular atrophy) or 'floppy strong' (an infant with central weakness and hence UMN signs, e.g. cerebral palsy).[20] **Cerebral palsy** is an umbrella term for a group of non-progressive clinical conditions, ranging in severity, whose key characteristic is that of **motor abnormalities** of tone, movement and posture. It occurs due to an abnormality or 'insult' in the developing brain.

Start by assessing tone in the arms and legs by moving the joints passively at the wrists, elbows, knees and ankles. As well as assessing for hypotonia, note any rigidity or spasticity. A few simple manoeuvres are particularly useful in demonstrating tone and strength in infants and small children, particularly when looking for reduced tone.[25] This is called the **180° examination** (see Fig. 37.29).

1. *The 180° examination:* Begin with the infant or small child lying supine on a firm surface.

   Note the resting posture and positioning and look for movement of the arms and legs (voluntary and involuntary), symmetry of movements and general level of alertness.

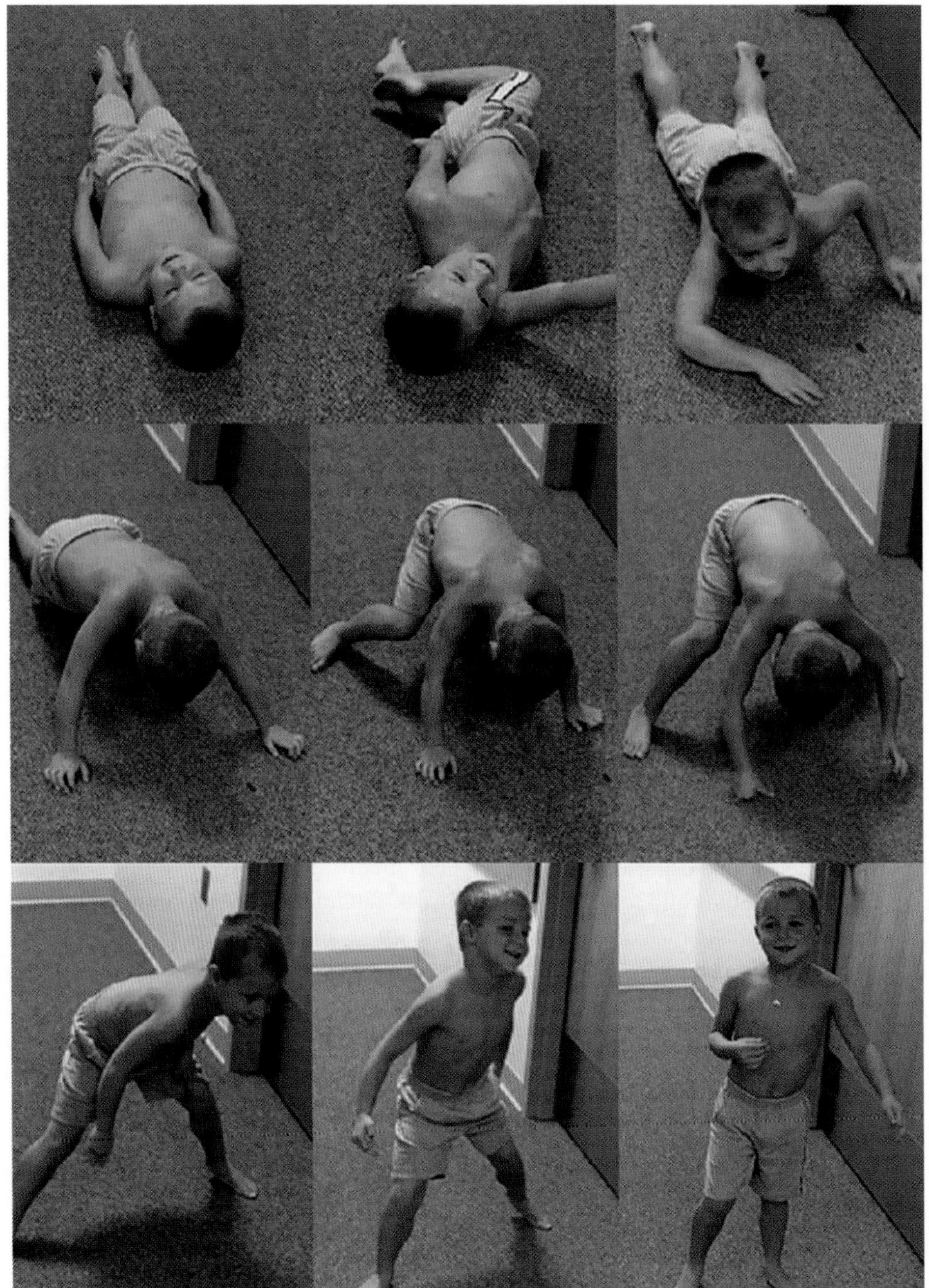

Gower's sign

(Menezes MP, North KN. Inherited neuromuscular disorders: pathway to diagnosis. *Journal of Paediatrics and Child Health* 2012; 48(6):458–465 © John Wiley & Sons.)

FIGURE 37.28

2. *'Scarf sign'*: take the child's hand and pull it (gently) across his or her chest so that the elbow is underneath the chin.

   This tests appendicular tone in the shoulders, but remember that this is also reflective of the child's level of alertness (a child in a deep sleep may appear to have lower tone).

   In the hypotonic child the elbow can be easily pulled beyond the middle line with minimal resistance.

3. *'Pull to sit'*: grasp the child's hands and pull the child gently into a sitting position.

   This tests axial tone of the neck and back and appendicular tone of the shoulder and arms.

   Normal newborns will have a head lag, but this should not be present after 2–3 months of age (always remember to use the corrected age for premature infants, who may have lower tone than term infants).

Measurers of hypotonia.

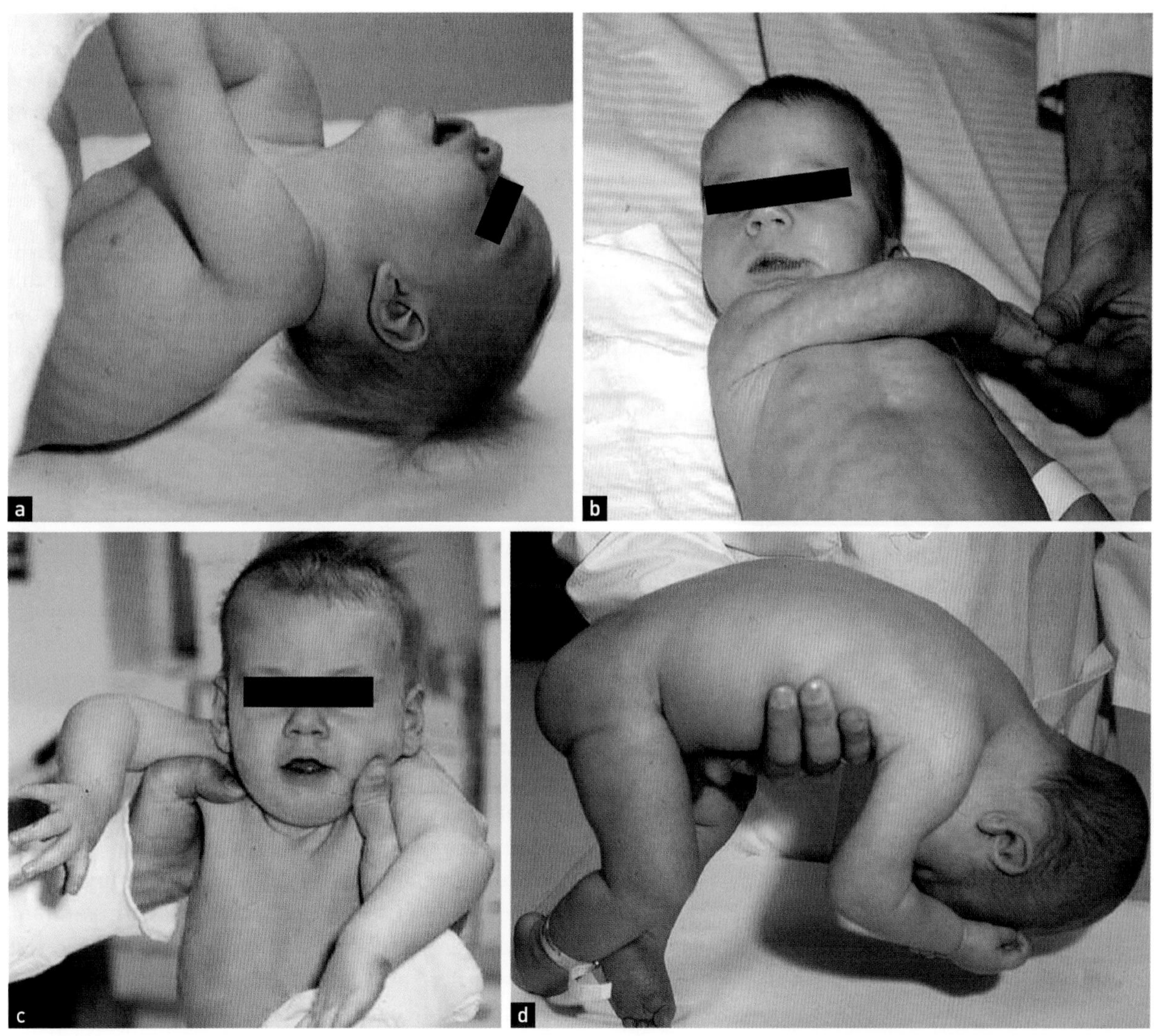

(a) 'Pull to sit', (b) scarf sign, (c) shoulder suspension and (d) ventral suspension

(From Bodensteiner JB. The evaluation of the hypotonic infant. *Semin Pediatr Neurol* 2008; 15(1):10–20.)

FIGURE 37.29

4. *'Shoulder suspension'*: lift the child up by holding him or her under the arms.

   This gives an indication of head control, appendicular tone and strength. It is also useful for looking for scissoring of the lower limbs, which is seen in cerebral palsy.

   The hypotonic child tends to slip through your hands (take particular care when performing this procedure).

   While performing this manoeuvre, it is also useful to 'stand' the child up on the flat surface. This helps to demonstrate hypotonia and weakness, but also inappropriate early weight-bearing, as seen in children with UMN lesions (as in cerebral palsy).
5. *'Ventral suspension'*: lift the child up and hold him or her with a hand under the chest and abdomen.

   Again, this gives an idea of head control and appendicular tone and strength.

   With severe hypotonia, the child adopts a floppy 'C' shape. Conversely, there may be increased extensor tone in children with UMN lesions (as in cerebral palsy).
6. Lay the child prone on a firm surface.

   Position in the classic 'tummy time' pose, with the child's hands placed palms down on the bed on either side of the shoulders, with elbows flexed.

   Once again, this gives an idea of head control, appendicular tone and strength.

Coordination can be tested in older children in a similar way to testing in adults, often by asking the child to touch your finger and then his or her nose. Remember to hold your finger at arm's length away from the child, so that any tremor can be seen.

Test for sensation in the upper and lower limbs in the older child as it is performed in adults; infants or young children are generally unable to understand and follow commands (or have a long enough attention span) for this to be feasible.

Testing deep tendon reflexes in infants and children is also essentially identical to that in adults. In the smaller child, many paediatricians place their finger over the tendon and tap on that with the tendon hammer, rather than risk hurting the child.

There are some excellent videos detailing the paediatric neurological exam at http://library.med.utah.edu/pedineurologicexam/html/introduction.html.

Developmental assessment

The developmental assessment is what truly differentiates the paediatric examination from examination of the adult. The developmental kit, with all its amusing toys and paraphernalia, clearly separates paediatric doctors from their adult colleagues with their boring briefcases (see Fig. 37.30).

Developmental assessment is increasingly important in paediatrics as it has evolved from acute care, particularly the treatment of infectious diseases, to 'a near revolution of successful preventive care measures that have improved the health and prognosis of children and created the expectation of longer, safer lives'.[26] Added to this are the increasing numbers of surviving extremely premature infants, for whom disability, ranging in severity, is not uncommon. The care of children with developmental disabilities remains a major challenge, requiring regular follow-up and early intervention to maximise outcomes.[27]

Although it is not expected that every doctor who examines children should be able to complete a full developmental assessment, it is imperative that doctors who regularly examine children are familiar with the common developmental milestones and can quickly and accurately assess for delay.

Remember that development progresses in an orderly fashion from cephalic to caudal: head control precedes trunk control, which in turn progresses to standing and eventually to locomotion. Many assessment tools are used to monitor development. Most extremely premature infants are now monitored at regular intervals using the Bayley Scales of Infant Development or the Griffiths Scale. These and many other assessment tools take into account four key fields: **gross motor**, **fine motor** (including vision), **speech** (including hearing), and **social and interpersonal** development. Delays in any of these areas should be cause for concern and require follow-up and possibly referral to appropriate services. Generally, however, manipulative or fine-motor development is more important than gross-motor development. A child's level of alertness and interest in his or her surroundings is most important in the assessment of **cognition**.[28]

Much of the developmental assessment can be completed by **observation**: watch how the child plays with toys; watch their interaction with other children, family and clinicians. In this way it can be easier to

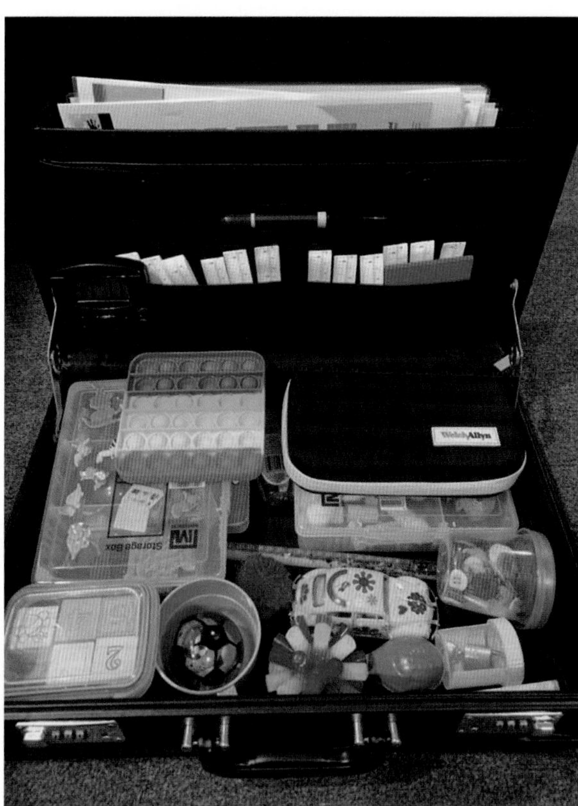

Inside a paediatrician's briefcase

(Photo courtesy of Dr Jacqui Pearson.)

FIGURE 37.30

gauge children's social development by the way they interact with their parents, with you and with their surroundings. **Listen** for any vocalisations or words that children make throughout the examination, whether they can follow any commands given and make note of any of their interactions with you (smiling, waving, pushing you away, etc.).

Developmental examination

Begin the formal part of the developmental assessment by testing vision and hearing, as the assessment will need to be modified extensively if these senses are impaired. Before starting, some developmental milestones may be elicited on history: can the infant roll, sit, crawl, pull to stand, cruise or walk independently? Can the infant suck his or her fist, reach for objects, swap objects from hand to hand, feed self, stack blocks, wave? Can the infant understand simple words like 'yes', 'no', 'milk', 'mummy'? How many words do infants have; can they put two or three words together; can they be understood by strangers? Do they make good eye contact, share things they are enjoying, socialise with other children? Do they know colours, animals, parts of the face? Do they point to things they want, things they are interested in, things they want to share with you? The answers to these questions can then guide the developmental examination.

Vision is relatively easy to assess: hold out a toy for a small child to fix on and follow. If the child's response appears normal, place much smaller items in the palm of your hand for the child to see, reach for and grasp (the classic is to use hundreds-and-thousands). For older children, ask him or her to read aloud from a book. Very young infants often prefer a face—yours or the parents'—rather than a toy.

Assessing **hearing** in an infant or a small child is a little more tricky and requires a cooperative child, preferably held in the parent's lap, and an assistant with a toy that makes a noise (like a bell or a squeaky toy). Have the assistant stand behind the child out of the child's line of sight. Distract the child using a toy that does not make any noise and, once you are sure you have the child's attention, hide this toy behind your back. The assistant should then make a sound with the noisy toy next to the child's ear. Note whether the child's expression changes or the child turns towards the sound. Check each ear in turn. In an older child, you should have an idea of the child's level of hearing from speaking and interacting with him or her throughout the examination.

Fine-motor skill is usually assessed next. If the child was able to grasp the hundreds-and-thousands in the visual test, this indicates that the child has a **pincer grip**. Watching the child play will also give you an idea of fine-motor skills: shaking a rattle, stacking blocks, threading beads on a string, rolling a ball and miming eating using a knife and fork are all good tests of fine-motor skills.

Moving on to **gross-motor skills**, consider checking the primitive reflexes in an infant (see Ch 38) and complete the *180° examination* described earlier. In an older child, the **standard gait examination** can be used to assess gross-motor skills.

Finally, summarise your findings and determine whether there is isolated delay or global delay. Remember to always ask the parents whether there are any particular areas of development that they are concerned about.

Table 37.8 is a general guideline for development over the first 5 years of life. It is included to give you a rough idea of the childhood development milestones expected at different ages. There is large variability in the range of normal for childhood development and these guidelines are not meant to be followed strictly. If there are any concerns about a child's development, formal testing using a verified scale (e.g. the Denver Developmental Screening Test or Bayley's scales) should be used.

Lymphatic and immune system

History: frequent coughs and colds (even up to 10 a year) in an otherwise normally developing, normally growing child may not necessarily signify an immune disorder but rather recurrent exposures to common childhood viruses that children often grow out of. Recurrent invasive bacterial infections, frequent hospitalisations, significant lethargy, night sweats, weight loss, bone or joint pain and rashes (e.g. petechiae) may herald more sinister diseases of the immune and haematopoietic systems.

Parents are often concerned about **adenoidal and tonsillar hypertrophy**. This is usually assumed to be the cause of a great variety of persistent ENT or respiratory problems but, except for obstructive sleep apnoea,[g] a causal relationship between these immune organs and illness is poorly established. Thus, always explore the sleeping history, particularly whether symptoms of obstructive sleep apnoea such as loud snoring and abnormal breathing or breathing efforts during sleep have been observed by the parents. This problem is sometimes associated with daytime somnolence and behavioural problems.

Examination: lymphadenopathy (small, <1 cm, non-tender, freely mobile lymph nodes) is *extremely* common in younger children, particularly in the head and neck region (see List 37.1).[29]

The location of the lymphadenopathy will often give a clue to its aetiology. Cervical lymph node enlargement is more commonly caused by infection, whereas supraclavicular lymphadenopathy, particularly when large and unilateral, is more likely to be malignant. If lymphadenopathy is localised, ensure that the region drained by the nodes is examined for evidence of infection or inflammation. Note the size, shape and

[g] Repeated cessation of breathing due to upper airway obstruction, particularly in rapid eye movement (REM) sleep.

CAUSES OF LYMPHADENOPATHY IN CHILDREN

- Viral, bacterial, protozoal or fungal infection
- Autoimmune disorders (systemic lupus erythematosus, sarcoidosis, Kawasaki's disease)
- Primary malignancy (lymphoma)
- Secondary malignant infiltration (much less common in children)

(Motyckova G, Steensma DP. Why does my patient have lymphadenopathy or splenomegaly? *Hematolol/Oncol Clin North Am* 2012; 26(2):395–408.)

LIST 37.1

A guide to developmental assessment

Age	Gross motor	Vision / fine motor	Hearing / speech	Personal / social
6 weeks	Symmetrical limb movements Ventral: head in line with body briefly Supine: fencing posture Automatic stepping and walking	Fixes and follows to 90° Turns to light Grasp reflex	Cries / coos Startles to noise	Smiles
3 months	Moves limbs vigorously No head lag Back: lumbar curvature only Prone: lifts upper chest up	Fixes and follows to 180° Plays with own hands Holds rattle placed in hand	Quietens to mother's voice Turns to sound	Laughs and squeals

TABLE 37.8

A guide to developmental assessment *continued*

Age	Gross motor	Vision / fine motor	Hearing / speech	Personal / social
6 months	Sits without support Lifts chest up on extended arms Grasps feet Rolls from front to back Downward parachute reflex	Palmar grasp Transfers objects Shakes rattle Mouths objects	Turns to quiet sound Says vowels and syllables	Laughs and screams Not shy
9 months	Tripod sits: rights self if pushed and can reach for toy steadily Rolls back to front Pulls to standing Stands holding on Forward parachute reflex (7 months)	Reaches for small objects Rolls balls Points with index finger Early pincer grip Looks for fallen objects Releases toys	Distraction hearing test Says 'mama', 'dada' non-specifically	Chews biscuit Stranger anxiety Plays 'peek-a-boo' Understands 'no' and 'bye-bye'
12 months	Cruises around furniture Walks if held, may take a few steps unsupported	Neat pincer grip Casting objects Bangs cubes together	Knows own name Understands simple commands Says a few words	Finger-feeds Waves 'bye' Finds hidden object
15 months	Broad-based gait Kneels Pushes wheeled toy	Sees small objects Builds tower of 2 bricks To and fro scribble	Speaks 2–6 words Communicates wishes and obeys commands	Uses cup and spoon
18 months	Steady purposeful walk Runs, squats Walks carrying toy Pushes / pulls Creeps downstairs	Circular scribble Points to pictures in book Turns pages of book Hand preference	Speaks 6–20 words	Points to named body parts Feeds independently Domestic mimicry Symbolic play alone Takes off socks and shoes
2 years	Kicks ball Walks up and down stairs holding on	Builds tower of 6 bricks Copies vertical line	Uses 2–3 word sentences Uses pivotal grammar Uses question words	Feeds with fork and spoon Begins toilet training Has temper tantrums
3 years	Walks up stairs one foot per step, down with two Walks on tip-toes Throws ball Pedals tricycle	Builds tower of 9 bricks Builds train and bridge with bricks if shown Copies circle	Gives first and last name Knows sex Recognises colours Pure tone audiometry	Washes hands and brushes teeth Eats with fork and spoon (+/− knife) Make-believe play Likes hearing and telling stories
4 years	Walks up and down stairs one foot per step Hops	Builds steps of bricks Copies cross Draws man	Counts to 10 or more	Able to undress
5 years	Skips Catches ball Runs on toes	Copies triangle	Asks 'how' and 'when' questions Uses grammatical speech	Uses knife and fork Able to put on clothes and to do up large buttons

(Stephenson T, Wallace H, Thomson A. *Clinical paediatrics for postgraduate examinations*. Edinburgh: Churchill Livingstone, 2003.)

TABLE 37.8

consistence of any enlarged node and whether it is tender or warm to touch. It is particularly important to determine whether the node is freely movable or fixed to underlying structures. Fixed nodes or groups of nodes matted together are particularly suspect and *less likely* to be benign.

You need to have a system for reviewing the different lymph node groups to ensure that none are forgotten. It is usually easiest to have the child in the parent's lap facing you.

Start at the head and examine bilaterally for the pre- and postauricular nodes, followed by the occipital and posterior cervical nodes at the back of the neck. Feel under the angle of the jaw for the superior cervical, submaxillary and submental nodes. Feel along the sternocleidomastoids bilaterally, followed by the supraclavicular nodes.

The axilla (see Fig. 37.31) is palpated next: feel high up into the apex and along the lateral, medial and pectoral surfaces. This usually elicits gales of laughter in most children and can be quite difficult if the child is ticklish. Feel for the epitrochlear nodes, although these are not commonly palpable in children. Ensure that the child's arm is bent at 90° and palpate around the head of the medial epicondyle of the humerus (see Fig. 37.31).

Palpate along the inguinal crease for any nodes and into the femoral triangle. It is not uncommon to be able to palpate small (<1 cm) nodes in the inguinal region, but it is less common to feel nodes in the femoral triangle.[7] Lastly, feel behind the knees for the popliteal nodes.

The spleen and the tonsils are also part of the lymphatic system and should be examined: these are covered in the abdominal examination and the ENT examination, respectively.

Respiratory and cardiovascular system

Common symptoms

Ask the parents or an older child what the main problem has been.

Establish with each symptom whether it is acute (less than 3 weeks' duration), chronic (more than 3 months' duration) or recurrent (with variable symptom-free episodes).

Respiratory noises (wheeze, stridor and/or grunting) are symptoms that are suggestive of some degree of respiratory disease or cardiovascular failure (see Table 37.9). The parents may have noticed laboured breathing, difficult feeding, weight loss, diaphoresis or rapid breathing.

Noisy breathing is extremely common but distinguishing the different noises from each other can be difficult when gathering the history from the parents.[30] Ascertain from the parents whether the noises occur episodically or continuously and are present acutely or chronically. Some parents can specify whether the respiratory noise is more pronounced during inspiration or expiration.

Cough is also very common (see Questions box 37.1) and in an otherwise healthy child may not warrant specific investigation unless prolonged (>3 weeks).[31]

History

A detailed history will help narrow the large list of differential diagnoses.

An episodic dry cough with wheeze and shortness of breath triggered by viruses, cold air exposure (winter, night-time), exercise, allergen exposure (house dust mites, pollen, animals) and/or weather change suggests asthma.

Pertussis should be considered when there is a more persistent spasmodic (paroxysmal: occurring in bouts), choking, repetitive cough with a whooping inspiratory sound, even if the child is vaccinated. Unvaccinated small babies with whooping cough often present with cyanotic coughing spells, which may terminate with life-threatening apnoeic episodes (cessation of respiration longer than 20 seconds).

A dry, honking and loud cough in the absence of any other symptoms that occurred after a non-specific chest infection and is not heard at night likely constitutes a psychogenic (habitual) cough.

Persistent cough (and wheeze) after a choking episode that has occurred after a child has had access to small objects (e.g. peanuts) suggests foreign body aspiration.

Many children have recurrent cough as the chief symptom of frequent episodes of respiratory infections. It is not uncommon for healthy preschoolers to have eight to ten mild respiratory infections ('common colds') per year.

However, a history of two or more bouts of lobar pneumonia in a short interval, confirmed by chest X-ray, suggests the possibility of aspiration, abnormal immune function or suppurative lung disease. Ask about associated problems, such as:

- poor weight gain, steatorrhoea (cystic fibrosis)
- severe infections of other tissues such as meningitis, skin, intra-abdominal abscesses or osteomyelitis (immunoglobulin deficiency)

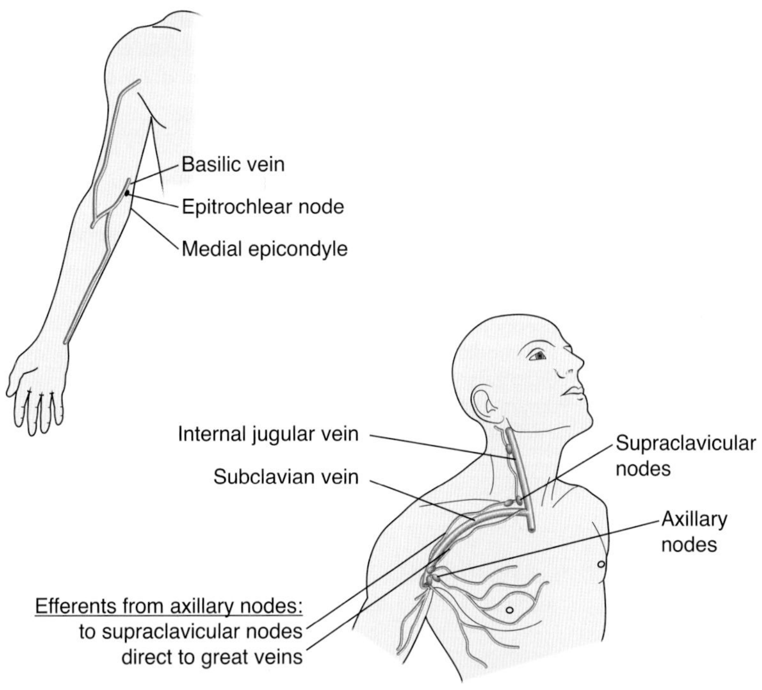

The epitrochlear and the axillary nodes

(From McGee S. *Evidence-based physical diagnosis*. 3rd edn. Philadelphia: Saunders, 2012, pp 215–226.)

FIGURE 37.31

- detection of unusual pathogens such as *Pneumocystis jiroveci (previously carinii)*, *Serratia marcescens*, *Candida* (e.g. cellular immune deficiency) and *Aspergillus*.

Ask about **rapid breathing** (tachypnoea) or **difficult breathing** (dyspnoea). These are important features of respiratory distress, which is a common indicator of a respiratory, cardiac or circulatory problem in children. In young infants particularly there may also be neurological and metabolic causes (see Ch 38). Respiratory distress may rapidly worsen and result in life-threatening respiratory failure (type 1: hypoxia with normocapnia; type 2: hypoxia and hypercapnia) or cardiocirculatory failure (inadequate tissue perfusion; see Table 37.10).

Ask the parents of small infants about feeding duration (normally less than 20 minutes), frequency (6–8 times per day in fully breastfed or bottle-fed babies) and fluid intake (normally 100–150 mL/kg per 24 hours of oral feeds in infants of less than 10 kg).

Parents may have noticed **squatting** (rare nowadays) in children with cyanotic heart defects because this position improves systemic oxygen saturation by reducing the right-to-left shunt. Ask about cyanosis, although this can be difficult for parents to recognise. Hypercyanotic (blue) spells are easily recognised medical emergencies and always require specialist involvement in the long-term management.

If **chest pain** has been the problem, careful questioning can help in the assessment (see Questions box 37.2).

Breathlessness during exercise raises the possibility of heart disease. If the onset is recent, a cardiomyopathy

QUESTIONS TO ASK THE CHILD AND PARENT(S) ABOUT COUGH

1. Is the cough dry or wet?
2. Does it occur at night or during exercise?
3. Does anything seem to bring it on?

QUESTIONS BOX 37.1

Site of origin and differential diagnoses of common respiratory breathing noises

Respiratory breathing noise	Site of origin	Differential diagnoses	
		Acute	**Chronic**
Expiratory wheeze or stridor	Intrathoracic	Virus-induced wheezy illness Bronchiolitis (infants) Viral pneumonitis Foreign body in lower airways Asthma attack	Asthma Tracheomalacia Bronchomalacia Chronic lung disease of prematurity (infants) Cystic fibrosis
Inspiratory or biphasic stridor	Extrathoracic or extra- and intrathoracic	Laryngotracheitis (infectious, pseudomembranous, spasmodic croup) Epiglottitis Foreign body in trachea / oesophagus	Laryngomalacia Tracheomalacia Vascular rings and slings Haemangioma Vocal cord paralysis Subglottic stenosis Laryngeal web Laryngeal warts Gastro-oesophageal reflux Rare congenital lesions of the larynx and trachea
Rattle (often confused with wheeze)	Intra- or extrathoracic or both	Upper and / or lower respiratory tract infection	Protracted bronchitis Aspiration Suppurative lung disease (cystic fibrosis, primary ciliary dyskinesia, immune deficiencies, bronchiectasis of unknown aetiology) Anatomical airway malformations
Snore (stertor)	Oronasopharynx	Tonsillitis Pharyngitis	Adenoidal / tonsillar hypertrophy
Snuffle / snort	Nasopharynx	Infectious rhinitis / head cold (coryza)	Allergic rhinitis
Grunt	Alveoli / lung parenchyma	Respiratory distress syndrome / hyaline membrane disease Pneumonia	Chronic lung disease Interstitial lung disease

(Modified from Mellis C. Respiratory noises: how useful are they clinically? *Pediatr Clin North Am* 2009; 56(1):1–17, ix.)

TABLE 37.9

or episode of myocarditis is a possibility. Gradually worsening symptoms may indicate congenital heart disease. Shortness of breath directly after physical activity in association with respiratory noises (cough, wheeze) is a typical symptom of exercise-induced asthma.

Fainting (syncope) and **dizziness** are not uncommon symptoms in older children (see Questions box 37.3).

Palpitations may have been noticed by the child, or the parents may have found an abnormal heart rate (see Questions box 37.4).

Most importantly, beware of the **three Cs** of serious infection and illness:

- Concerns from the parents that the current illness is different from previous illnesses (if a parent says the child is sick, the child is sick)
- Changes in behaviour by the child (e.g. crying, drowsiness, moaning or inconsolability)
- your Clinical instinct that something is wrong.

Examination

The respiratory and cardiovascular examination is of particular significance in paediatrics because it can detect clinical features that identify a seriously ill child (see Table 37.10). Note that some important warning signs are already found in the history and on careful inspection. **Palpation** (starting with the hands and proceeding in an opportunistic fashion) and **auscultation** are usually done next. Sometimes, in a quiet, sleeping infant, *auscultation* may be done first. **Percussion** and particularly inspection of the oral cavity may upset a young child, so these are best left until last.

Look at the child carefully to pick up unusual posturing or body habitus (see List 37.2).

Inspect the chest for:

- signs of respiratory distress such as chest in-drawings (intercostal or subcostal recessions), tracheal tug and nasal flaring
- abnormally shaped chest (e.g. bell-shaped, unilateral or bilateral lung hypoplasia; see Ch 38)
- symmetrical expansion and any deformities such as a pectus excavatum or pectus carinatum (see Ch 10)
- signs of hyperinflation (e.g. barrel chest with increased anterior–posterior chest diameter)
- a horizontal groove along the lower border of the thorax corresponding to the insertion of the diaphragm (Harrison's sulcus), which signifies increased contractile activity of the diaphragm (e.g. in chronic asthma) or rachitic rosary as a result of vitamin D deficiency
- left-sided chest prominence, which can be due to cardiac enlargement.

Look out for any thoracic scars (including on the back) that may indicate previous surgery. A midline sternotomy scar suggests complex surgery for congenital heart disease in the past, whereas a left-sided thoracotomy scar may indicate persistent ductus arteriosus, aortic coarctation repair, or—similar to a right-sided thoracotomy—pulmonary artery banding (palliative reduction of excessive pulmonary blood flow), Blalock–Taussig[h] shunt (palliative systemic-to-pulmonary shunt to increase impaired pulmonary blood flow) or non-cardiac surgery (e.g. removal of congenital pulmonary airway malformation).

Assess for the presence of acrocyanosis (nailbeds) or central cyanosis (mouth and tongue at the end of the examination in young children; see also Ch 38). Cyanosis may be present only in the lower extremities in patients with aortic coarctation or a persistent ductus arteriosus complicated by pulmonary hypertension and reversal of the shunt.

[h] In 1938 Helen Taussig, a paediatric cardiologist, approached Alfred Blalock, the Chief of Surgery at Johns Hopkins, to create a ductus-like anastomosis between the left subclavian and pulmonary artery. Coincidentally, a young surgical technician named Vivien Thomas in Dr Blalock's laboratory had already performed this work successfully in dogs. He stood behind Blalock during the first surgery performed in a 15-month-old girl with tetralogy of Fallot in 1944 to provide procedural advice. The technical oversight of Vivien Thomas contributed to one of the most dramatic progresses in 20th century paediatric cardiology.

QUESTIONS TO ASK THE CHILD AND PARENT(S) ABOUT CHEST PAIN

1. What is the pain like? Is it sharp and worse when you take big breaths? (Pleuritic or sometimes muscular pain) Is it stabbing? (Musculoskeletal) Is it dull and heavy? (Myocardial ischaemia—very rare in children)
2. Where do you feel the pain? (Left- or right-sided pain is unlikely to be cardiac)
3. Does the pain go to anywhere else? (To the back with aortic dissection or musculoskeletal pain)
4. How bad is it? Does it keep you awake at night?
5. Does it come on with exercise?
6. Are you sore to touch anywhere on the chest?

QUESTIONS BOX 37.2

Arrange for the measurement of oxygen saturation employing pulse oximetry if available or you are in doubt, and expose to 100% oxygen (hyperoxygenation test; see Ch 38). Check for dental caries and pallor while inspecting the oral cavity. Pallor can also be detected by inspecting the conjunctivae and palmar creases. Common causes of pallor include:

- low haemoglobin levels (with increased pulse rate)
- poor cardiac output (weak pulse, prolonged capillary refill and sometimes bradycardia).

There may be koilonychia if the cause is iron deficiency, hypertension if the cause is renal disease, or a recent history of erythema infectiosum ('fifth disease') with bone marrow suppression.

Clubbing is present when there is an increase in the angle between the nail and the skin overlying the distal phalanx (>160°).[7] This is caused by proliferation of subungual tissue at the root of the nail and can easily be detected when it exceeds 180° by holding both thumbs back to back with the fingertips and interphalangeal joints aligned. With clubbing, the elongated, diamond-shaped opening that is normally apparent is lost (Schamroth's sign, p 80). Applying

QUESTIONS TO ASK THE CHILD AND PARENT(S) WHO HAS BEEN DIZZY OR SYNCOPAL

1. Did you black out altogether? (Syncope) Did you get any warning? What did you feel before you blacked out? Did you notice an odd sensation or a funny smell? (Aura) Did you hurt yourself?
2. Did anyone see it happen? Did you notice any funny shaking movements in your child? (Seizure)
3. Did you bite your tongue or pass urine while you were blacked out? (Seizure)
4. Did you feel strange or sleepy when you woke up? (Postictal symptoms)
5. Did it come on after you stood up suddenly? (Postural hypotension)
6. Did you feel sick in the stomach or sweaty before it happened? (Vasovagal episode)
7. Had you just seen something upsetting, like an accident? (Vasovagal)
8. Had you been coughing badly just before it happened? (Tussive syncope)
9. Is your child diabetic? (Hypoglycaemia)
10. Was there a feeling of spinning or turning? (Vertigo)

QUESTIONS BOX 37.3

QUESTIONS TO ASK THE CHILD AND PARENT(S) ABOUT PALPITATIONS

1. Do you think you can feel your heart beating abnormally?
2. Is it beating fast? A bit faster than normal, or faster than it has ever gone before? (Supraventricular tachycardia)
3. Does it seem to be steady or is it missing and jumping? (Ectopic beats or, if fast, atrial fibrillation)
4. Have you or your parents ever counted how fast it is?
5. Does it start very suddenly? (Supraventricular tachycardia, which often begins in teenagers)
6. Do you feel dizzy or faint when it happens?
7. Have you had any other problems with your heart? (Congenital heart disease is associated with atrial and ventricular arrhythmias)
8. Is there a history of sudden death in your family? (Inherited *channelopathies*, e.g. long QT interval syndrome)

QUESTIONS BOX 37.4

pressure onto the root of a clubbed nail produces movement towards the bone ('floating nail').

Look out for rarities such as splinter haemorrhages and Osler's nodes (infective endocarditis), tuberous and tendon xanthomata (familial hypercholesterolaemia), absent thumbs (Holt–Oram syndrome) or absent radii. Bending of the fifth finger (clinodactyly) occurs in many genetic conditions (Russell-Silver syndrome, Down syndrome, pseudohypoparathyroidism) but is also seen in the general population.

BODY HABITUS ABNORMALITIES TO NOTE ON GENERAL INSPECTION

- Marfanoid (risk of aortic dilation, dissection)
- Cushingoid (hypertension)
- Dysmorphic features (webbed neck, short stature and commonly cardiac malformations in Turner syndrome)
- Developmental delay (supravalvular aortic stenosis with Williams–Beuren syndrome)

LIST 37.2

Heart and circulation

Feel the brachial pulses in the antecubital fossa of both upper limbs using your first and second index fingers. Determine:

- rate (see Table 37.11)
- rhythm (regularly irregular: coupled extrasystoles; irregularly irregular: ectopic beats [more common], atrial fibrillation [less common])

Respiratory distress and associated signs and symptoms

Impaired function	Possible signs / symptoms	Aetiology
Cardiac / circulatory	Tachypnoea, sweating, fatigue, impaired tolerance to physical activity, poor feeding, failure to thrive, cyanosis, pallor, weak pulses, prolonged capillary refill, low / high blood pressure, tachycardia / bradycardia, murmur, subcostal recessions	Congenital heart disease: left-to-right shunt causing fluid overload (e.g. ventricular septal defect, persistent ductus arteriosus) right-to-left shunt causing cyanosis (e.g. tetralogy of Fallot, transposition of the great arteries) stenoses causing obstruction (e.g. coarctation of the aorta, aortic stenosis, pulmonary stenosis) Acquired heart disease, e.g.: Kawasaki disease (myocardial infarction) rheumatic fever (mitral stenosis) drug-induced cardiomyopathy cardiac tamponade pericarditis myocarditis Cardiac arrhythmias, e.g.: pre-excitation syndromes (Wolff–Parkinson–White syndrome) supraventricular tachycardia AV block Circulatory, e.g.: hypertension dehydration blood loss anaphylaxis septicaemia neurogenic
Respiratory	Respiratory noises, reduced or prolonged or added breath sounds, tachypnoea / dyspnoea, tachycardia, subcostal recessions, failure to thrive, tracheal tug, nasal flaring	Obstructive lung disease (airway resistance increased [reduced airway patency]): upper airway (e.g. croup, epiglottitis, choanal atresia, piriform aperture stenosis, adenoidal hypertrophy) lower airways (e.g. bronchiolitis, wheezy illness, asthma, cystic fibrosis) Restrictive lung disease (lung compliance reduced [stiff lungs]): respiratory distress syndrome pneumonia hypersensitivity / viral pneumonitis interstitial lung disease / lung fibrosis scoliosis / kyphosis neuromuscular disease pulmonary oedema (mixed cardiac and respiratory) Other: pneumothorax trauma (flail chest)

TABLE 37.10

- volume (full: persistent ductus arteriosus, aortic regurgitation; shallow: left ventricular outflow tract obstruction, cardiac / circulatory failure)
- presence of pulsus paradoxus, which is an exaggeration of the physiological decrease in systolic blood pressure during inspiration (greater than 10 mmHg). On palpation, the pulses are fainter during inspiration and this can be found with severe airways obstruction (e.g. in asthma or croup) or reduced left ventricular filling (e.g. cardiac tamponade or pericarditis). It must be quantified with a stethoscope and blood pressure cuff.

The femoral pulses must be checked at some stage but in chubby babies this requires patience. Thus, feel the groins only towards the end of the examination. Absence of the femoral pulses or a radiofemoral delay raises suspicion of the presence of aortic coarctation.

Test the capillary refill time by pressing your index finger onto the child's chest for 5 seconds. This inhibits skin perfusion and leaves a pale area, which should regain its colour (refill) within 2–3 seconds. A prolonged capillary refill indicates poor peripheral perfusion, which is most commonly caused by:

- septicaemia
- dehydration, or
- heart failure.

Assess the location and quality of the impulse of the apex beat, which should be located in the fourth intercostal space approximately on the left midclavicular line. Feel for a vibration under your right hand held onto the left lower sternal border (ventricular septal defect, VSD) and left upper sternal edge (pulmonary valve stenosis). A parasternal impulse may be felt when there is right ventricular hypertrophy (e.g. tetralogy of Fallot). In infants you can feel for impulse and thrill by pressing the first and second digits of your right hand onto the left lower sternal border (next to the xiphoid process) and the second intercostal space (above the pulmonary valve area). Next, place your index finger into the suprasternal notch to search for a thrill caused by aortic stenosis.

Proceed to auscultation of heart sounds using the diaphragm of a good-quality paediatric stethoscope and then make your way backwards with the bell to search for murmurs of low frequency. At least four praecordial areas should be auscultated:

- apical or mitral area (fourth intercostal space between the midclavicular and anterior axillary lines)
- tricuspid area (left lower sternal border [LLSB] in the fourth intercostal space)
- pulmonary area (left upper sternal border [LUSB] in the second intercostal space)
- aortic area (right upper sternal border [RUSB] in the second intercostal space).

If a murmur is present, then assess as follows using the mnemonic **CARDIO**:

C haracter of the sound or murmur
A rea where the sound is the loudest
R adiation of the sound into other areas
D egree or **I**ntensity of the loudness of the sound or murmur
O ccurrence of the sound or murmur in the cardiac cycle.

Character of the sound or murmur

Normal

The first heart sound (S_1) marks the closure of the mitral and tricuspid valves and is louder than the second heart sound (S_2). S_1 is not split except above the tricuspid area where it may be closely split. S_2 is produced by closure of the aortic (A_2) and pulmonary (P_2) valves. S_2 is split in inspiration but there is no split or only a close split in expiration above the pulmonary area.

Innocent systolic (between S_1 and S_2) vibratory ejection murmurs are common (Still's murmur) and have a musical character (like twanging a piece of tense string). There are also systolic flow ejection murmurs, which are not musical (medium-pitched) but they are never harsh or coarse. They may be innocent if S_2 is normal. They are also heard with atrial septal defect (ASD) (p 106), but then there is also a fixed splitting of S_2.

Proposed normal values for heart rate per minute

Age range (years)	Pediatric advanced life support, American Heart Association	Advanced paediatric life support, Advanced Life Support Group
0–1	100–190*	110–160
1–2	100–190	100–150
2–5	60–140	95–140
5–10	60–140	80–120
10–12	60–100	80–120
12–18	60–100	60–100

**PALS provides separate ranges for infants up to 3 months, and for those between 3 months and 2 years of age.*

(American Heart Association; Ralston M, Hazinski FM, Zaritsky AL, Schexnayder FM. *PALS provider manual.* Dallas: American Heart Association, 2006; Advanced Life Support Group (Manchester England). *Pre-hospital paediatric life support: a practical approach to the out-of-hospital emergency care of children.* Oxford: BMJ Books/Blackwell, 2005.)

TABLE 37.11

Abnormal

1. *Heart sounds.* If the intensity of S_1 varies from beat-to-beat variation, there may be complete atrioventricular heart block present. This causes dissociation between closure of the valve leaflets and ventricle contractions. This sign can be useful in distinguishing complete heart block from sinus bradycardia.

   An absent or faint S_1 is found when the PR interval is prolonged. A fixed split of S_2 is found with ASD and pulmonary valve stenosis. However, ASD is associated with a systolic flow murmur (medium-pitched), while pulmonary valve stenosis leads to a systolic obstructive murmur (low-pitched, harsh, coarse).

   A third heart sound (S_3) can be found in normal children with hyperdynamic circulation, but a fourth heart sound (S_4) is always abnormal.
2. *Murmurs.* A systolic regurgitant murmur is non-musical and has a high-pitched sound character like breath sounds or blowing. A systolic ejection murmur due to valvular stenosis is also non-musical but low-pitched, meaning it sounds harsh or coarse, and is usually quite loud and easily heard. Almost any diastolic murmur or continuous murmur is pathological except for a venous hum. A venous hum arises from the neck and disappears when the patient is supine or when gentle pressure is applied to the base of the neck.
3. *Clicks and rubs.* Clicks at the beginning of systole directly after S_1 are generated by the opening of the heart valves and are heard in aortic or pulmonary stenosis. A midsystolic click is pathognomonic for mitral valve prolapse.

   A pericardial friction rub is a scratchy sound heard at the left sternal border and usually has one systolic and two diastolic components. It can occur with pericarditis or after cardiac surgery. A mediastinal crunch (Hamman's sign: a crackly, crunchy, bubbly sound) can be heard with mediastinal emphysema[i] after chest injury or thoracic surgery.

[i] Air in the mediastinum.

Area where the sound is the loudest

The suggested sequence of auscultation is the mitral, tricuspid, pulmonary and aortic areas with the diaphragm of the stethoscope first to detect high- and medium-pitched murmurs and then in the reverse direction with the bell for low-pitched murmurs.

Radiation of the sound into other areas

A thrill in the suprasternal notch may be palpable in aortic stenosis. The harsh systolic obstructive murmur found with pulmonary valve stenosis radiates into the back, whereas the high-pitched blowing systolic regurgitant murmur with mitral valve regurgitation may be auscultated in the axilla.

Degree or intensity of the loudness of the sound or murmur

This can be measured by grading the loudness from 1 to 6 for systolic and 1 to 4 for diastolic murmurs. For instance, a grade 1 murmur is extremely faint, whereas a grade 3 murmur is loud. With a grade 4 murmur a thrill is also palpable and with a grade 6 murmur you would not need a stethoscope to hear it. Importantly, innocent murmurs are not loud and never have a thrill (see below).

Timing of the occurrence of the sound or murmur in the cardiac cycle

A systolic regurgitant murmur (usually high-pitched, blowing) commences immediately *with* S_1 and concludes only with S_2 (pan- or holosystolic); for example, it is observed in mitral or tricuspid valve regurgitation. In contrast, systolic obstructive ejection murmurs (low-pitched, harsh) commence *after* S_1 (small pause between S_1 and murmur). They have a crescendo–decrescendo occurrence, meaning that their intensity increases and then decreases before S_2. Ejection murmurs can occur in early, mid or late systole and are heard with, for instance, aortic and pulmonary valve stenosis. Diastolic regurgitant murmurs commence *with* S_2 and are high-pitched with aortic regurgitation (high pressure gradient) and low-pitched with pulmonary regurgitation (low pressure gradient) but they are not pandiastolic. In contrast, diastolic obstructive murmurs commence *after* S_2 and have a crescendo–decrescendo occurrence. In mitral valve stenosis, they occur in late diastole and have a low-pitched rumbling character. There are also occasionally short mid-diastolic flow murmurs (medium-pitched) in severe VSD, ASD, tricuspid or mitral valve regurgitation due to markedly increased flow volume.

Many healthy children have a heart murmur and several types of **innocent murmurs** are reported (see Table 37.12). Innocent murmurs are not harsh and occur in systole but are not pansystolic. They are not loud and they may further diminish in intensity in different positions. Usually they are localised with no radiation except for the pulmonary branch murmur of infancy. Patients with murmurs with these characteristics can usually be reassured, especially if there are no cardiac symptoms. In neonates, however, the absence of a murmur never excludes structural heart disease.

Pathological murmurs may be due to congenital or acquired heart defects (<1% in the general population). If they are not recognised and treated they can lead to progressive limitation and premature death. Consider the following features suggestive of pathological murmurs:

- harsh character
- loud (grade 3 or more)
- pansystolic, diastolic or continuous (if not disappearing in supine position)
- associated with ejection clicks
- associated with abnormal S_2 sound
- associated with other abnormal cardiac findings.

Table 37.13 summarises potential auscultation notes for some more common structural heart defects in childhood (see also Ch 38 for ventricular and atrial septal defect and persistent ductus arteriosus, which are equally relevant to older children).

Mitral valve prolapse is common (2–3% in children) and may be associated with connective tissue disorders (Marfan syndrome, Ehlers–Danlos syndrome, Stickler syndrome) or other structural abnormalities. On auscultation the characteristic feature is of one or more midsystolic clicks best heard at the cardiac apex. These become louder when the child stands up and may be followed by a murmur of mitral regurgitation.

During auscultation decide again whether the cardiac rhythm is regular or irregular. Count the heart rate over 15 seconds and check the normal range (see Table 37.11).

Measure the blood pressure (also lower extremities if there is no femoral pulse or radiofemoral delay) and liver size (see below) and assess for periorbital, sacral and pretibial oedema to complete the cardiovascular examination.

Lungs

Respiratory rate

Count the respiratory rate over one full minute by assessing both chest movements and breath sounds. Although percentile charts are published (see Fig. 37.1), it is more common in clinical practice to employ the proposed ranges of normal that are best suited to a specific region and are endorsed by local policy (see Table 37.14).

Rapid breathing (tachypnoea) and reduced breathing (hypopnoea, apnoea) are signs of respiratory failure. They are red flags indicating severe illness. List 37.3 outlines important differential diagnoses of rapid breathing often associated with **type 1 respiratory failure** where there is a ventilation / perfusion mismatch and a fall in oxygenation. List 37.4 outlines important differential diagnoses of reduced breathing often associated with **type 2 respiratory failure** where there is inadequate ventilation and a fall in oxygenation is associated with a rise in carbon dioxide levels.

Trachea and chest wall

Verify the position of the trachea in the midline with your index finger by gently palpating the trachea in the suprasternal (jugular) notch while placing your first finger and third finger onto the clavicles on either side of the clavicular notch of the manubrium sterni. Shifting of the trachea signifies an increase in the intrathoracic pressure, which may be the result of:

- air (a tension pneumothorax, congenital lobar emphysema, congenital pulmonary airway malformation)
- fluid (a volume increase due to effusion, haemorrhage in the contralateral hemithorax)
- collapse (a volume decrease [atelectasis] on the same side [the ipsilateral hemithorax]).

Check the chest wall for subcutaneous air (pneumomediastinum +/− pneumothorax), which results in crackling under the skin with palpation.

Auscultation

Next auscultate the lung sounds in a pragmatic fashion:

1. anterior: compare right versus left upper sternal border (upper lobes), lower sternal border (middle lobe right, lingular segment left) and lateral lower chest (lower lobes)
2. posterior: compare right versus left in the upper (upper lobes), median and lower chest (between spine and scapula)
3. laterally (all lower lobes).

Characteristics of innocent murmurs in childhood

Origin (term)	Character	Area	Radiation	Degree / intensity	Occurrence
Left ventricular outflow tract (Still's murmur)	Non-harsh	LLSB	No	Less than grade 3	Early systole, diminishes with inspiration, sitting, standing
Right ventricular outflow tract (pulmonary flow murmur)	Non-harsh	LUSB	No	Less than grade 3	Early systole, diminishes with inspiration, sitting, standing
Pulmonary branch murmur of infancy	Non-harsh	LUSB RUSB	Axillae and back	Less than grade 3	Early systole
Supraclavicular arterial / carotid bruit	Non-harsh	Neck	No	Less than grade 3	Early systole, diminishes with neck extension
Superior vena cava (cervical venous hum)	Machinery-like	Right infraclavicular	No	Often grade 3	Continuous, disappears with supine position or light pressure on jugular vein

TABLE 37.12

Lung sounds are bronchovesicular in young infants. They are of medium pitch and volume and equal in expiration and inspiration. In older children they are vesicular. Vesicular breath sounds are low-pitched and soft and louder and longer in inspiration. Listen for reduced breath sounds (for causes see Ch 38). Bronchial breath sounds are high-pitched, loud and more prominent in expiration. They can normally be heard over the trachea but not over healthy lung areas. They may be heard over consolidated lungs.

Prolonged expiration is a sign of lower airway obstruction and is characteristic of asthma. **Prolonged inspiration** is characteristic of viral croup (infectious laryngotracheitis). These children also have stridor due to upper airway obstruction and collapse (for other causes of stridor, see Ch 38).

If **stridor** is audible during inspiration and expiration, it is an ominous sign indicating severe obstruction or obstruction at multiple sites with the potential to progress rapidly to complete airway obstruction and death.

Grunting is produced at the start of expiration when air is forced against a closed glottis to prevent small-airway collapse. It is heard in association with respiratory distress. **Wheeze** is more high-pitched and musical sounding and may be monophonic or polyphonic. Wheeze is usually heard during expiration and is associated with lower airway obstruction (e.g. asthma in older children). If an infant presents with wheeze, coryza, signs of respiratory distress and inspiratory fine crackles it is suggestive of a virus-induced infection of the terminal airways (**bronchiolitis**), which causes small-airway obstruction, lung hyperinflation and collapsed lung areas. These are often mistaken for consolidation.

The diagnosis of asthma is difficult to make in young children, even if they present with apparently typical features (episodic wheeze, cough and shortness of breath). First, young children are more prone to wheeze when they have a respiratory virus infection (e.g. bronchiolitis in the first 2 years of life). Half of them will outgrow this predisposition by the age of 3 years. Second, children born with hypoplastic lungs and airways as a result of maternal smoking during pregnancy or of prematurity are prone to these symptoms but improve as their lungs grow. Third, there are many other causes of wheeze in early life, including structural airway anomalies such as broncho- and tracheomalacia, and cystic fibrosis. Thus, it is sensible to consider a wide range of differential diagnoses if severe and frequent wheezy illnesses occur, unless a compelling case for asthma can be made based on clinical presentation and response to specific treatment.[1]

Auscultation findings in common structural heart diseases

Cause	CARDIO	
Pulmonary valve stenosis (0.8:1000 [50% with other lesions])	C	Ejection click, murmur low pitch, harsh
	A	Left upper sternal border
	R	Back
	D	Variable
	I	
	O	Crescendo–decrescendo (ejection) midsystolic murmur (the later the peak intensity, the greater the obstruction), S_2 widely split proportionate to severity of obstruction (P_2 delayed)
Aortic valve stenosis (1:2500–1:25,000)	C	Ejection click, murmur low pitch, harsh
	A	Right upper sternal border
	R	Into the neck, thrill suprasternal notch
	D	Variable, usually grade 4 or more
	I	
	O	Crescendo–decrescendo (ejection) midsystolic murmur, S_2 narrowly split proportionate to severity of obstruction (A_2 delayed) Early diastolic regurgitation murmur common
Mitral valve stenosis (rare)	C	Low-pitched, rumbling
	A	Apex in left lateral decubitus position
	R	None
	D	Grade 1 to 2
	I	
	O	Diastolic murmur
Mitral valve regurgitation	C	High-pitched, blowing
	A	Apex
	R	Axilla
	D	Less than grade 3
	I	
	O	Pansystolic murmur, soft/absent S_1, loud S_2 (with pulmonary hypertension), diastolic flow murmur (in severe cases) due to increased flow volume

(Keane JF, Lock JE, Fyler DC, Nadas AS. *Nadas' pediatric cardiology*. Philadelphia: Saunders, 2006.)

TABLE 37.13

IMPORTANT DIFFERENTIAL DIAGNOSES OF RAPID BREATHING OFTEN ASSOCIATED WITH TYPE 1 RESPIRATORY FAILURE

- Structural (pleural / lung / abdomen) abnormalities (pneumothorax, pleural effusion, ascites, interstitial lung disease, diaphragmatic hernia / paresis)
- Infection and inflammation (pneumonia, pneumonitis, bronchitis, tracheitis, bronchiolitis, asthma)
- Cardiocirculatory failure (congenital heart disease, arrhythmias, pneumomediastinum, pericardial effusion, septicaemia, metabolic disease, severe anaemia)

LIST 37.3

IMPORTANT DIFFERENTIAL DIAGNOSES OF REDUCED BREATHING OFTEN ASSOCIATED WITH TYPE 2 RESPIRATORY FAILURE

- Obstruction of upper / lower airways (infection [croup, epiglottitis], inflammation [asthma], congenital / anatomical)
- Central hypoventilation (CNS infections, respiratory infections in young infants, extreme obesity, apnoea of prematurity [diagnosis of exclusion], head trauma, brainstem compression, metabolic disturbances)
- Neuromuscular impairment (congenital / genetic diseases, drugs / intoxication, metabolic disturbances)

LIST 37.4

Proposed normal values for respiratory rate per minute

Age range (years)	Pediatric advanced life support, American Heart Association	Advanced paediatric life support, Advanced Life Support Group
0–2	30–60	30–40
2–3	24–40	25–35
3–5	24–40	25–30
5–12	20–24	20–25
12–18	12–20	15–20

(American Heart Association; Ralston M, Hazinski FM, Zaritsky AL, Schexnayder FM. *PALS provider manual.* Dallas: American Heart Association, 2006. Advanced Life Support Group (Manchester England). *Pre-hospital paediatric life support: a practical approach to the out-of-hospital emergency care of children.* Oxford: BMJ Books/Blackwell, 2005.)

TABLE 37.14

Crackles are non-musical interrupted lung sounds of short duration that may occur at any time during inspiration or expiration. Crackles may be high-pitched (fine) or of variable pitch (coarse). They are produced by abrupt opening of closed airways during inspiration.[32] This means that crackles heard during early inspiration originate from the abrupt opening of larger airways, whereas those generated during late inspiration come from the terminal bronchioli or alveoli and are a sign of bronchiolitis, pneumonitis or pneumonia.[33] Place your stethoscope on the child's neck to distinguish coarse lung crackles from conducted upper airway sounds due to upper airway secretions if they are heard in both lungs.

Percussion, chest expansion and vocal fremitus

Percussion can be very helpful in localised processes of the lung to describe the extent of dullness. Dullness to percussion can be the result of consolidation, collapse (atelectasis) or fluid in the pleural space. An increased percussion note (hyperresonance) suggests unilateral hyperinflation due to a unilateral pneumothorax; when associated with wheeze it may be the result of a foreign body in the main bronchus.

Chest expansion is not routinely measured but may be assessed by percussion (p 95).

Vocal fremitus can be tested in older children.

The respiratory examination is completed with an assessment of the ear, nose and throat (see above).

Gastrointestinal system: abdomen

Examination of the abdomen is central to assessment of the gastrointestinal system. Remember, however, that examination of other systems can provide very important (and sometimes the only) clues to pathologies that are primarily localised in the abdomen. Assessment of nutrition is part of the abdominal and gastrointestinal examination. This includes a medical history (see Table 37.15) and a physical examination focused on detecting significant loss of subcutaneous fat (face, arms, chest, buttocks), muscle wasting (temples, shoulders, thighs, knees, calves) and peripheral oedema (pretibial, sacral).

Positioning the patient

Ask the child to lie flat in the supine position with the arms placed alongside their body and the feet together. The abdomen and inguinal region should be fully exposed; use a sheet to cover the external genitalia in older children. The external genitalia should be inspected routinely in young children so that important abnormalities such as testicular torsion, undescended testes and penile malformations are not missed. A toddler may be unwilling to lie flat and may become upset if you (or the parent) try to insist. Young children may, however, sit quietly in the parent's lap and let the parent proceed with undressing them. Remember that rather than the crying agile toddler, it is the unusually quiet child with paucity of movements and suspected illness who is of greatest concern and who requires most urgent assessment.

Inspection

Begin with inspection. Imagine a vertical line and a perpendicular horizontal line running through the umbilicus to 'divide' the abdomen into four quadrants (right upper, right lower, left upper, left lower) and describe the location of any abnormality. The abdomen often appears as if it is generally distended in toddlers owing to their physiological lumbar lordosis. Abdominal distension may be observed with the following:

- ascites (liver disease, cardiac failure, malnutrition, protein-losing enteropathy)
- malabsorption (coeliac disease, food allergy, lactase or sucrase–isomaltase deficiency and intolerance, glucose–galactose malabsorption)
- maldigestion (pancreatic insufficiency in cystic fibrosis and Shwachman–Diamond syndrome, impaired bile flow in chronic liver disease)

- solid organomegaly (hepatic or haematological or infectious splenic disorders)
- urogenital malformations (obstructive uropathy due to urethral valves)
- tumours (haemangioma, nephroblastoma, neuroblastoma)
- cysts (polycystic kidney disease), abscess (paratyphoid in appendicitis)
- mechanical (bowel obstruction due to impacted meconium or stool, intussusception, malrotation with volvulus, intestinal atresias, inflammatory or postsurgical adhesions) or paralytic ileus (infections [gastroenteritis, appendicitis], postsurgery, ischaemia, electrolyte imbalances [low potassium])
- umbilical hernia and diastasis recti (separation of the left and right rectus abdominis muscles).

Epigastric peristalsis may be visible owing to hypertrophic pyloric stenosis, which typically manifests after the neonatal period with projectile vomiting and life-threatening dehydration. A paucity of abdominal wall movements during respiration may be due to significant abdominal pain. A depressed abdomen with bowel sounds in the chest indicates a congenital or acquired (trauma) diaphragmatic defect. Assess for the asymmetry caused by an abdominal mass and the bulging flanks that result from ascites. If inguinal swelling is observed, it is commonly—but not always—caused by a hernia (see Ch 38). Carefully attempt to reduce the hernia at the end of the examination. A hernia is an indication for prompt surgical review (and if not reducible this is urgent). Note any abdominal scars indicating past surgical operations that may be relevant to the current major problem. Carefully inspect the skin for jaundice, discoloration, rashes, petechiae, bruising and spider naevi (see also Ch 38).

Auscultation

Auscultation of the abdomen is usually performed to assess bowel sounds and to listen for vascular bruits. It is generally felt that auscultation should take place before palpation, as this may alter bowel sounds. There is a lack of evidence that palpation alters bowel sounds but conventions in medicine are hard to alter. Auscultation requires patience, cooperation from the child (and the parent) and, in the case of bruits, a quiet room.

Nutrition-focused medical history

Domain	Indicators of potential impairment in nutritional status
Growth	Below third percentile Crossing percentiles downwards in serial measurements (may be normal in first 2 years of life and puberty if shifting towards fiftieth percentile) Reduced weight-to-length percentile ratio Unintentional weight loss (5–10% moderate; >10% severe) Rapid weight loss
Dietary intake	Appetite ('fussy' eater) Frequency (decreases with age) and amount (increases with age) of food Feeding problems (uncoordinated swallow) Restrictions (parent-perceived food intolerance versus specialist-diagnosed allergy)
Functional impairment	Activity Power/strength
Metabolic stress	Infection (gastroenteritis, sepsis, pneumonia) Inflammation (pancreatitis) Endocrine disorders (hyperthyroidism, diabetes) Trauma Surgery (bowel resection)
Abdominal symptoms	Frequent vomiting Gastro-oesophageal reflux Constipation Pain Nausea Diarrhoea

TABLE 37.15

Begin by listening in the right upper quadrant over the liver for bruits or rubs. Bruits can occasionally be heard in children with hepatic haemangiomas. Bowel sounds from the overlying segments of bowel will often be heard in all quadrants. Next, move to the left upper quadrant to similarly listen over the spleen for bruits or rubs. Auscultate the left and right lower quadrants for inguinal bruits, before moving to the periumbilical region, where aortic and renal bruits are most commonly heard.[7] If a renal bruit is suspected, listen within 2 centimetres of the midline, halfway between the umbilicus and the xiphoid process. Remember that a renal bruit may be associated with hypertension as a result of renal artery stenosis so measure the blood pressure. Bruits are caused by turbulent flow through major blood vessels. Aortic bruits are usually heard only in systole, whereas **venous hums** are continuous.

To conclude that no bowel sounds can be heard, you need to have listened for several minutes and in several different areas of the abdomen. **Bowel sounds** that can be heard without a stethoscope are referred to as borborygmi. The complete absence of bowel sounds in the setting of abdominal pathology is an ominous sign that usually implies a paralytic ileus.[34] Increased or 'active' bowel sounds may be heard in patients with gastroenteritis, and when obstruction is present they often have a high-pitched or 'tinkling' quality.

Although auscultation is a commonly practised part of the paediatric abdominal examination, there is very little evidence of its value in the literature. Thankfully, what evidence can be found shows that bowel sounds have high specificity but low sensitivity in diagnosing abdominal obstruction.[35] This means that if abnormal sounds are heard, obstruction is likely, *but* the presence of normal bowel sounds will not accurately exclude bowel obstruction.

Palpation

Occasionally it is helpful to flex the knees or put a cushion under the neck in older children. This may help relax the abdominal muscles. First palpate all abdominal quadrants superficially and away from any tenderness. Remember to look at the child's face—not your hands—for any sign that the examination is painful. There is little you can do about a child's giggling during palpation except to try to divert his or her attention to something else. Giggling at least suggests that the examination is not painful. Next palpate more deeply with slow rather than poking movements. If you can feel a mass, assess it for tenderness and size and try to define its borders. This can also be done by percussion. Feel the surface and decide whether it is flat or nodular and whether the texture is soft or firm. If not completed previously, listen for bruits. A firm mass deep in the right lower abdominal quadrant (iliac fossa) is often due to faecal loading. This will disappear after bowel movements.

To palpate the **liver**, begin in the right iliac fossa using one hand in toddlers and infants and, if preferred, both hands in older children. Advance towards the right hypochondrium, which is the area below the right costal margin, and then across to the epigastrium to feel the liver edge, which is usually palpable just below the costal margin in older children or 1–2 centimetres below in younger children. The liver edge can be confirmed and the liver span can be determined with percussion using a tape measure. This may help you to decide whether the liver is enlarged (hepatomegaly) or pushed downwards (liver ptosis) by lung hyperinflation or a pleural effusion.

To palpate the **spleen**, begin in the *left* iliac fossa and advance towards the left costal margin. This is different from the adult examination. Remember that an enlarged spleen in older children (as in adults) can extend into the right iliac fossa. An enlarged spleen may be painful upon palpation so be very gentle. The tip of the spleen can often be felt in normal young children just below the left costal margin, particularly during inspiration, and in the right lateral decubitus position. If splenomegaly is suspected, it is important to ensure that you cannot palpate over the mass in the cranial direction, that you can feel a notch along the medial border and that the percussion note is dull.

Next palpate for **kidney enlargement** or cysts. Causes include hydronephrosis due to obstructive uropathy, polycystic kidneys and tumours such as nephroblastoma and neuroblastoma. Palpation is performed with two hands, one positioned beneath the flank and the other anteriorly in line with the first hand. The kidney may be felt during inspiration and can be trapped (ballotted) by pushing up with the hand under the flank and catching the kidney as it rises with the other hand.

Percussion

In children, abdominal percussion is used mostly to assess organ size and to check for ascites, but it is also useful in detecting mass lesions and areas of tenderness. Generally, fluid such as ascites or urine in the bladder or mass lesions will elicit a dull sound, whereas an air-filled structure like gas within the bowel will elicit a resonant note on percussion. Techniques are not different from those used in adults (see Ch 14), but be gentle, sensible and opportunistic in your approach.

Genitourinary system

Genitourinary examination is not routinely performed in children, and in many instances, including suspected child sexual abuse, should be carried out only by a clinician who is well trained in this area. For small children, the parent should always be present; if an

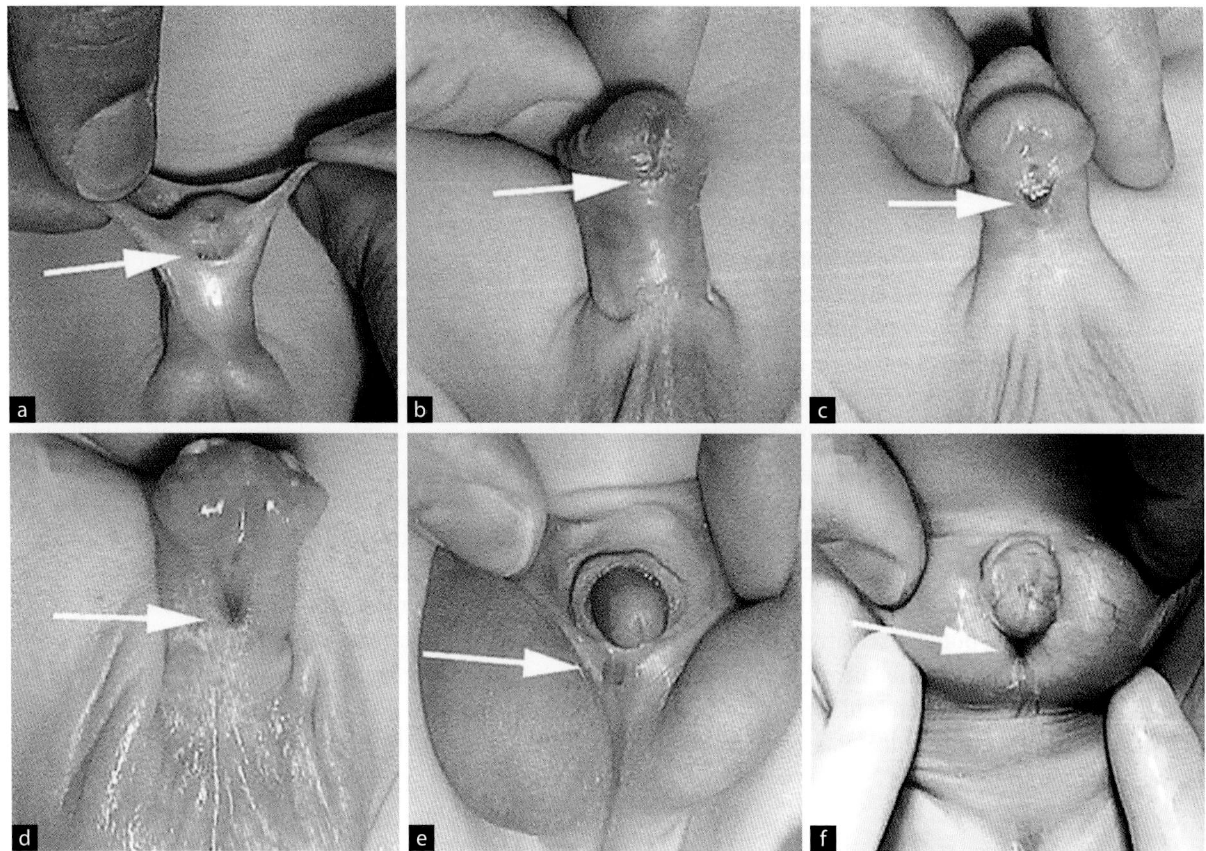

Hypospadias with the abnormal displaced urethral opening located in (a) the glans, (b, c) distal end of the penile shaft, (d) midshaft, (e) scrotum and (f) perineum

(From Baskin LS. Hypospadias and urethral development. *J Urol* 2000; 163:951–956.)

FIGURE 37.32

older child or adolescent is uncomfortable having the parent act as a chaperone, another appropriate chaperone should be provided. The examination for ambiguous genitalia is covered briefly in Chapter 38.

Genital examination in males

Check that the scrotum contains both testes, which should also be of similar size. Orchidometer beads can be used to estimate testicular size. Examine the skin for any unusual lesions and visualise the urethral meatus. Examine the glans for hypospadias (see Fig. 37.32): in this condition, the urethral meatus may be displaced ventrally, anywhere within the glans, the shaft of the penis, the scrotum or even the perineum.

Palpate the scrotum for hernias, abnormal masses such as a varicocele or testicular enlargement (e.g. as a result of acute lymphoblastic leukaemia), and ensure that there is no pain or swelling of the testes that would suggest torsion. If a hydrocele is suspected, transilluminate the scrotum (see Fig. 18.11 on p 324). Check bilaterally for **inguinal hernia. Penile length** should be assessed as part of Tanner staging (see p 699). Care should be taken to ensure that the examination is not painful.

Genital examination in females

Proper visualisation of the female genitalia is usually easiest with the patient lying supine with the legs abducted at the hips. Again, care should be taken to ensure that this examination is not painful. If necessary, the labia can be separated to review the clitoris, the urethral meatus and the vaginal introitus. If clitoral enlargement is present, consider androgen stimulation as a result of congenital adrenal hyperplasia or disorders of sex development. Examine for labial adhesions and soft-tissue masses such as urethral prolapse, prolapsed ectopic ureterocele or paraurethral cysts. Check to ensure that the patient does not have an imperforate hymen or the associated hydrocolpos.

Internal examination (using a speculum) is almost never indicated in young girls and specialist advice should be sought before attempting this, even in the postpubertal female.

Anal and rectal examination

Anal and rectal examination is fairly similar for all age groups. Check for an anteriorly placed anus, skin tags, haemorrhoids (uncommon in children) and anal fissures, which can be caused by constipation or inflammatory bowel disease. Although inspection can be very important and informative, rectal examination is almost never indicated in children.

ADOLESCENT HISTORY AND EXAMINATION

Adolescence is the phase of life between childhood and adulthood, ranging approximately from ages 10 to 24. It is a unique stage of human development characterised by dynamic brain development; in which the interaction with the social environment shapes the capabilities that an individual will take forward into adult life.[36] During these years, adolescents acquire the physical, cognitive, emotional, social and economic resources that are the foundation for later life health and wellbeing. These same resources define trajectories into the next (and any subsequent) generations. Investments in adolescent health and wellbeing bring benefits today, but more importantly for the children of the future for decades to come.[37]

Tanner staging and pubertal assessment

Puberty generally refers to the physical maturation that occurs during adolescence – most obviously changes in height and development of secondary sex characteristics, but also including changes in body composition, achievement of fertility and changes in most body systems (see Table 37.16). The timing of puberty will vary widely among individuals of a given sex and ethnic background, although most adolescents will follow a predictable path through pubertal maturation.

There is growth in all body parts during puberty (except for the tonsils, adenoids and thymus). The linear growth in puberty accounts for approximately 20% of adult height,[38] and growth in weight accounts for approximately 50% of 'ideal' adult weight.[39] In early puberty the limbs will accelerate before the trunk, while in later puberty the growth spurt is mainly truncal.[40] The majority of the height and weight increases in puberty occurs during a 36-month period, with peak growth occurring about 18–24 months earlier in females.[39] Bone mass and muscle mass will increase in parallel with epiphyseal fusion being one of the last changes of puberty. Height and weight should be plotted on the appropriate charts. Gender-specific, height-for-age, weight-for-age and head-circumference charts for ages 5 to 19 are shown in Fig. 37.33.

Terms associated with puberty	
Gonadarche	Activation of the gonads by the pituitary hormones—luteinising hormone (LH) and follicle-stimulating hormone (FSH)
Adrenarche	Increase of androgens by the adrenal cortex
Thelarche	Appearance of breast tissue, which is primarily due to the action of oestradiol from the ovaries
Menarche	First menstrual bleed, typically caused by the effects of oestradiol on the endometrial lining (often not associated with ovulation)Oestradiol and progesterone produced by the ovaries lead to regular menstrual cycles
Spermarche	First sperm production, due mainly to the effects of FSH along with a contribution from LH-induced testosterone productionTypically starts with nocturnal sperm emissions and the appearance of sperm in urine
Pubarche	Appearance of pubic hair, primarily due to the effects of androgens from the adrenal gland. Also applies to the first appearance of axillary hair, apocrine body odour and acne
Precocious puberty	Pubertal onset at an age 2–3 standard deviations below the mean age of onset of puberty—for example, breast development before the age of 8 years in girls and testicular enlargement before the age of 9 in boys
Delayed puberty	The absence of signs of puberty by an age 2–3 standard deviations above the mean age of onset of puberty—for example, 12–13 years for girls' breast development and 13–14 years for testicular enlargement in boys

TABLE 37 16

Text continued on p 706

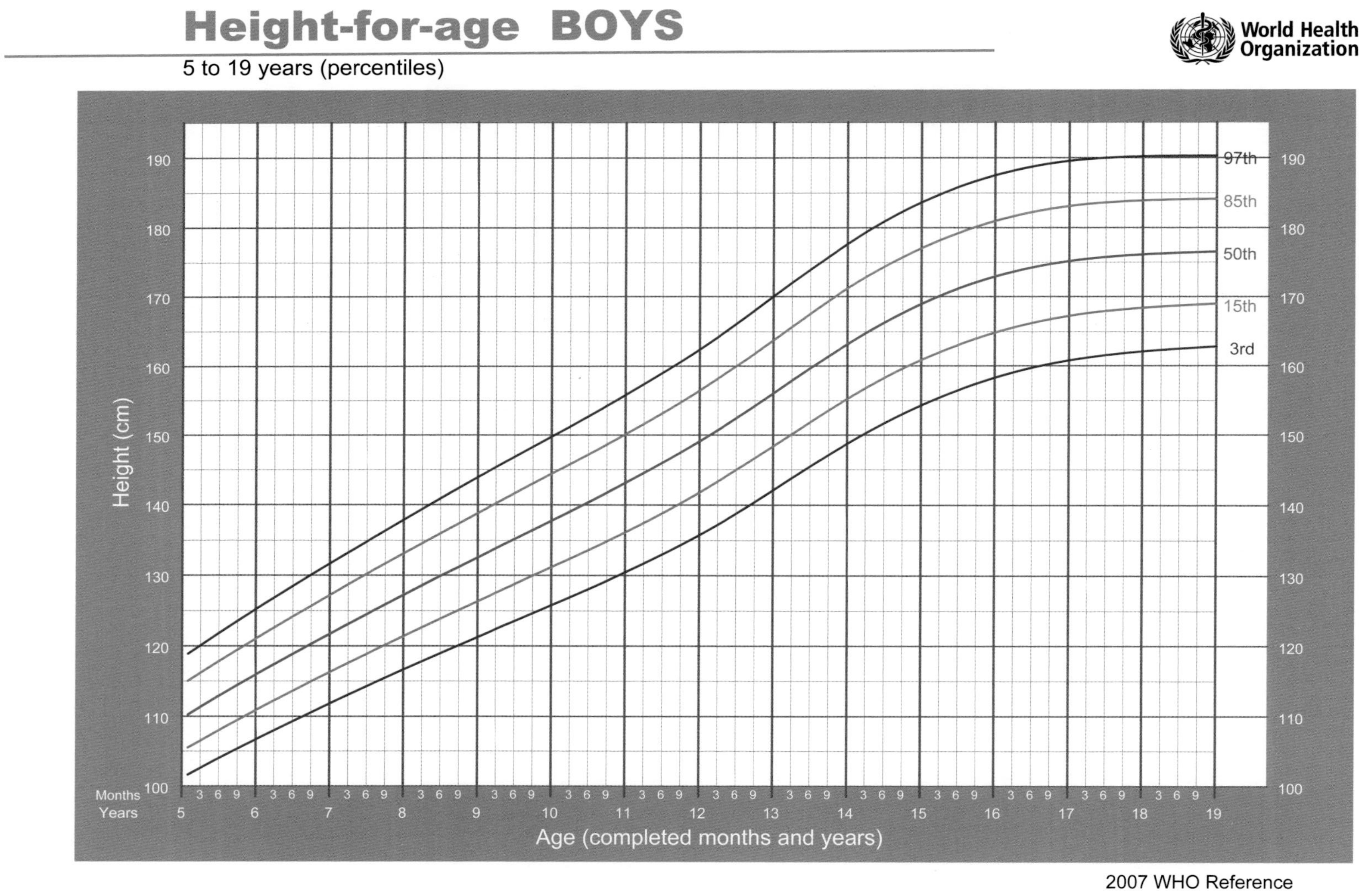

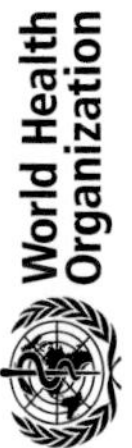

Growth charts from 5 to 19 years

(Reprinted from World Health Organization Child Growth Standard Charts https://www.who.int/tools/growth-reference-data-for-5to19-years/indicators.)

FIGURE 37.33

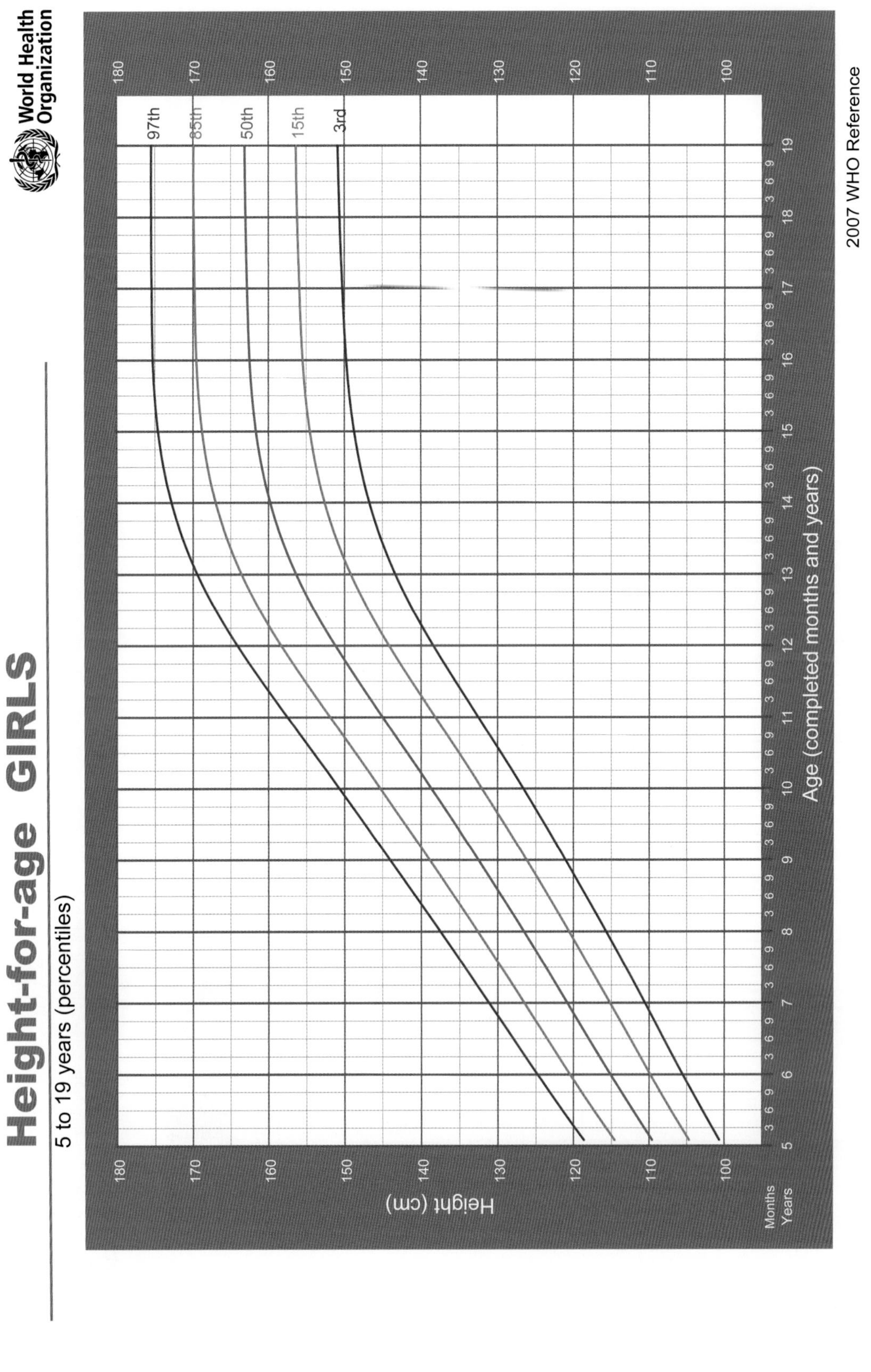

Height-for-age GIRLS

5 to 19 years (percentiles)

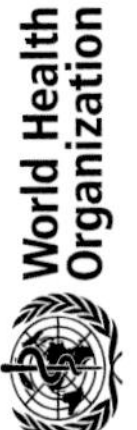

Height (cm)

180 170 160 150 140 130 120 110 100

97th
85th
50th
15th
3rd

Months
Years
5 6 7 8 9 10 11 12 13 14 15 16 17 18 19

Age (completed months and years)

2007 WHO Reference

FIGURE 37.33, cont'd

Continued

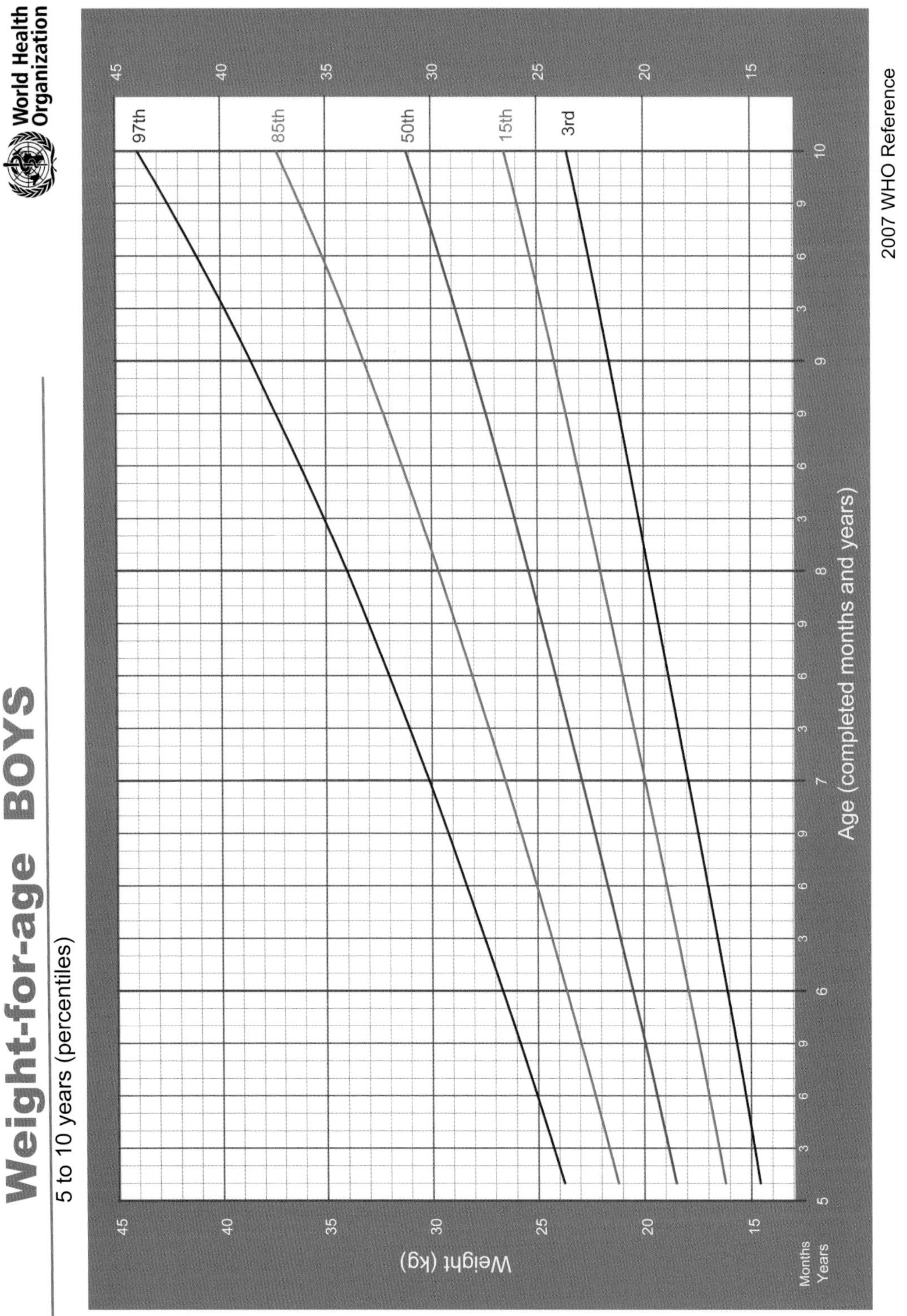

Weight-for-age BOYS

5 to 10 years (percentiles)

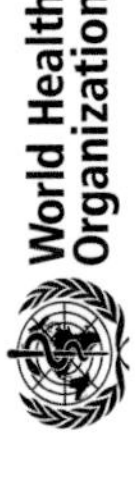

Weight (kg)

45
40
35
30
25
20
15

97th
85th
50th
15th
3rd

Months
Years

5 3 6 9 6 3 6 9 7 3 6 9 8 3 6 9 9 3 6 9 10

Age (completed months and years)

2007 WHO Reference

FIGURE 37.33, cont'd

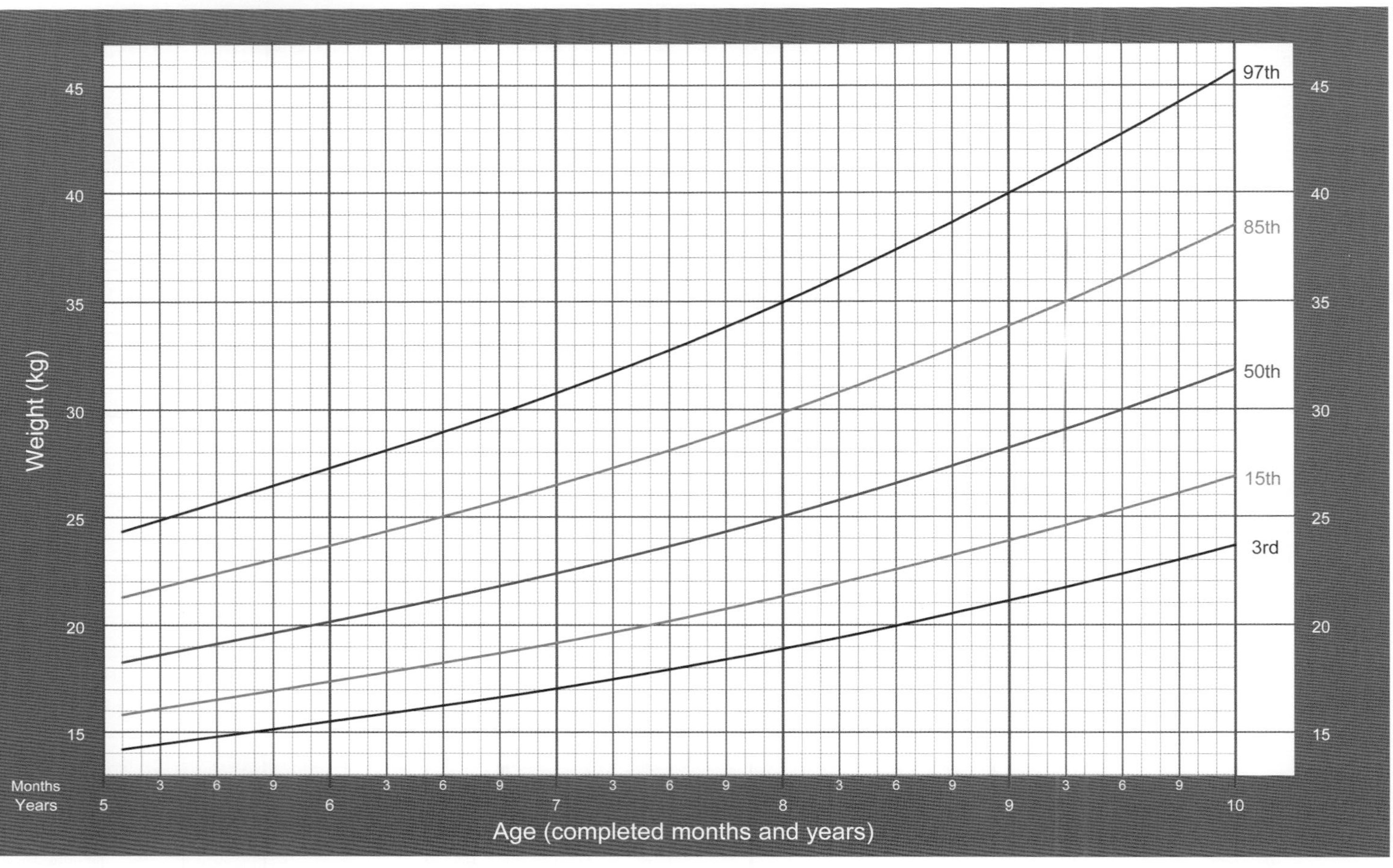

FIGURE 37.33, cont'd

Continued

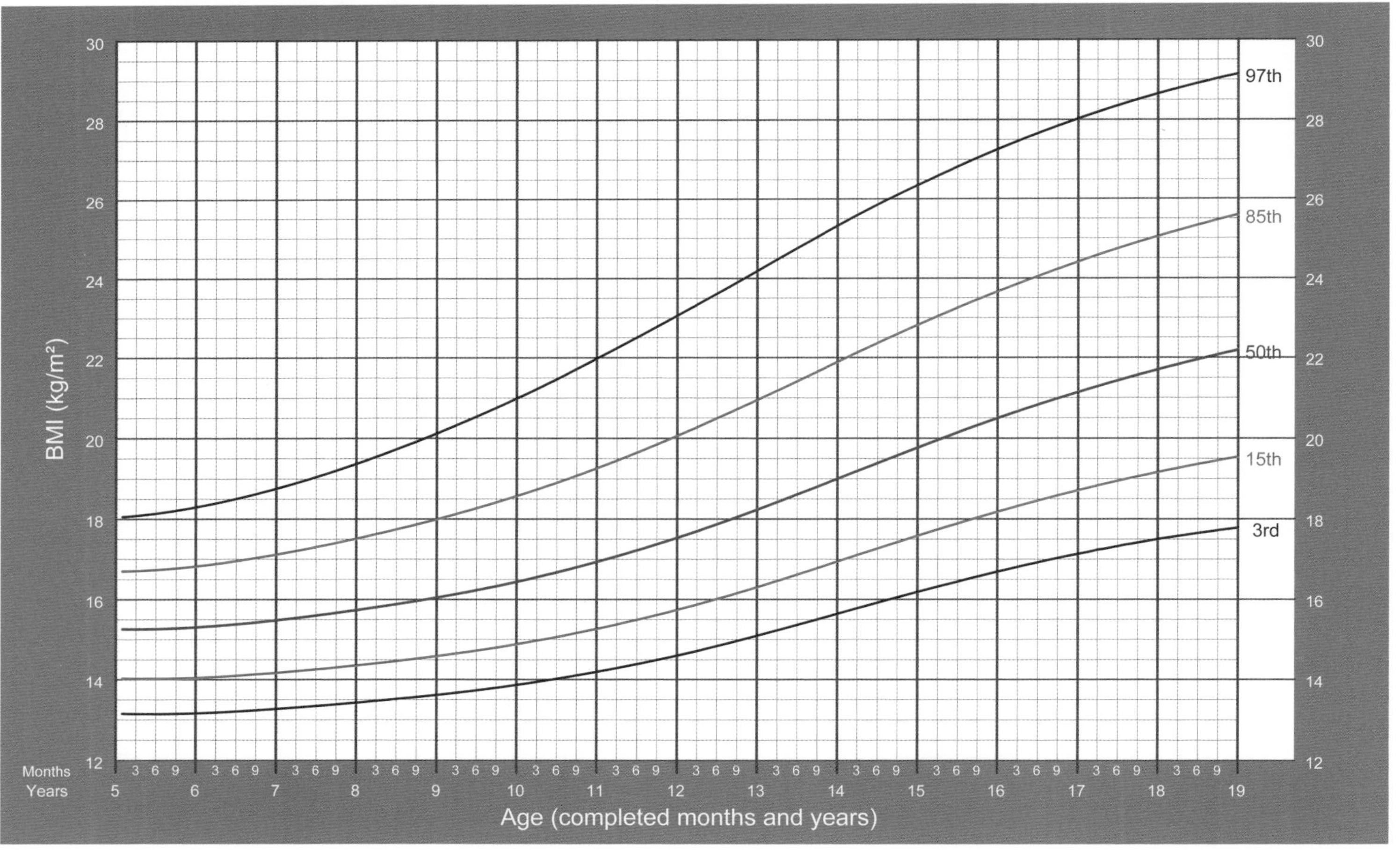

FIGURE 37.33, cont'd

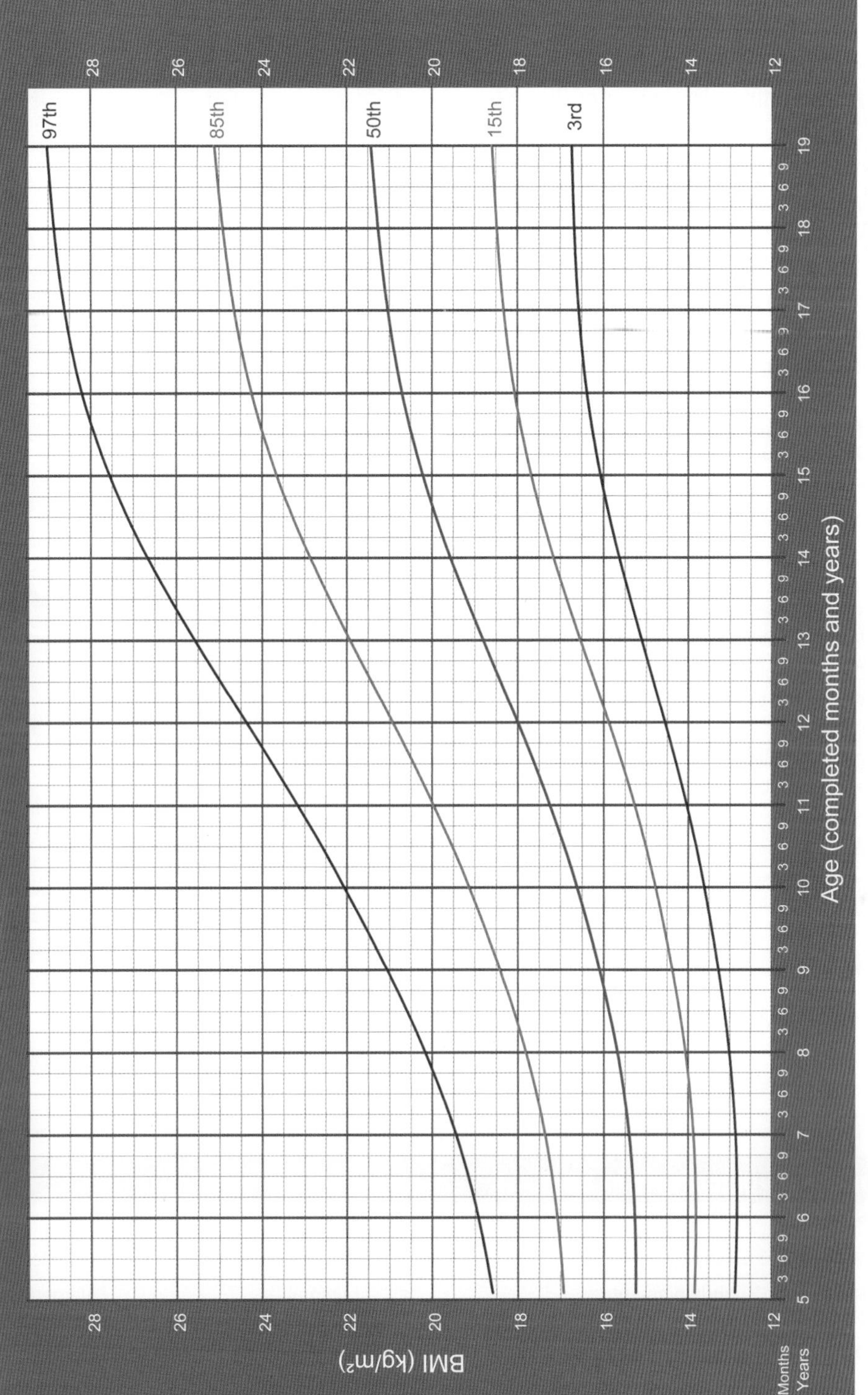

FIGURE 37.33, cont'd

Continued

In the 1960s, Tanner and colleagues developed a staging system that is still used today to assess progression through puberty in both sexes (see Tables 37.17 and 37.18). Generally, enlargement of the testes is the first physical evidence of puberty in males (≈98%) and the appearance of palpable breast tissue under the areola is the first physical evidence of puberty in females (≈80%; see Fig. 37.34). In the remainder of adolescents, pubic hair is the first physical evidence (see Fig. 37.35). Additionally, there is growth of axillary hair in both sexes, and in males the lowering of the voice and development of facial hair.

Classification of sexual maturity in girls

SMR stage	Pubic hair	Breasts
1	Preadolescent	Preadolescent
2	Sparse, lightly pigmented, straight, medial border of labia	Breast and papilla elevated as small mound; diameter of areola increased
3	Darker, beginning to curl, increased amount	Breast and areola enlarged, no contour separation
4	Coarse, curly, abundant, but less than in adult	Areola and papilla form secondary mound
5	Adult feminine triangle, spread to medial surface of thighs	Mature, nipple projects, areola part of general breast contour

SMR = sexual maturity rating.

(Republished with permission of John Wiley & Sons Inc, from Tanner JM. *Growth at adolescence*, 2nd edn. Oxford, Blackwell Scientific/Wiley, 1962, permission conveyed through Copyright Clearance Center, Inc.)

TABLE 37.17

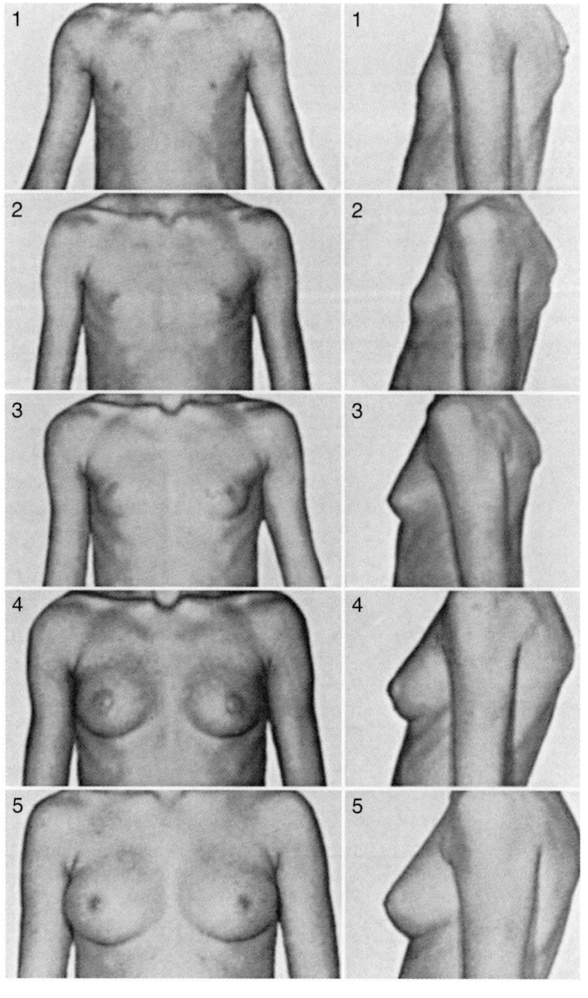

Sexual maturity ratings (1–5) of breast changes in adolescent girls

(From Behrman RE, Kliegman RM, St Geme JW et al. *Nelson textbook of pediatrics*, 17th edn. Philadelphia: Saunders, 2004.)

FIGURE 37.34

Classification of sexual maturity in boys

SMR stage	Pubic hair	Penis	Testes
1	None	Preadolescent	Preadolescent
2	Scanty, long, slightly pigmented	Minimal change/enlargement	Enlarged scrotum, pink, texture altered
3	Darker, starting to curl, small amount	Lengthens	Larger
4	Resembles adult type, but less quantity; coarse, curly	Larger; glans and breadth increase in size	Larger, scrotum dark
5	Adult distribution, spread to medial surface of thighs	Adult size	Adult size

SMR = sexual maturity rating.

(Republished with permission of John Wiley & Sons Inc, from Tanner JM. *Growth at adolescence*, 2nd edn. Oxford, Blackwell Scientific/Wiley, 1962, permission conveyed through Copyright Clearance Center, Inc.)

TABLE 37.18

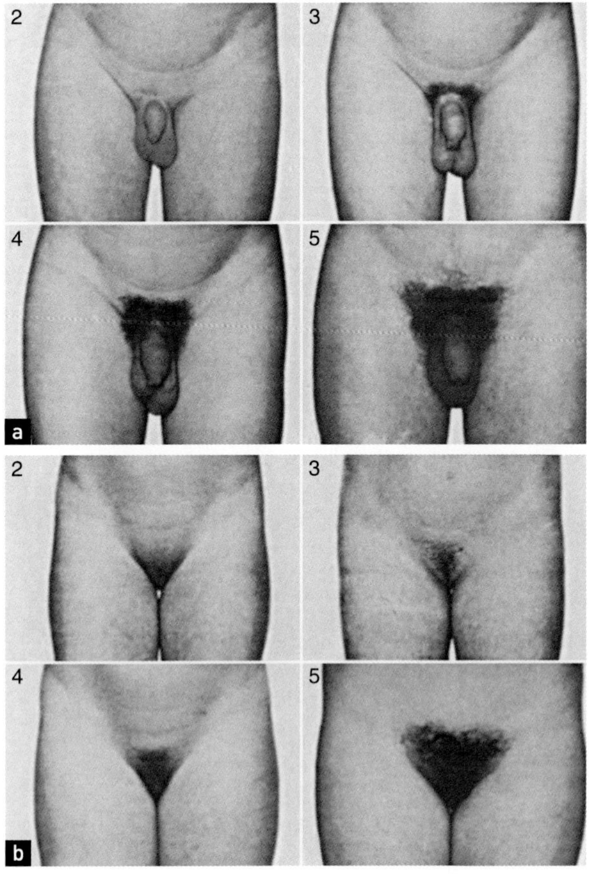

Sexual maturity ratings (2–5) of pubic hair changes in adolescent (a) boys and (b) girls

(From Behrman RE, Kliegman RM, St Geme JW et al. *Nelson textbook of pediatrics*, 17th edn. Philadelphia: Saunders, 2004.)

FIGURE 37.35

HINT BOX

For a quick screening, it is often sufficient to show children the Tanner staging illustrations and ask where they see their current stage best represented.

Psychological development of adolescents

In addition to the physical growth of adolescence, there is the complex process of psychological, sexual, social and cognitive maturation which, again, can show significant variation between individuals and, in contrast to the relentless progression of physical changes, can regress or progress depending on environmental stressors. Puberty does not affect cognitive function or development, but it can have a significant impact on psychological and social issues. In particular, a mismatch between pubertal development and chronological age may have an especially negative psychological impact (this seems to be most prevalent in early-maturing females and late-maturing males[41]). It is also crucial to remember that young people come from a wide range of social and cultural backgrounds, and health services need to ensure that services provide culturally responsive healthcare. This may include[42]:

- taking a non-expert position that facilitates all young people in being open about their particular situation, whatever their background or circumstances;
- acknowledging customs of the individual's and family's culture of origin;
- understanding differences in inter-family relating (e.g. youth relationships with parents and with other authority figures) and the possibility of religious and spiritual factors; and
- having a basic knowledge about the challenges facing young people in the community who experience mental health problems at a disproportionate rate in comparison with their peers (e.g. First Nations youth, young people from a sexual minority and gender diverse group, refugee and homeless youth).

First Nations

Particular issues for First Nations communities need to be considered in the provision of culturally sensitive adolescent psychological and mental health services. Additional risk factors in these patients may include poor general health and socioeconomic deprivation, high rates of suicide particularly in young males, racism and discrimination, poverty, underemployment, and alcohol and other substance misuse.[43] Considerations of mental health in this population needs to be placed within a social and historical context that takes into account the traditional holistic understanding of health (see Text box 37.3).[42]

Depression screening

Many guidelines (including the Bright Futures and American Academy of Paediatrics) suggest universal screening for depression annually in adolescents,

Factors that may assist in improving access to services for specific sociocultural groups

Aboriginal and Torres Strait Islander youth (Hayman et al 2009)

- Employing Aboriginal and Torres Strait Islander staff as health workers, on reception and as liaison officers
- Ensuring cultural responsiveness of healthcare professionals (AHMAC 2004)
- Providing culturally appropriate resources (including local adaptation of materials)
- Providing a culturally appropriate waiting room (e.g. culturally appropriate posters and artefacts)
- Disseminating information about services available within the health service
- Promoting intersectoral collaboration

Youth from a sexual minority and gender diverse group (VMACGLBTIHW 2009)

- Educating staff about issues that may affect individuals from a sexual minority and gender diverse group and ways to facilitate staff-client communication
- Recommending procedures for confidentiality and sexual minority and gender diverse inclusive documentation
- Developing and reviewing a directory of appropriate or specific counselling services, medical services and support groups to which young people can be referred as needed

Refugee youth

- Providing social support, for example through ethnic-specific cultural liaison officers
- Ensuring cultural responsiveness among health professionals
- Providing education, including linguistically appropriate information
- Developing culturally appropriate resources, including resources in spoken format for young people who lack literacy in their own languages, and access to interpreter services during appointments

Young people leaving foster care or who are homeless

- Investigating ongoing developmental and financial support for young people leaving formal care
- Providing specific teams/centres for young people at risk of homelessness or who are homeless

(From *Cultural competency in health: a guide for policy, partnerships and participation*. Canberra: NHMRC, 2006; for references see original source.)

TEXT BOX 37.3

HEEADSSS assessment	
Home	Who, where, recent moves, relationships, violence
Education and employment	Where, attendance, year, performance, relationships, supports, recent moves, bullying, disciplinary actions, future plans, work details
Eating	Weight (heaviest, lightest, recent changes), dieting, exercise, menstrual history, restricted eating, binging, purging
Activities	Outside of school: sport, organised groups, clubs, parties, TV / computer use
Alcohol and drugs	Cigarettes, alcohol and illicit drug use by friends, family and patient, patterns and frequency of use, regrets from using substances, how use is financed, problems it has caused
Sexuality	Close relationships, sexual experiences, number of partners (total and in the last 3 months), gender of sexual partners (don't assume sexual preferences), uncomfortable situations / sexual abuse, risk of pregnancy and previous pregnancies (relevant to males as well as females), contraception, condoms, sexually transmissible infections (STIs)
Suicide, depression and self-harm	Presence and frequency of feeling down or sad as well as current feelings (e.g. 'How do you feel in yourself at the moment on a scale of 1 to 10?'), actions when down, supports, self-harm (thoughts and actions), suicide (thoughts, attempts, plans and means), hopes for future
Safety from injury and violence	Serious injuries, use of safety gear for sports and driving, riding with an intoxicated driver, exposure to violence at school and in neighbourhood, online (cyber) safety; for high-risk youths: carrying or use of weapons, other criminal behaviour, incarceration of family or friends

(Royal Children's Hospital, Melbourne, Australia, *Clinical Practice Guideline on Engaging with and assessing the adolescent patient*, [Internet]. Available from: https://www.rch.org.au/clinicalguide/guideline_index/Engaging_with_and_assessing_the_adolescent_patient/#HEEADSSS.)

TABLE 37.19

particularly given that there is a significant body of evidence that these patients are particularly reluctant to disclose sensitive information without being prompted.[44] The most frequently reported reasons for delayed help-seeking by young people are lack of recognition that they have a mental health problem and lack of knowledge about how and where to seek help,[45] but some of this reluctance may be due to anxiety about confidentiality,[44] as well as the stigma of mental health disorders.[43] (Also see the Chapter 46 The psychiatric history and mental health examination.)

One of the most commonly used screening assessments for adolescents is the HEEADSSS assessment (see Table 37.19). More comprehensive questions and suggestions can be found in the *NSW Health Kids and Families Youth Health Resource Kit—an essential guise for workers* (https://www.health.nsw.gov.au/kidsfamilies/youth/Publications/youth-health-resource-kit.pdf) and the Contemporary paediatrics website (https://www.contemporarypediatrics.com/view/heeadsss-30-psychosocial-interview-adolescents-updated-new-century-fueled-media).

Sexuality and sexual identity

One of the tasks of healthy adolescent development is the acquisition of a mature and responsible sexual identity. Adolescent sexuality, partly because of its serious health consequences, has long been equated with risk and danger, but we are seeing the growing acceptance that adolescent sexuality is a normal and expected aspect of human development.[46] This can be particularly complex for adolescents from sexual minorities (including lesbian, gay, bisexual, pansexual, intersex as well as identities and expressions that defy labels) and transgender and gender diverse (TGD) individuals. Healthcare professionals providing care for adolescents should integrate developmentally appropriate conversations around gender and sexuality into their education and counselling. Again, it is important to understand that there are significant cultural differences in concepts of gender (see Fig. 37.36).

Some TGD individuals may present for the first time in adolescence, and the physical changes of puberty may be usually exceptionally difficult for these patients. Feelings of gender dysphoria may increase in intensity during puberty with the development of unwanted

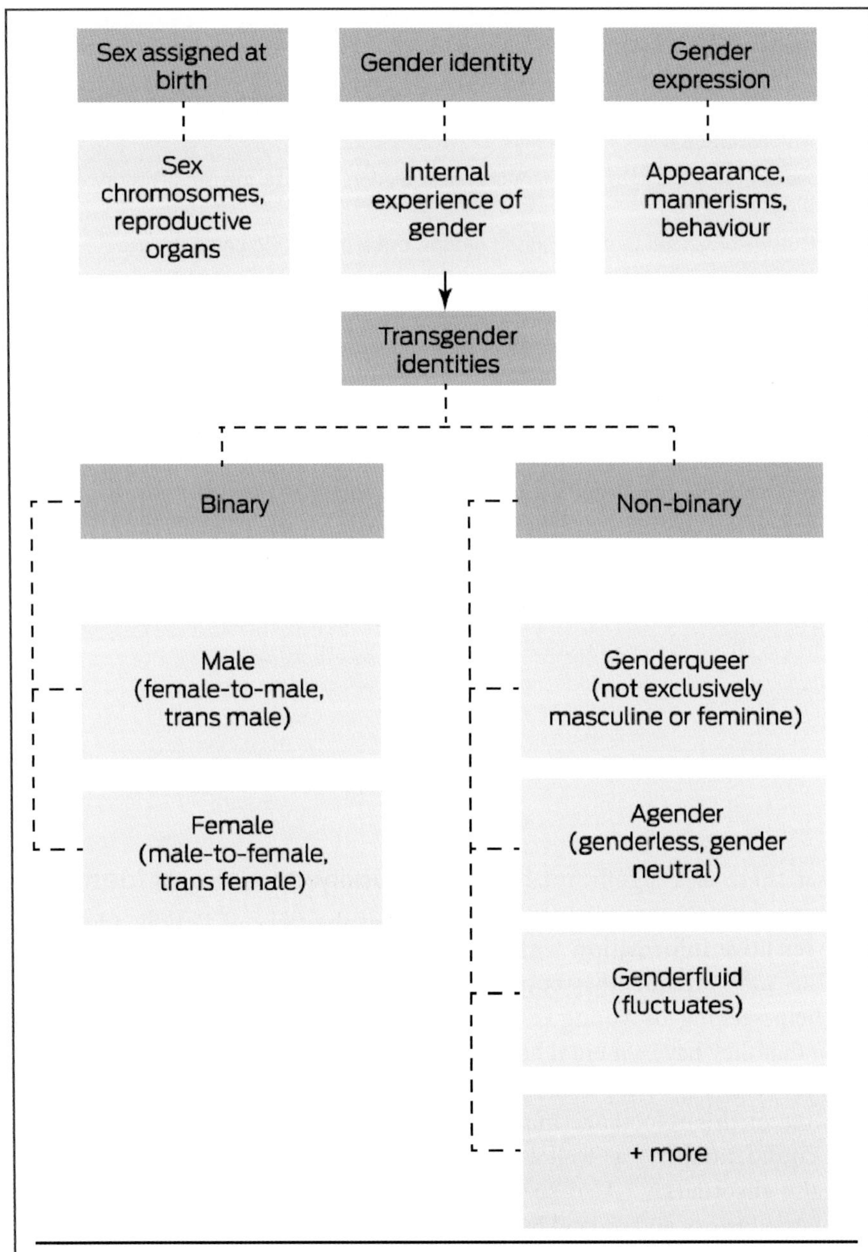

Gender identity and gender expression are distinct from biological sex. Although there are many gender identities,[7] transgender and gender diverse identities can be roughly separated into binary (ie, trangender male, transgender female) and non-binary. The term non-binary is used here as a broad umbrella category to describe identities which are outside of the binary; however, non-binary is also a specific gender identity. ◆

Distinction between gender identity, gender expression and sex assigned at birth

(From Cheung AS, Wynne K, Erasmus J et al. Position statement on the hormonal management of adult transgender and gender diverse individuals. *Med J Aust* 2019; 211: 127–133. https://doi.org/10.5694/mja2.50259.)47.))

FIGURE 37.36

secondary sexual characteristics.[48] For such youths, the addition of the incongruence of designated sex to the physical, social and emotional changes of adolescence can be overwhelming, leading to isolation, anxiety, depression, suicidality and dangerous behaviours.[49] Conversely, healthcare provider recognition and validation of the gender continuum and acceptance of individuals no matter where on the spectrum they identify may help to increase tolerance in families and communities.[50]

Eating disorders

Eating disorders are moderate to severe illnesses that are characterised by disturbances in thinking and behaviour around food, eating and body weight or shape.[51] The DSM-5 has specific psychological, behavioural and physiological characteristics for the diagnosis of these disorders (see Table 37.20).[52]Refer to Mental Health Chapter page 879.

Eating disorders can be associated with significant psychiatric and medical morbidity. Early detection and

Summary of DSM-5 diagnostic criteria for eating disorders	
Anorexia nervosa	**Bulimia nervosa**
a. Restriction of energy intake resulting in a significantly low body weight; or a less than minimally expected weight (based on age, sex or developed trajectory) b. Intense fear of gaining weight; or persistent behaviour that interferes with weight gain, despite low weight c. Disturbance in body image; or persistent lack of recognition of the seriousness of the current low body weightSubtypes: Restricting type, binge-eating/purging type	a. Recurrent episodes of binge eating (this involves eating an excessive amount of food in a discrete period of time AND a sense of lack of control) b. Recurrent inappropriate compensatory behaviours to prevent weight gain, such as vomiting, laxatives, diuretics, fasting or excessive exercise c. Frequency of at least once per week for three months d. Self-evaluation unduly influenced by body shape and weight e. Absence of anorexia nervosa
Binge eating disorder	**Other specified feeding or eating disorder (OSFED)**
a. Recurrent episodes of binge eating b. Associated with symptoms such as eating more rapidly, feeling uncomfortably full, not feeling hungry, eating alone due to embarrassment and/or feelings of self-disgust c. Marked distress regarding binge eating d. Frequency of at least once per week for three months e. Absence of compensatory behaviours, anorexia nervosa and bulimia nervosa	Eating disorders causing significant distress but not meeting criteria for other diagnostic categories Examples: • Atypical anorexia nervosa - 'normal weight anorexia nervosa' • Bulimia nervosa (of low frequency and/or limited duration) • Subthreshold binge-eating disorder • Purging disorder • Night eating syndrome
Avoidant/restrictive food intake disorder (ARFID)	**Unspecified feeding or eating disorder (UFED)**
a. Eating or feeding disturbance with persistent failure to meet nutritional needs associated with either significant weight loss (or growth failure), significant nutritional deficiency, dependence on enteral/supplemental feeding or marked interference with psychosocial functioning b. Not explained by lack of available food or culturally sanctioned practice c. Absence of anorexia nervosa, bulimia nervosa or body image disturbance d. No intercurrent medical illness	Presentations in which clinically significant symptoms occur but do not meet full criteria for other eating disorders. Includes situations where the clinician chooses not to specify the reason criteria are not met or where this may be unknown (eg emergency room setting)
(From Rowe E. Early detection of eating disorders in general practice. *Aust Fam Physician* 2017; 46:833–838.)[53]	

TABLE 37.20

intervention may improve treatment outcomes, so it remains important that appropriate treatment and care of affected children/adolescents encourage close collaboration between clinicians working in the psychiatric and medical settings.[52]

This history and examination, where possible, should be carried out only by a clinician who is well trained in this area. For younger children, the parent should always be present; if an older child or adolescent is uncomfortable having the parent act as a chaperone, another appropriate chaperone may be appropriate.

It is imperative to remember that the interview process (see Text box 37.4) may be difficult for many young people with eating disorders and will depend, in part, on their level of insight as well as their medical and psychological status at the time.[51] Parent or carer input may be required to validate or supplement some of the interview findings. Additionally, during the examination, the patient will be exposing their body (often a disliked aspect of themselves) to an unfamiliar person. Try to ensure that t he physical examination is carried out with sensitivity, tact and privacy (see Text box 37.5).

Clinical interview

Identifying abnormal thinking about weight, body image, diet and exercise

Suggested questions to help explore attitudes towards weight control:

- What do you think is your healthy weight?
- What would you like to weigh?
- Do you think you need to lose more weight?
- Are you afraid of gaining weight?
- Are you unhappy with your body shape?
- Is there any part of your body that you are especially unhappy with?
- Do you eat in front of others? If not, when did you stop doing this and why?
- How frequently do you weigh yourself?
- How have you tried to control your weight?
- What type of exercises do you do?
- How much exercise do you do, how often, level of intensity?
- What sorts of foods and drinks do you avoid, and when did you start avoiding them?
- Do you have any ritualised eating habits?
- Do you prefer to eat alone?
- Do you count calories/fat/carbohydrates?
- When young people eat large amounts quickly we call this a binge. Do you ever binge on food? If so how often? What do you binge on? How much of that would you eat?
- Sometimes when young people are trying to control their weight they use medications or other methods to get rid of food, either by making themselves vomit or by going to the toilet a lot. Have you ever tried this? (If so, enquire about frequency, amount, and timing in relation to meals.)

Family and social history

- Family history: obesity, eating disorders, depression, other mental illness (especially anxiety disorders and obsessive-compulsive disorder), substance abuse by parents or other family members.
- Social history: home life, school life, friends, activities, sexual history.

Menstrual history

- Age at menarche, regularity of cycles, last menstrual period.

Additional history

- Use of cigarettes, drugs, alcohol (heavy use of alcohol increases the requirements for B vitamins)
- Use of anabolic steroids (especially in boys)
- Use of stimulants
- Involvement with websites or other forms of social media that are proanorexia ('pro-ana') or probulimia ('pro-mia')
- History of trauma
- Previous therapies (type, duration and outcomes)

(From *Assessment and treatment of children and adolescents with eating disorders in Queensland*. Document Number: QH-GDL-961:2020.)

TEXT BOX 37.4

Adolescent physical examination in a possible eating disorder case

Pubertal development
- Assessment and documentation of pubertal stage
- Signs of delayed or interrupted pubertal development

Signs of recurrent vomiting/purging
- Gingivitis and dental caries (erosion of enamel, gum recession and friable gums)
- Hypokalaemia and/or elevated bicarb
- Loss of enamel on surfaces of teeth
- Callouses on dorsum of the hand (Russell's sign)
- Subconjunctival haemorrhage

Mental health
- Flat or anxious affect
- Functional decline
- Comprehensive risk assessment including suicidality and self-harm
- Severe family stress or strain
- Symptoms of depression, anxiety and obsessive-compulsive disorder or other co-morbid conditions

Other features of severe malnutrition
- Lanugo hair
- Dull thinning scalp hair
- Dry skin
- Skin breakdown and/or pressure sore
- Bruising/abrasions over the spine related to excessive exercises
- Muscle wasting (can be proximal and distal)
- Muscle weakness on testing
- Bones, including carefully assessing for lumber crush fractures
- Arrhythmias on Electrocardiogram
- Cardiomyopathy, cardiac failure
- Postural hypotension
- Postural tachycardia
- Bradycardia
- Peripheral oedema
- Hypothermia
- Constipation
- Amenorrhoea

TEXT BOX 37.5

PHYSICAL EXAMINATION FOR SUSPECTED CHILD ABUSE (SEE TEXT BOX 37.6)

Unfortunately, child abuse is one of the leading causes of injury-related mortality in infants and children,[54] and those of us who regularly examine children need to be able to recognise potentially abused children (see Table 37.21 and List 37.5) and treat them at first presentation to prevent significant morbidity and mortality.

Physical abuse should always be a differential for injuries in children. Suspicion may be raised during history taking, particularly if the caregiver has no explanation for the child's injuries, the explanation changes over time or there is a delay in seeking care.

Always remember that when children disclose about abuse they are almost never lying. As clinicians, it is our duty to protect children from potential harm and act accordingly.

As part of routine paediatric practice, children are sometimes referred for examination by an order of a child welfare agency. These children require complete examination, rather than focusing on the area in question (e.g. bruising). Bear in mind that in preverbal children a physical examination is insufficient, and imaging (e.g. skeletal survey) and other investigations (e.g. blood tests) are usually required.

The rationale for physical examination is three-fold:

1. to assess the extent of the injury and to formulate a management plan
2. to provide a sense of safety for the child
3. to provide documentation that may be used as evidence.

Start (as always) by documenting the child's growth parameters, and ensure that appropriate documentation is completed (including clinical photography if indicated). Use a bodygram (see Fig. 37.37) if photography is not being performed to document any visible findings. Note the child's appearance, hygiene, nutritional status, affect

Assessing for suspected child abuse: a suggested method

1. Observe hygiene status, nutritional status, affect and behaviour.
2. Look carefully for bruising, lacerations, abrasions, scars, soft-tissue swelling and musculoskeletal deformities.
3. Palpate fontanels.
4. Inspect the oral cavity for dental caries, palatal petechiae and injuries to the lip and lingual frenula.
5. Inspect the eyes for subconjunctival haemorrhage and consider fundoscopy.
6. Palpate for bony pain or callus formation.
7. Perform the abdominal examination for tenderness or guarding.
8. Perform the genitourinary examination if required.
9. Complete the neurological examination.
10. Assess development.
11. Perform otoscopy.
12. Document meticulously.

TEXT BOX 37.6

Risk factors for child maltreatment

Caregiver factors	Criminal history, inappropriate expectations of the child, mental health history, misconceptions about child care, misperceptions about child development, substance abuse
Child factors	Behaviour problems, medical fragility, non-biological relationship to carer, prematurity, special needs
Family and environmental factors	High local unemployment rates, intimate partner violence in the home, poverty, social isolation or lack of support

(Reprinted with permission from Child Abuse: Approach and Management, January 15, 2007, Vol 75, No 2, American Family Physician Copyright © 2007 *American Academy of Family Physicians.* All Rights Reserved.)

TABLE 37.21

(e.g. frightened, friendly) and behaviour throughout the examination. Also make note of the parent's behaviour during the examination, if present.

Examine the child for:

- bruising
- lacerations
- abrasions
- scars
- soft-tissue swellings
- musculoskeletal deformities.

Document the size and location of any abnormality seen. It is mandatory to check for lesions that may be present under the child's clothes and do not forget to move the hair to visualise the scalp. Remember that it can be quite difficult to differentiate bruising from other, innocent,

CLUES IN THE EVALUATION OF NON-ACCIDENTAL TRAUMA IN CHILDREN

Suspect non-accidental trauma if the answer is 'yes' to any of the following questions

- Is there an unusual distribution or location of lesions?
- Is there a pattern of bruises or marks?
- Can a bleeding disorder or collagen disease be ruled out as a cause of the lesions?
- If there is a bite or handprint bruise, is it adult size?
- If there is a burn, are the margins clearly demarcated with uniform depth of burn?
- If there is a burn, is there a stocking and glove distribution?
- Are there lesions of various healing stages or ages?
- Is the reported mechanism of injury inconsistent with the extent of trauma?

(McDonald KC. Child abuse: approach and management. *Am Fam Physician* 2007; 75(2):221–228.)

LIST 37.5

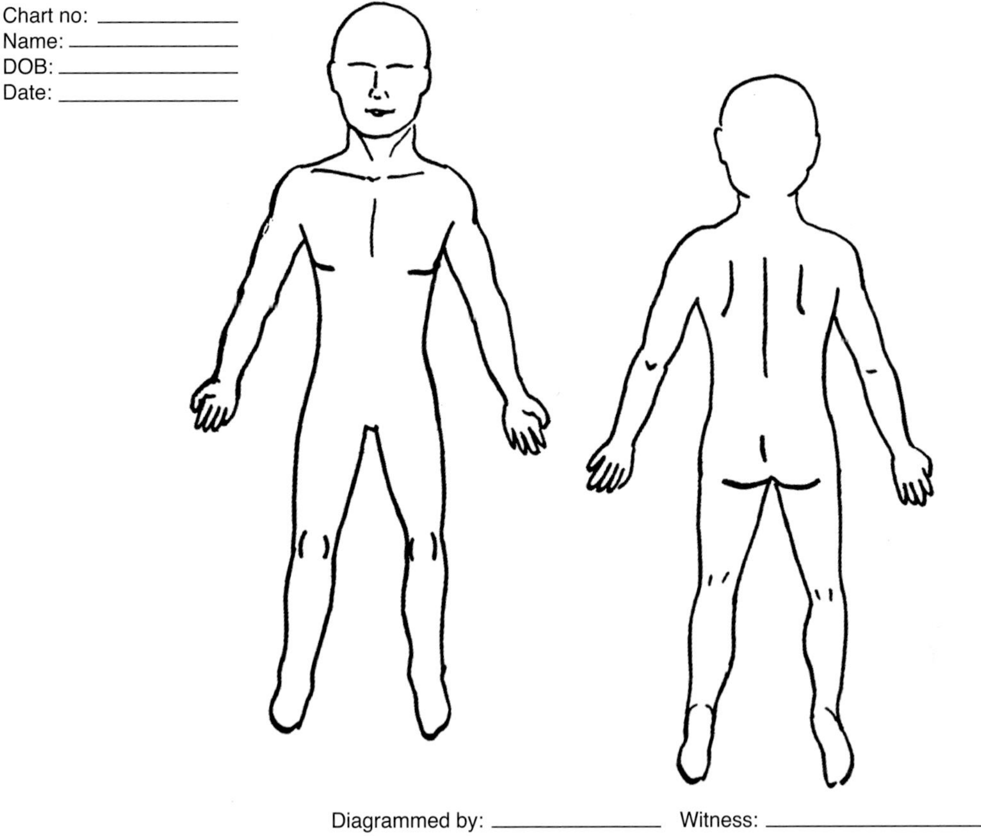

Bodygram

(From Legano L, McHugh MT, Palusci VJ. Child abuse and neglect. *Curr Probl Pediatr Adolesc Health Care* 2009; 39(2):e26–e31.)

FIGURE 37.37

skin discolorations (e.g. café-au-lait spots, pigmented birthmarks); when in doubt, reschedule a repeat examination for several days later. Palpate along the limbs for any tenderness or swelling. Look for redundant skinfolds secondary to weight loss, poor muscle bulk and other signs of malnutrition and neglect such as severe nappy rash.

Palpate the fontanel in infants, as an intracranial haemorrhage or cerebral oedema may present with a bulging or tense fontanel. Examine the oral cavity for dental caries, palatal petechiae and injuries to the lip and lingual frenulum. Examine the eyes for subconjunctival haemorrhage. Examine the retina by fundoscopy and consider whether dilated indirect fundoscopy (usually performed by an ophthalmologist) is required. Perform otoscopy looking for haemotympanum or a perforated eardrum and check over the mastoids for bruising.

Palpate over the chest (particularly looking for callus formation and crepitus due to rib fractures) and perform an abdominal examination noting any tenderness or guarding. Genitourinary examination may need to be performed, but kept minimally invasive. External examination is sufficient in girls; and the penis and scrotum should be visualised in boys to check for injuries or bruising.

Perform a neurological examination, but be aware that further imaging is required in very young children if intracranial haemorrhage is to be ruled out. Perform a developmental examination in any child suspected of being neglected.

T&O'C ESSENTIALS

1. *Children are not simply little adults: history taking and physical examination need to be tailored to their specific needs.*
2. *Much information can be gathered by observing the child.*
3. *Be gentle and opportunistic but as thorough as possible in conducting the examination.*
4. *Do not make up clinical signs or disregard them if they are detected with appropriate certainty.*
5. *Perform less-pleasant assessments (e.g. ear, nose, throat) at the end of the examination.*
6. *Height, weight and head circumference should always be assessed and recorded.*
7. *Differentiate between physiological conditions often seen in childhood (e.g. lumbar hyperlordosis) and pathological conditions (e.g. scoliosis).*
8. *Careful inspection of the face, eyes, ears and oral cavity may reveal the presence of a syndromic or genetic abnormality.*
9. *The majority of the neurological examination in smaller children is best performed using a combination of observation and play.*
10. *The respiratory and cardiovascular examinations are of particular significance in paediatrics because they can identify a seriously ill child.*
11. *The genitourinary examination is not routinely performed in children.*
12. *Adolescence is a unique stage of human development characterised by dynamic brain development; in which the interaction with the social environment shapes the capabilities that an individual will take forwards into adult life.*
13. *Physical abuse should always be a differential for injuries in children.*

OSCE REVISION TOPICS – **THE PAEDIATRIC HISTORY AND EXAMINATION**

Use these topics, which commonly occur in the OSCE, to help with revision.

1. This child's parent is concerned that he is much shorter than his brother was at the same age. Please examine him. (p 645)
2. This child has an unusual-shaped head. Please examine her. (p 666)
3. Please perform a developmental assessment on this child and give an estimate of the child's developmental age. (p 681)
4. The community nurse is concerned that this child is 'floppy'. Please perform a 180° examination. (p 680)
5. Please examine this child's cranial nerves. (p 675)
6. A general practitioner has noticed that this child has clubbing. Please examine her. (p 685)
7. Please examine this child who has been noted to have a murmur. (p 689)
8. This child's teacher has noticed some unusual bruising. Please examine the child. (pp 661, 703)
9. This child's parent has noticed that his abdomen is more distended than usual. Please examine the child. (p 693)
10. Please examine this child's ears as his parents have noticed some purulent discharge. (p 669)

Meticulously document all your findings and arrange any medical treatments that may be required. Be aware that this documentation may be required as evidence in child protection and even criminal investigations.

References

1. Cook DE, Andringa CL, Hess KL. et al. School health examinations. *Pediatrics* 1981; 67(4):576–577.
2. Riley M, Locke AB, Skye EP. Health maintenance in school-aged children: Part I. History, physical examination, screening, and immunizations. *Am Fam Physician* 2011; 83(6):683–688.
3. Committee on Practice and Ambulatory Medicine. The use of chaperones during the physical examination of the pediatric patient. *Pediatrics* 1996; 98(6):1202.
4. Britto MT, Tivorsak TL, Slap GB. Adolescents' needs for health care privacy. *Pediatrics* 2010; 126(6):e1469–e1476.
5. Watts K, Bell LM, Byrne SM et al. Waist circumference predicts cardiovascular risk in young Australian children. *J Paediatr Child Health* 2008; 44(12):709–715.
6. Owen GM. Measurement, recording, and assessment of skinfold thickness in childhood and adolescence: report of a small meeting. *Am J Clin Nutr* 1982; 35(3):629–638.
7. Walker HK, Hall WD, Hurst JW (eds). *Clinical methods: the history, physical, and laboratory examinations*. Oxford: Butterworth–Heinemann, 1990.
8. US Dept of Health and Human Sciences. The fourth report on the diagnosis, evaluation, and treatment of high blood pressure in children and adolescents. *Pediatrics* 2004; 114(2 suppl 4th report):555–576.
9. National High Blood Pressure Education Program Working Group on Hypertension Control in Children and Adolescents. Update on the 1987 task force report on high blood pressure in children and adolescents: a working group report from the national high blood pressure education program. *Pediatrics* 1996; 98(4):649–658.
10. Kavey RE, Daniels SR, Flynn JT. Management of high blood pressure in children and adolescents. *Cardiol Clin* 2010; 28(4):597–607.
11. Kaelber DC, Pickett F. Simple table to identify children and adolescents needing further evaluation of blood pressure. *Pediatrics* 2009; 123(6) e972–e974.
12. Fouzas S, Priftis KN, Anthracopoulos MB. Pulse oximetry in pediatric practice. *Pediatrics* 2011; 128(4):740–752.
13. Devrim I, Kara A, Ceyhan M et al. Measurement accuracy of fever by tympanic and axillary thermometry. *Pediatr Emerg Care* 2007; 23(1): 16–19.
14. El-Radhi AS, Barry W. Thermometry in paediatric practice. *Arch Dis Child* 2006; 91(4):351–356.
15. Fabry G. Clinical practice. Static, axial, and rotational deformities of the lower extremities in children. *Eur J Pediatr* 2010; 169(5):529–534.
16. Fabry G. Clinical practice: the spine from birth to adolescence. *Eur J Pediatr* 2009; 168(12):1415–1420.
17. Houghton KM. Review for the generalist: evaluation of low back pain in children and adolescents. *Pediatr Rheumatol* 2010; 8(28):1546–1696.
18. Foster HE, Jandial S. pGALS – paediatric Gait Arms Legs and Spine: a simple examination of the musculoskeletal system. *Pediatr Rheumatol* 2013; 11:44. A good resource for paediatric musculoskeletal exam.
19. Hohenleutner U, Landthaler M, Hamm H, Sebastian G. Hemangiomas of infancy and childhood. *J Dtsch Dermatol Ges* 2007; 5(4):334–338.
20. Menezes MP, North KN. Inherited neuromuscular disorders: pathway to diagnosis. *J Paediatr Child Health* 2012; 48(6):458–465.
21. Forrest CR, Hopper RA. Craniofacial syndromes and surgery. *Plast Reconstr Surg* 2013; 131(1):86e–109e.
22. Rothman R, Owens T, Simel DL. Does this child have acute otitis media? *JAMA* 2003; 290(12):1633–1640.
23. Park YW. Evaluation of neck masses in children. *Am Fam Physician* 1995; 51(8):1904–1912.
24. Toriello HV. Role of the dysmorphologic evaluation in the child with developmental delay. *Pediatr Clin North Am* 2008; 55(5):1085–1098, xi.
25. Bodensteiner JB. The evaluation of the hypotonic infant. *Semin Pediatr Neurol* 2008; 15(1):10–20.
26. Miller JW. Screening children for developmental behavioral problems: principles for the practitioner. *Prim Care* 2007; 34(2):177–201; abstract v.
27. Wood NS, Marlow N, Costeloe K et al. Neurologic and developmental disability after extremely preterm birth. EPICure Study Group. *N Engl J Med* 2000; 343(6):378–384.
28. Stephenson T, Wallace H, Thomson A. *Clinical paediatrics for postgraduate examinations*. Edinburgh: Churchill Livingstone, 2003.
29. Motyckova G, Steensma DP. Why does my patient have lymphadenopathy or splenomegaly? *Hematol Oncol Clin North Am* 2012; 26(2):395–408.
30. Mellis C. Respiratory noises: how useful are they clinically? *Pediatr Clin North Am* 2009; 56(1):1–17, ix.
31. Shields MD, Bush A, Everard ML et al. BTS guidelines: Recommendations for the assessment and management of cough in children. *Thorax* 2008; 63:iii1–iii15.
32. Forgacs P. Crackles and wheezes. *Lancet* 1967; 2(7508):203–205.
33. Nath AR, Capel LH. Inspiratory crackles and mechanical events of breathing. *Thorax* 1974; 29(6):695–698.
34. Goldbloom RB. *Pediatric clinical skills*. Philadelphia: Saunders, 2010.
35. Böhner H, Yang Q, Franke C et al. Simple data from history and physical examination help to exclude bowel obstruction and to avoid radiographic studies in patients with acute abdominal pain. *Eur J Surg* 1998; 164(10):777–784.
36. Blakemore, S-J, & Mills, KL. Is adolescence a sensitive period for sociocultural processing?. *Ann Rev Psychol* 2014; 65(1): 187–207.
37. Patton, GC, Sawyer, SM, Santelli, JS, et al. Our future: a *Lancet* commission on adolescent health and wellbeing. *Lancet* 2016; 387(10036), 2423–2478.
38. Abbassi, V. Growth and normal puberty. *Pediatrics* 1998; 102(2 Pt 3), 507–511.
39. Barnes, HV. The adolescent patient. In HK Walker, WD Hall, & JW Hurst (eds.), *Clinical methods: the history, physical, and laboratory examinations* (3rd edn). Oxford: Butterworth-Heinemann, 1990.
40. Bass, S, Delmas, PD, Pearce, G, et al. The differing tempo of growth in bone size, mass, and density in girls is region-specific. *J Clin Invest* 1999; 104(6), 795–804.
41. Striegel-Moore, RH, McMahon, RP, Biro, FM, et al. Exploring the relationship between timing of menarche and eating disorder symptoms in Black and White adolescent girls. *Int J Eat Disord* 2001; 30(4), 421–433.
42. McDermott, BM, Chanen, A, Fraser, L, et al. beyondblue Expert Working Committee (2010) clinical practice guidelines: depression in adolescents and young adults. Melbourne: beyondblue, 2011.
43. Paterson, K, Jones, J, Dagg, B, et al.Getting in early: a framework for early intervention and prevention in mental health for young people in New South Wales. *N S W Public Health Bull*, 2001; 12(5), 137.
44. Cheng, TL, Savageau, JA, Sattler, AL, et al. Confidentiality in health care. A survey of knowledge, perceptions, and attitudes among high school students. *JAMA*, 1993; 269(11), 1404–1407.
45. Wright, A, & Jorm, AF. Labels used by young people to describe mental disorders: factors associated with their development. *Aust N Z J Psychiatry*, 2009; 43(10), 946–955.
46. Michielsen, K, De Meyer, S, Ivanova, O, et al. Reorienting adolescent sexual and reproductive health research: reflections from an international conference. *Reprod Health*, 2016; 13(1), 3.

47. Cheung, AS, Wynne, K, Erasmus, J, et al. Position statement on the hormonal management of adult transgender and gender diverse individuals. *Med J Aust*, 2019; 211(3), 127–133.
48. Winter, S, Diamond, M, Green, J, et al. Transgender people: health at the margins of society. Lancet, 2016; 388(10042), 390–400.
49. Grossman, AH, & D'Augelli, AR Transgender youth and life-threatening behaviors. Suicide Life Threat Behav, 2007; 37(5), 527–537.
50. Turban, J, Ferraiolo, T, Martin, A, et al. Ten things transgender and gender nonconforming youth want their doctors to know. *J Am Acad Child Adolesc Psychiatry*, 2017; 56(4), 275–277.
51. NSW Government. NSW eating disorders toolkit: a practice-based guide to the inpatient management of children and adolescents with eating disorders. Sydney: NSW Ministry of Health; 2018.
52. Hay, P, Chinn, D, Forbes, D, et al. Royal Australian and New Zealand College of Psychiatrists clinical practice guidelines for the treatment of eating disorders. *Aust N Z J Psychiatry*, 2014; 48(11), 977–1008.
53. Rowe, E. Early detection of eating disorders in general practice. *Aust Fam Physician*, 2017; 46, 833–838.
54. McDonald KC. Child abuse: approach and management. *Am Fam Physician* 2007; 75(2):221–228.

CHAPTER 38

The neonatal history and examination

Joerg Mattes and Bryony Ross

The important thing is to make the lesson of each case tell on your education. The value of experience is not in seeing much, but in seeing wisely. SIR WILLIAM OSLER (1849–1919)

Neonates are very different from adult and even paediatric patients. They are very fragile, cannot cooperate in their examination and cannot give you a history. The usual systematic approach to the history taking and examination is often not possible and an *opportunistic* method must be adopted. This means that history taking may have to wait until the parents, hospital staff or relatives are available and the examination must be fitted around the infant's feeding schedule, need for sleep and mood.

THE HISTORY

In many cases, history taking begins with a review of the maternal and infant medical records (if available) and the gathering of information from clinical staff, and then progresses to an interview with the parents. As with history taking for the adult, your approach needs to be methodical. There may not be a presenting complaint, but asking about problems that may have occurred during the pregnancy or delivery is an important aspect of the history taking.

Remember that this is usually a happy but anxious time for new parents. They must be approached with understanding and patience. Allow enough time for the interview and respect their privacy and sensitivities of various sorts. Parents' worries must always be taken seriously and dealt with respectfully, even when they seem insignificant from a medical point of view.[a]

First, introduce yourself to the parents and congratulate them on the birth of their child. Explain the reasons for the neonatal assessment and tell them how it will be carried out. Ask for their consent wherever possible.

Maternal health

Assemble a comprehensive history by asking about the mother's current and past medical and surgical history. This should identify any chronic illnesses that could affect the baby's health (see Table 38.1). If the mother has an acute or a chronic illness, ask questions around the mnemonic **SIC**:

Symptoms (severity, frequency, triggers, treatments)
Investigations
Complications.

A maternal illness may affect the mother's ability to look after her baby and directly affect the baby's health.

Next, ascertain the mother's health, lifestyle and psychosocial background using the mnemonic **HeLP**:

Health status
Lifestyle
Psychosocial background.

Of particular relevance is substance use (see Table 38.2). Also assess nutrition and immunisation status and possible mental health problems. Ask tactfully what the parents know about neonatal health and safety by keeping in mind the mnemonic **CARE**:

Coping with parenthood (e.g. understanding the baby's nutritional needs and sudden infant death syndrome [SIDS] risk factors)

[a] Experienced parents' opinions should always be taken seriously.

Mother's medical and surgical history

Mother	Effect on baby
Endocrine system, e.g:	
Diabetes[2]	Macrosomia (birth weight >4000 g), birth trauma, jaundice, seizures (hypoglycaemia, hypocalcaemia), plethora (polycythaemia), birth trauma, major congenital anomalies, cardiomyopathy
Hypo / hyperthyroidism[3]	Premature birth, SGA, thyroid enlargement
Immune system, e.g:	
Lupus erythematosus[4]	Stillbirth, neonatal deaths, premature birth, SGA, thrombotic events
Asthma[5]	Premature birth, low birth weight
Inborn errors of metabolism, e.g:	
Hyperphenylalaninaemia[6]	Microcephaly,* murmurs / cyanosis (congenital heart disease)
Cardiovascular / renal system, e.g:	
Hypertension	Pulmonary complications, sepsis, prematurity
Medications, e.g:	
Valproate[7]	Neural tube defects, hypospadias,** cardiac defects and oral clefts
SSRIs[8]	Respiratory, motor, central nervous system and gastrointestinal symptoms (SSRI neonatal behaviour syndrome)

**Small head size.*
***An abnormality of the urethra such that it opens on the ventral surface of the penis or on the perineum or into the vagina.*
SGA = small for gestational age; SSRIs = selective serotonin reuptake inhibitors.

TABLE 38.1

A ccess to healthcare practitioners and social support
R elationships and conflicts
E ffects of illness on the child.

Other family history

Ask briefly about serious or possibly inherited illnesses in other family members, particularly siblings.

QUESTIONS TO ASK THE MOTHER ABOUT HER PREGNANCY AND DELIVERY

1. What type of antenatal screening did you have? (Ultrasound, amniocentesis)
2. Did you have problems with high blood pressure during your pregnancy? Was pre-eclampsia diagnosed?
3. Did you have any blood group incompatibility problems?
4. Did you have any bladder or kidney infections?
5. Was your baby delivered at full term?
6. How was your baby's health during delivery?
7. Was there any mention of meconium staining during delivery? (A sign of fetal distress)
8. Did you have a vaginal delivery or a caesarean section?

QUESTIONS BOX 38.1

History of the pregnancy, labour and delivery

This should include questions about:

- antenatal screening (e.g. serology, ultrasound, amniocentesis), pregnancy
- birth-related complications and operations (e.g. pre-eclampsia [hypertension and proteinuria], rhesus / ABO incompatibility [blood group])
- infections (urinary tract infections, group B *Streptococcus* colonisation)
- fetal wellbeing (blood-flow patterns, biophysical profiles such as cardiotocography)
- vaginal bleeding, amniotic fluid (amount and aspect) and type of delivery (vaginal or caesarian section)—see Questions boxes 38.1 and 38.2.

Enquire about the baby's health status at birth (Apgar score [see Table 38.3], any resuscitation required, medical support, treatments, birth weight, length, head circumference), immunisation status and

Mother's health, life and psychosocial background (HeLP)

Mother	Effect on baby
Infections[9–13]*, e.g:*	
HIV	Increased risk of sepsis and infections if HIV positive
Toxoplasmosis	Hepatosplenomegaly, lymphadenopathy, chorioretinitis, seizures, hydrocephalus, SGA
Syphilis	Stillbirth, hepatomegaly, lymphadenopathy, maculopapular / vesicular rash, rhinitis
Rubella	Sensorineural hearing loss, ocular abnormalities (glaucoma, retinopathy, cataract), congenital heart disease, central nervous system abnormalities, SGA
Cytomegalovirus	Hepatosplenomegaly, petechiae, microcephaly, chorioretinitis, sensorineural hearing loss, SGA
Parvovirus B19 (fifth disease)	Non-immune fetal hydrops,* myocarditis, hepatitis
Varicella-zoster	Skin scarring, eye defects, limb hypoplasia, premature birth, SGA
Listeriosis	Pneumonia, sepsis or meningitis
Herpes simplex	Local skin, eye and mouth infections with vesicular lesions, CNS infections
Obesity (BMI >30 kg / m^2)	Macrosomia / LGA, premature birth, neural tube defects, congenital heart disease, omphalocele**
Antenatal drug use[14] Nicotine	SIDS, SGA, asthma, ADHD
Marijuana	Decreased self-quieting ability, fine tremors, increased hand-to-mouth activity, sleep pattern changes
Methadone	Strabism,*** NAS: respiratory distress increased tone, tremors, seizures poor feeding, vomiting, regurgitation, diarrhoea sweating
Heroin	NAS, increased perinatal mortality, SGA, ADHD
Cocaine	Genitourinary malformations, CNS symptoms, SGA
Amphetamines	Congenital CNS, cardiovascular, limb defects, oral clefts, neurobehavioural effects
Hallucinogens	Congenital cardiovascular and kidney defects
Alcohol	Fetal alcohol spectrum disorder with developmental delay, ADHD, characteristic facial appearance, SGA (small eyes, flattened nasal bridge, maxillary hypoplasia, shortened palpebral fissures, short upturned nose, smooth philtrum, small upper lip)

**Increased amniotic fluid, a sign of fetal heart failure.*
***A hernia into the umbilical cord and then umbilicus.*
****Squint.*
ADHD = attention deficit hyperactivity disorder; BMI = body mass index; HIV = human immunodeficiency virus; LGA = large for gestational age; NAS = neonatal abstinence syndrome; SGA = small for gestational age; SIDS = sudden infant death syndrome.

TABLE 38.2

prophylaxis (hepatitis B, vitamin K) and current nutrition (breastfed / bottle-fed, frequency, amounts, weight gain).

Any bilious vomiting warrants immediate further investigation. Meconium should be passed within the first 48 hours. This pasty green substance consists of desquamated epithelial cells, mucus, bile, lanugo (fine hair that covers the fetus and is swallowed as it falls off before birth) and vernix caseosa (a white cheesy material that coats the fetal skin), which collects in the fetal bowel and is passed after birth. When meconium is passed in utero it may be a sign of fetal distress or hypoxia.

Predictors of severe illness in the medical history of the newborn include a history of difficult feeding, reduced feeding ability, weak sucking, lethargy,

QUESTIONS TO ASK THE PARENT(S) ABOUT THE BABY'S HEALTH AT BIRTH AND EARLY LIFE

! denotes a potentially serious symptom

1. Do you know your baby's Apgar score?
2. What was your baby's birth weight?
3. Has your baby been given vitamin K or any vaccinations yet?
4. Are you breastfeeding? How are you managing?
5. ! Is your baby able to suck strongly?
6. ! Has your baby had any convulsions?
7. ! Does your baby seem breathless when feeding?
8. ! Has your baby had any bilious vomiting? (Bowel obstruction)

QUESTIONS BOX 38.2

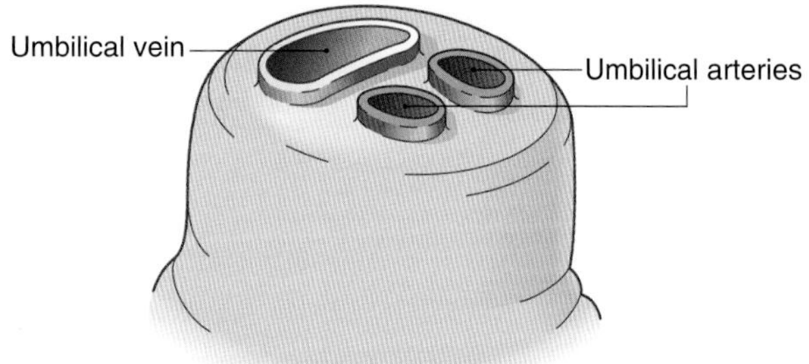

Normal umbilical cord vessel configuration with two arteries on the right and one vein on the left

(From Harding S. *Rennie & Roberton's textbook of neonatology.* Philadelphia: Elsevier, 2012.)

FIGURE 38.1

One- and five-minute Apgar values*	
Appearance	0=blue or pale 1=blue extremities only 2=pink (no cyanosis)
Pulse	0=absent 1=less than 100 beats per minute 2=more than 100 beats per minute
Grimace	0=no response when stimulated 1=grimace when stimulated 2=cry/pull away when stimulated
Activity	0=no muscle tone 1=flexor tone 2=flexor tone resisting extension
Respiration	0=absent 1=irregular/gasping 2=regular/crying

**Rapid assessment of the newborn immediately after birth (1 minute and 5 minutes after birth and each 5 minutes thereafter in a severely depressed neonate) was devised by Dr Virginia Apgar (1909–74), leading to a drastic reduction in infant mortality.*[15]

(Apgar V. A proposal for a new method of evaluation of the newborn infant. *Curr Res Anesth Analg* 1953; 32(4):260–267; republished *Anesth Analg* 2015; 120(5):1056–1059.)

TABLE 38.3

convulsions, fast or difficult breathing and abnormal behaviour.[16–18]

Obtain results of the placental examination (size, membranes, vessels, infarcts, clots) and umbilical cord, which usually has two arteries and one vein (see Fig. 38.1). If the cord has only one of each (1% of all deliveries), there is a 60% increased risk of associated anomalies in major organ systems (most commonly the kidneys).[19] Most of this information can be gathered by reviewing the mother and baby's medical records or by consultation with clinical staff.

THE PHYSICAL EXAMINATION

It is generally accepted that all neonates should have an immediate health check after birth, followed by a more detailed physical examination in the first 3 days of life.[20] Repeat physical examination is recommended at 6–8 weeks of age. The principal aims of the neonatal examination are to:

1. detect congenital anomalies and illnesses, insufficient perinatal adaptation to extrauterine life and adverse effects resulting from birth
2. discuss the results and limitations of the assessment with the parents in a tactful and sympathetic manner
3. arrange for appropriate follow-up examinations and management.

Examination of the neonate: a suggested method

1. **Preparation**
   Wash your hands and put on gloves if indicated.
   Undress the baby to the nappy but make sure that he or she is kept warm.
   Never leave the baby unattended on the examination table.
   Explain to parents what you are doing.
2. **Measurements**
   Weigh the baby without the nappy or weigh the nappy separately and subtract.
   Measure the baby's length (called height in adults).
   Measure the baby's head circumference.
   Plot these on the appropriate growth charts.
   Take the baby's temperature.
3. **Inspection**
   Posture and spontaneous movements
   Muscle fasciculations
   Dysmorphic features: face, hands and feet
   Asymmetry: muscles, limbs, leg creases
   Jaundice
   Cyanosis
   Skin
   - Naevi
   - Erythema or vesicles (suggesting infection)
   - Skin tumours

   Head and spine
   - Shape
   - Sutures
   - Fontanels
   - Signs of spina bifida

   Eyes
   - Size
   - Sclerae
   - Pupils
   - Movements
   - Dysmorphic features

   Ears
   - Abnormal position
   - Skin tags
   - Auditory canal

   Nose
   - Asymmetry
   - Nasal flaring or respiratory distress
   - Nasal cavity

   Mouth
   - Jaw size
   - Tongue size
   - Cleft palate or lip

   Neck
   - Torticollis
   - Abnormal skinfolds

   Chest
   - Deformity
   - Stridor, wheezing or grunting
   - Apex beat and heart sounds
   - Lung sounds

   Abdomen and genitals
   - Inspection, distension, umbilicus
   - Palpation
   - Auscultation
   - Hernias
   - Testes and scrotum
   - Penis
   - Female genitalia
   - Anus

   Limbs
   - Symmetry
   - Deformity
   - The hips

   Central nervous system
   - Posture
   - Tone
   - Developmental reflexes

TEXT BOX 38.1

A method for the examination of the neonate is given in Text box 38.1.

Preparing for the physical examination

A structured yet flexible head-to-toe approach is essential for the identification of serious pathologies and for differentiating them from benign variations or from what is expected during the physiological transition from intra- to extrauterine life. The newborn should not be examined immediately after a large feed, as this may cause vomiting, or when hungry as the baby is likely to cry. Exposure to bright light and cold environments may cause discomfort to the neonate.

Before you start the examination, remove your jewellery and/or watch and roll up your sleeves to above the elbow. Hand hygiene is crucial for the prevention of cross-infection and nosocomial infection in newborn infants.[21] Clean your hands and forearms with soap and water or an ethanol-based hand disinfectant before and after contact with the baby, before and after any

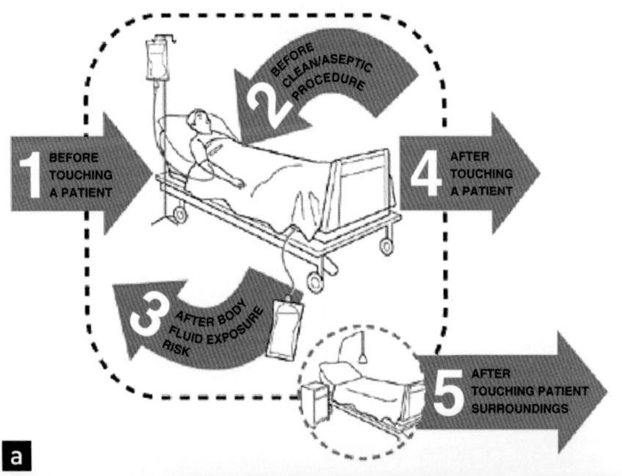

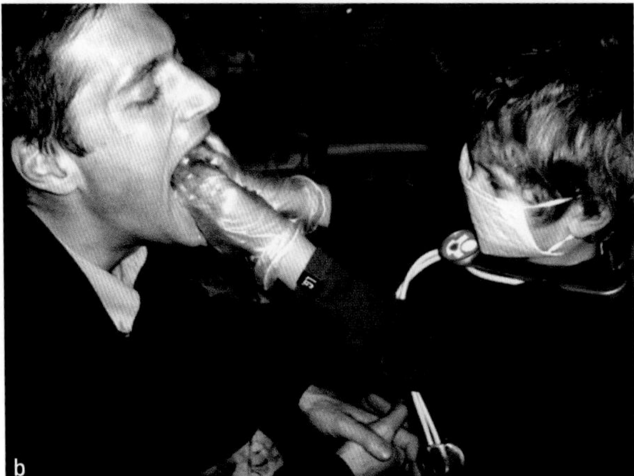

(a) The five moments for hand hygiene, and (b) use of personal protective equipment as indicated are extremely effective measures to prevent cross-infection

((a) Based on 'My 5 moments for hand hygiene', www.who.int/gpsc/5may/background/5moments/en/index.html, ©World Health Organization, 2009.)

FIGURE 38.2

procedure or exposure to bodily fluids, and after touching the baby's surroundings (see Fig. 38.2(a)). Wear examination gloves and other personal protective equipment when indicated to avoid cross-infection (see Fig. 38.2(b)). Clean your examination tools (e.g. stethoscope) thoroughly with the appropriate antimicrobial agents before and after use.

Usually, newborns cannot turn but they may be able to move rather dangerously sidewards on the examination table. This should be explained to the parents. It is imperative to create barriers on both sides of the baby (e.g. the wall and yourself) or to secure the baby gently with your hand during the examination. Never step away without asking someone else to watch the infant. Alternatively, carry the baby with you.

Measurements

Measurements of weight, length and occipitofrontal head circumference are important for the detection of serious pathologies and for monitoring growth and development. To obtain the bare weight, fully undress the neonate (including the nappy) and use an electronic baby scale. Never leave the baby unattended on the scales as they may fall off and injure themselves. If the room is too cold, use a heating lamp. Alternatively, you can measure the baby covered with a preweighed towel.

Use a newborn stadiometer (also called a head-board) to measure length. To obtain exact measurements a helper is required. Hold both the neonate's feet on the footpiece with one hand, fully extend the neonate's legs gently and slide the headpiece horizontally to rest (gently) on top of the neonate's head.

To measure head circumference use a non-stretching tape measure around the neonate's head at the widest point. This is usually achieved by placing the end of the tape measure on the middle of the forehead just above the palpebral fissures, then wrapping it around the temporal bones beneath the auricular helices and the most posterior portion of the occipital bone. Occipitofrontal circumference measurements should be taken until there is a variation of less than 0.5 centimetres between two repeated measurements.

Plot the results on growth charts that are most suitable for your location. The WHO *Child growth standards* (2006) charts (see Fig. 38.3) are based on data from term, breastfed and healthy infants born to non-smoking mothers in six countries (United States, Norway, India, Ghana, Brazil and Oman) and may be appropriate for term babies (see www.who.int/childgrowth/en/). The Fenton growth charts may be suitable for premature neonates (see www.biomedcentral.com/1471-2431/3/13/figure/F2). Note that other growth charts are available for premature babies (e.g. Babson and Benda,[22] Lubchenco et al.[23] and Dancis et al.[24]) and for infants with specific genetic conditions (e.g. for trisomy 21[25]).

Text continued on p 731

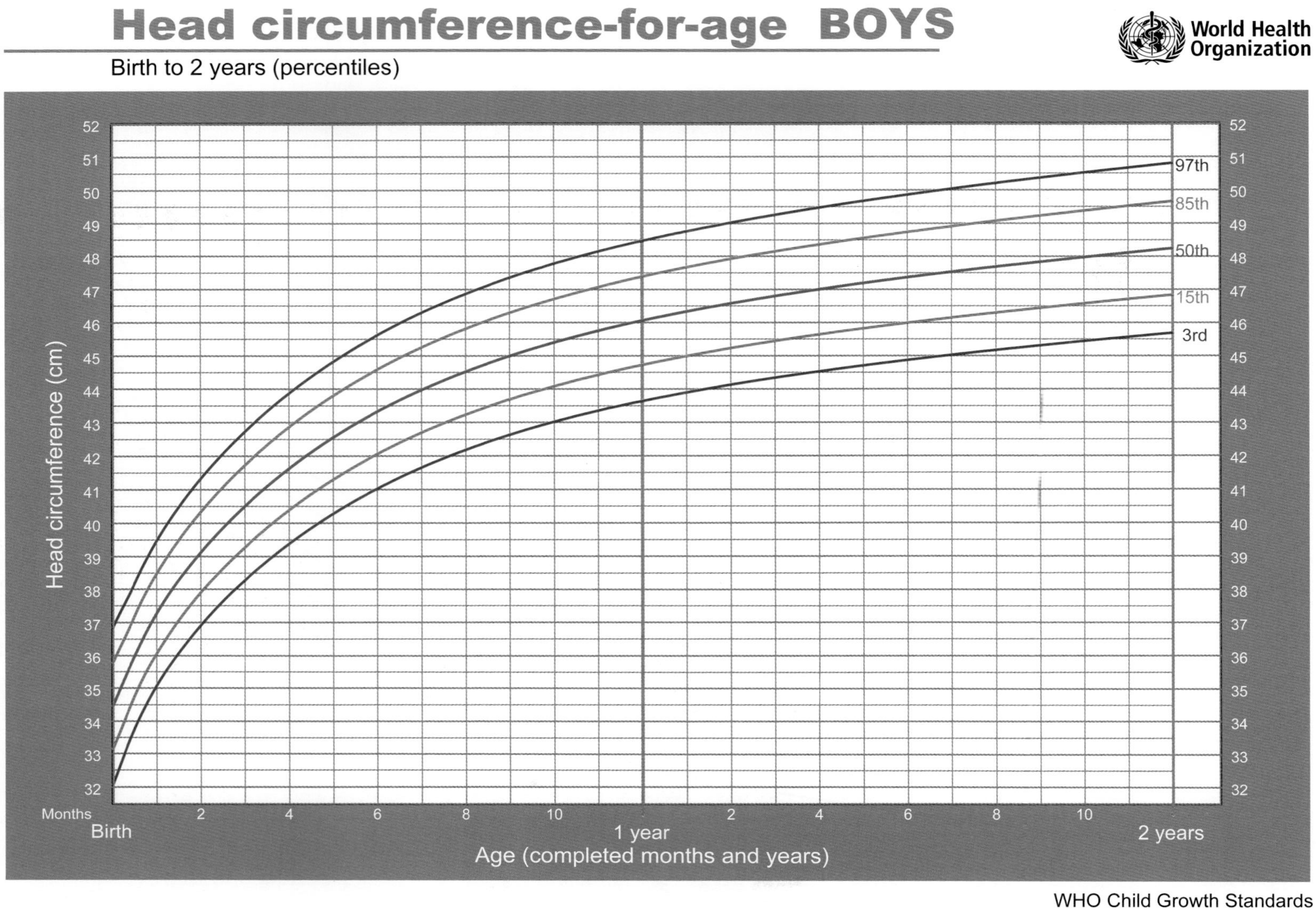

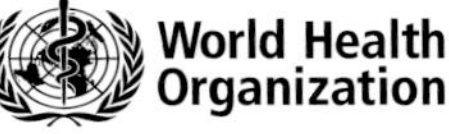

Growth charts for term infants

(Reprinted from World Health Organisation Child Growth Standard Charts, http://www.who.int/childgrowth/standards/en/.)

FIGURE 38.3

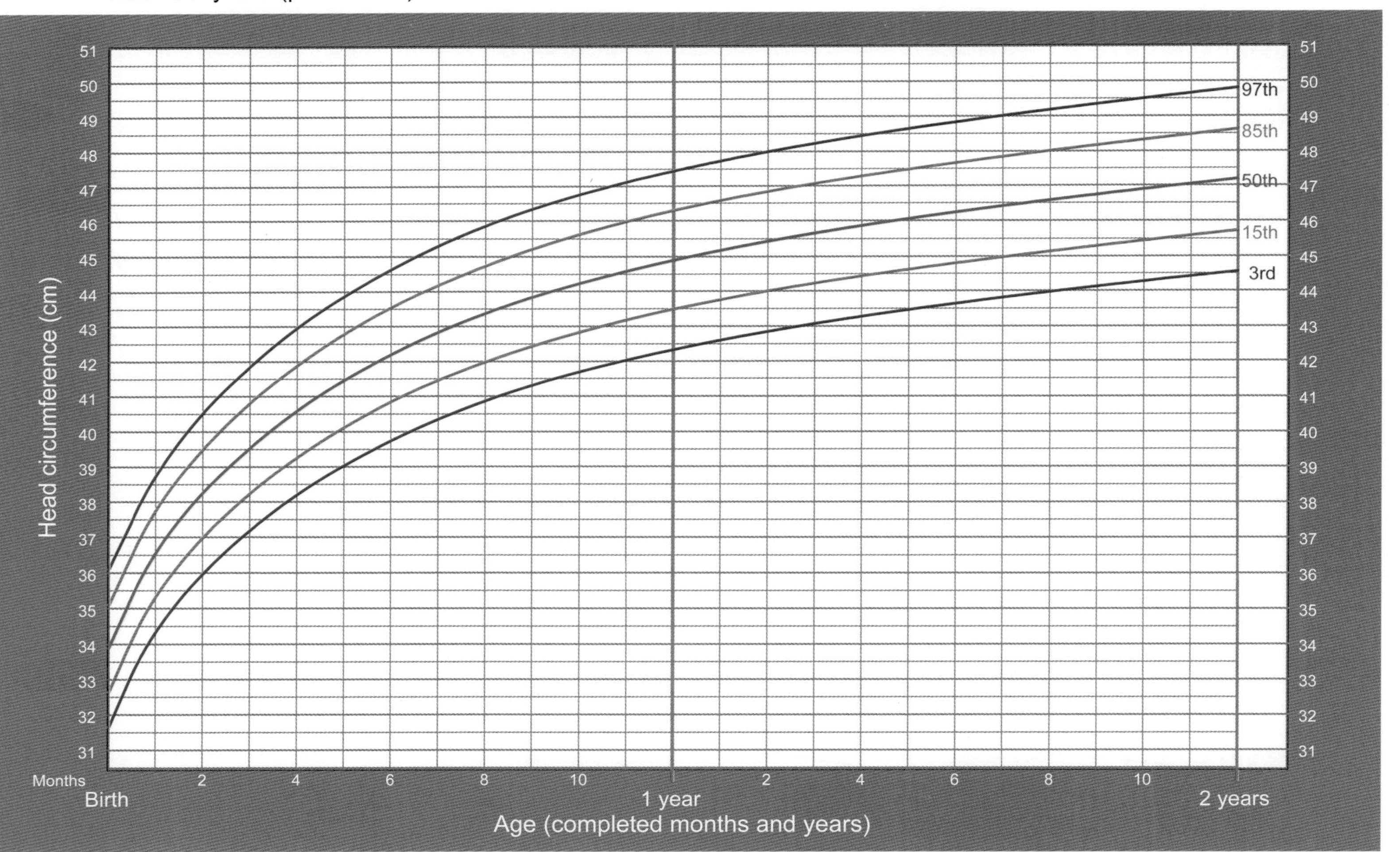

FIGURE 38.3, cont'd

Continued

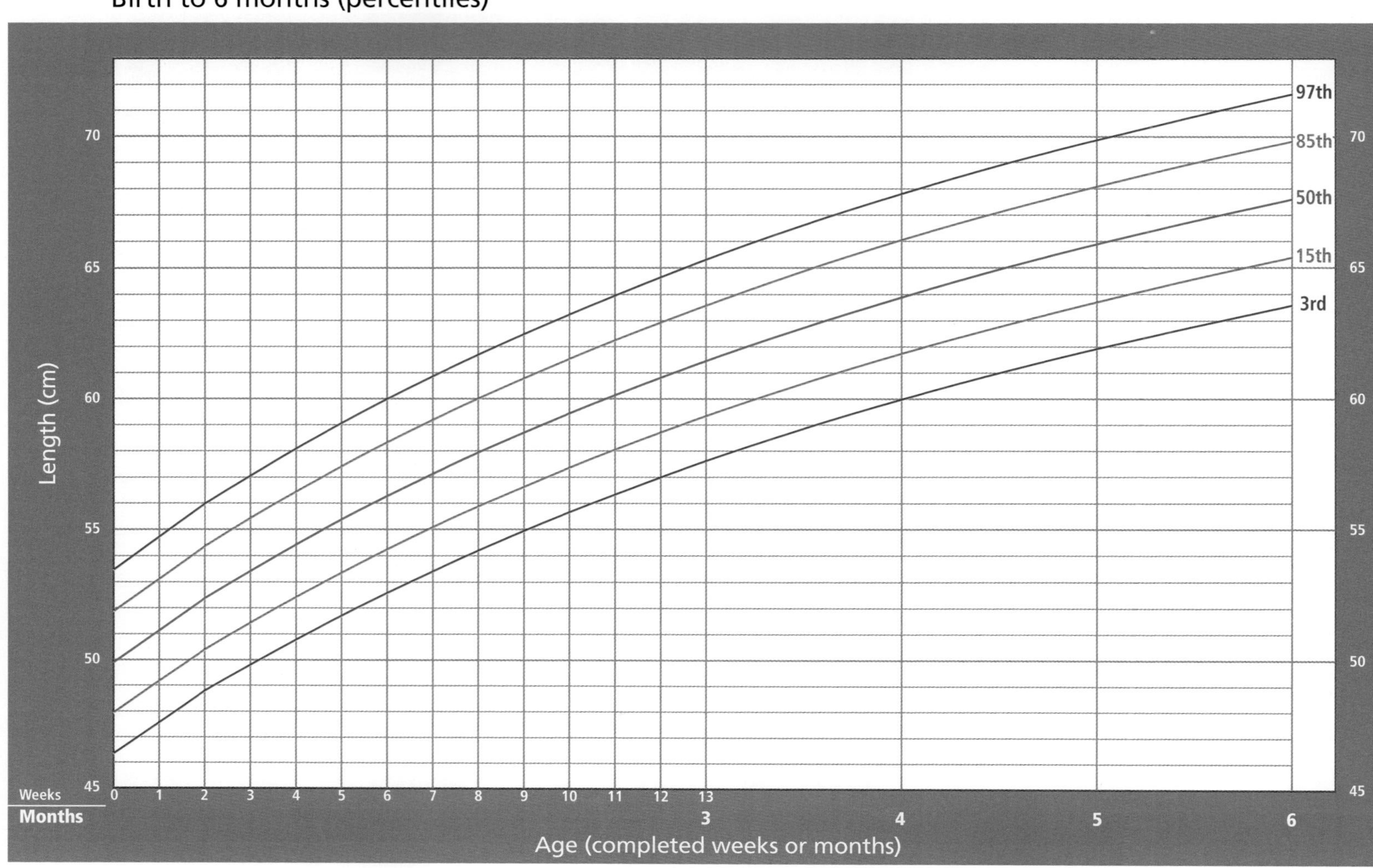

FIGURE 38.3, cont'd

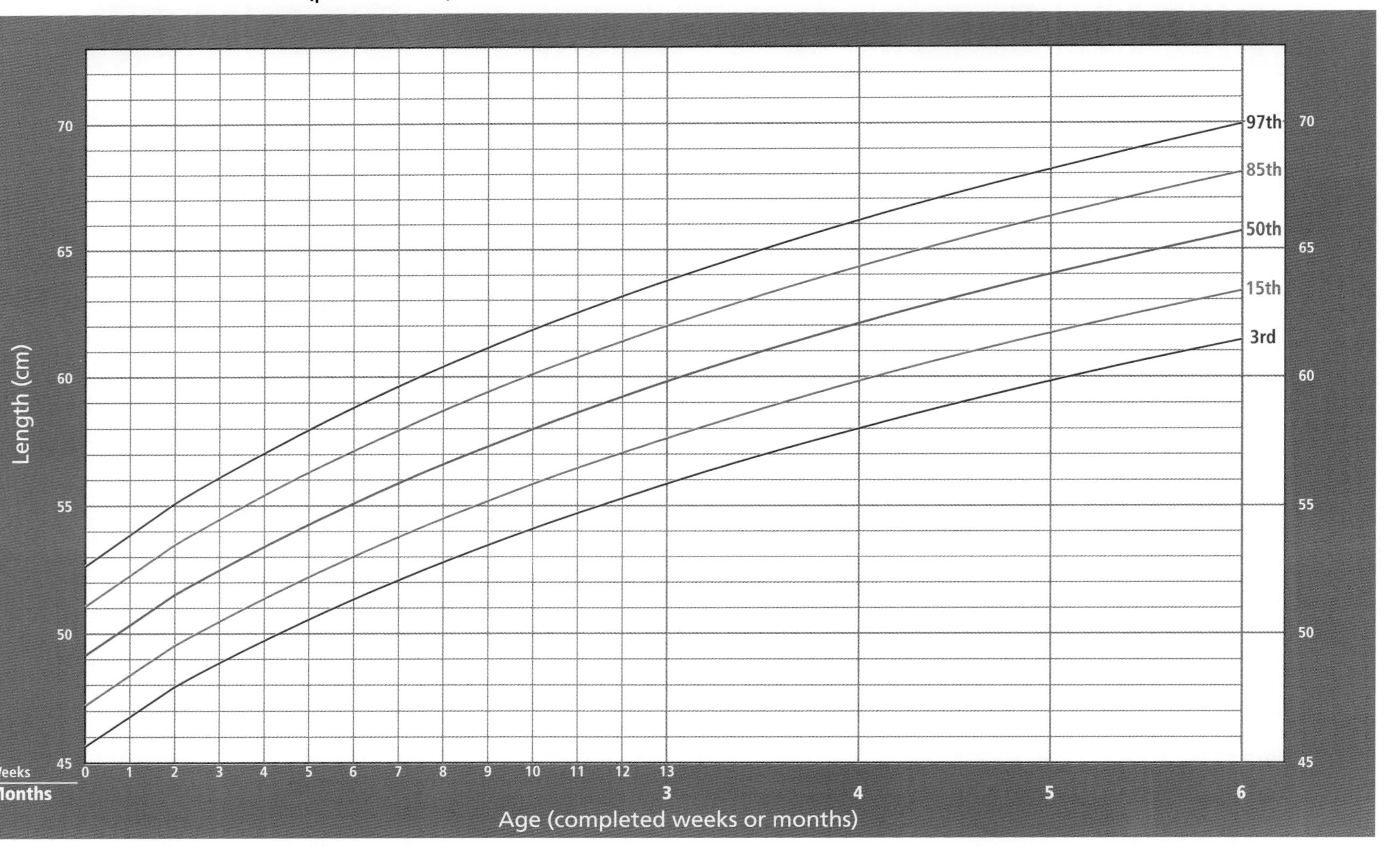

FIGURE 38.3, cont'd

Continued

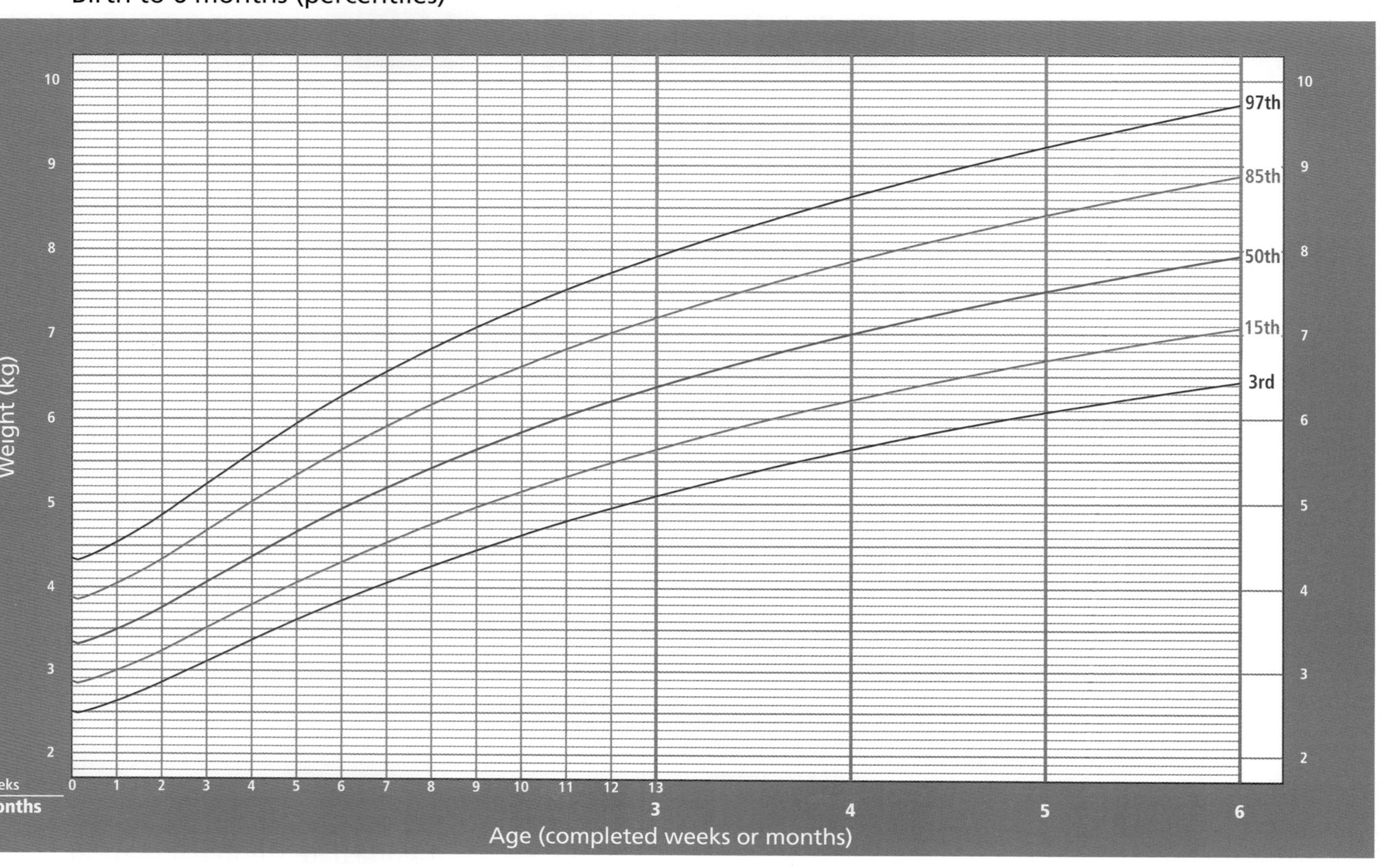

FIGURE 38.3, cont'd

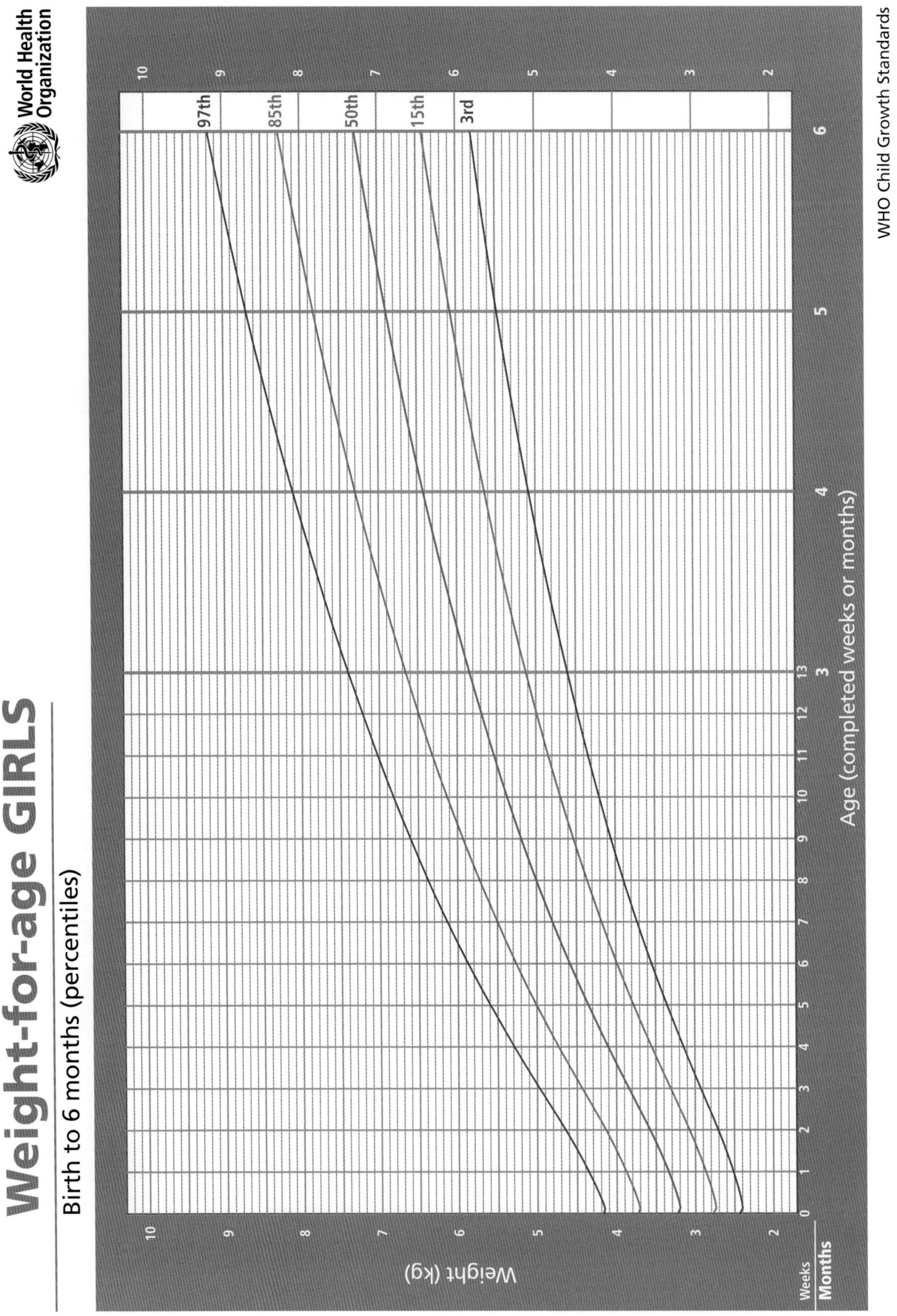

Weight-for-age GIRLS

Birth to 6 months (percentiles)

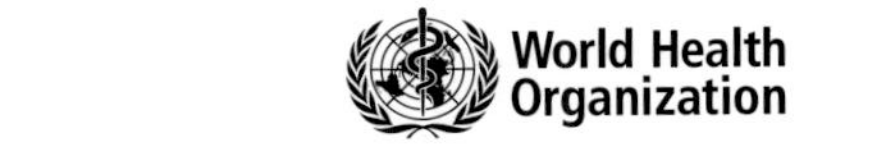

Weight (kg)

97th
85th
50th
15th
3rd

Weeks 0 1 2 3 4 5 6 7 8 9 10 11 12 13

Months 3 4 5 6

Age (completed weeks or months)

WHO Child Growth Standards

FIGURE 38.3, cont'd

Small for gestational age (**SGA**) is most commonly defined as a birth weight below the tenth percentile, whereas large for gestational age (**LGA**) is defined as a birth weight above the ninetieth percentile corrected for gestational age. A baby can be constitutionally small (e.g. small parents) or pathologically small (fetal, maternal, placental factors). If pathological SGA is potentially present, determine whether the newborn has symmetrical intrauterine growth restriction (weight, length and head circumference <tenth percentile). This indicates slow growth development throughout pregnancy present from a very early stage. Common causes are:

- intrauterine infections
- maternal drug abuse
- anaemia
- chromosomal abnormalities in the fetus.

Thus, symmetrical SGA is often associated with other clinical signs and serious long-term sequelae (see Tables 38.1 and 38.2). In contrast, asymmetrical intrauterine growth restriction leads to a disproportionate reduction in weight only (<tenth percentile) and indicates impaired growth development in the third trimester. Common causes are:

- pre-eclampsia
- placental insufficiency
- multiple gestation
- maternal age >35 years.

As the subcutaneous fat layer is underdeveloped, these neonates are at increased risk of hypoglycaemia, hypocalcaemia, polycythaemia, fetal distress and hypoxia.

A common cause of LGA is gestational diabetes, which has the potential to lead to serious complications if not recognised and managed appropriately (see Table 38.1).

Head-to-toe assessment

Posture and spontaneous movements

Observe the baby's posture and any spontaneous movements. Newborns perform flexion in the upper and lower limbs and symmetrical alternating movements involving all extremities. Deviation from this pattern may indicate birth injuries, deformities, or neurological or genetic abnormalities. A lack of spontaneous movements, which occur only on stimulation, is associated with a marked risk of severe illness.[18]

CAUSES OF UPPER MOTOR NEURONE WEAKNESS IN INFANTS

Generalised

- Hypoxic encephalopathy due to birth asphyxia
- Metabolic disturbances, infections
- Chromosomal abnormalities

Asymmetrical

- Cerebrovascular accident or haemorrhage
- Intracranial
- Spinal malformation

LIST 38.1

Generalised paucity of movements

If the baby is in a frog-leg position and there is a paucity of limb movements, this suggests reduced muscle tone and power (floppy infant). A history of polyhydramnios[b] and poor fetal movements may indicate congenital hypotonia and a problem with motor neurones that travel from the anterior horn of the spinal cord to the muscles (lower motor neurone lesions such as spinal muscular atrophy), motor end plate (e.g. congenital myasthenia gravis, botulism), or muscles (congenital myopathy, muscular dystrophy, infections).

Look for muscle fasciculations, especially of the tongue, and remember to test for a lack of tendon reflexes (biceps, triceps, brachioradialis, knee and ankle) that is suspicious for a lower motor neurone lesion. In the first 6 months of life upper motor neurone abnormalities are often associated with reduced muscle tone rather than spasticity (see List 38.1). The presence of increased muscle tone ('stiff limbs') indicates the possibility of severe illness in the newborn.[18] In older babies, an upper motor neurone lesion should be suspected if there is scissoring of the lower limbs and flexion of the thumbs.

Localised paucity of movements

Asymmetry in power and tone may indicate a focal upper or lower (e.g. brachial plexus palsies) motor

[b] Increased amniotic fluid volume.

Neonatal brachial plexus palsies

Brachial plexus palsy	Brachial trunk/spinal root	Clinical signs
Duchenne–Erb	Upper/C5–C6	'Waiter's tip' posture with arm adducted and internally rotated, elbow extended, forearm pronated, wrist and fingers flexed
Middle trunk	Middle/C7	Elbow flexed
Klumpke	Lower/C8–T1	'Claw hand' posture with arm supinated, elbow flexed, wrist extended, hyperextension of the metacarpophalangeal joints, flexion of the interphalangeal joints
Complete	Upper+middle+lower/C5–T1	'Flail limb' (all above) plus possibly Horner syndrome

(Adapted from Alfonso I, Alfonso DT, Papazian O. Focal upper extremity neuropathy in neonates. *Semin Pediatr Neurol* [Review] 2000; 7(1):4–14; Klumpke A. Klumpke's paralysis. 1885. *Clin Orthop Rel Res* [Biography Classical Article Historical Article Portraits] 1999; (368):3–4.)

TABLE 38.4

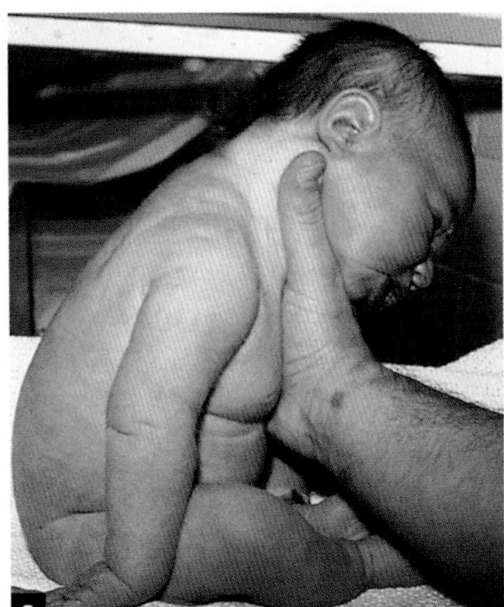

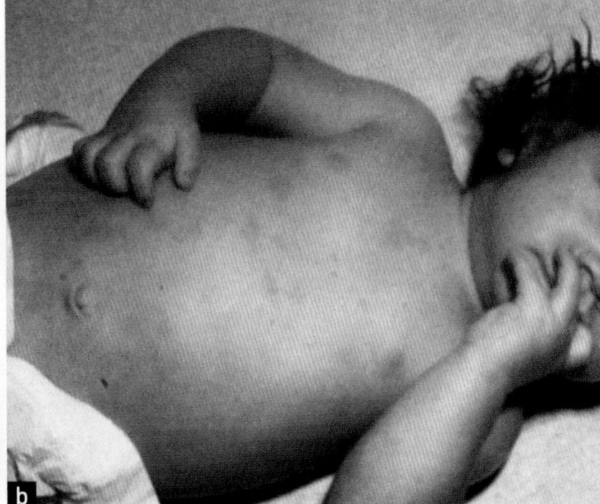

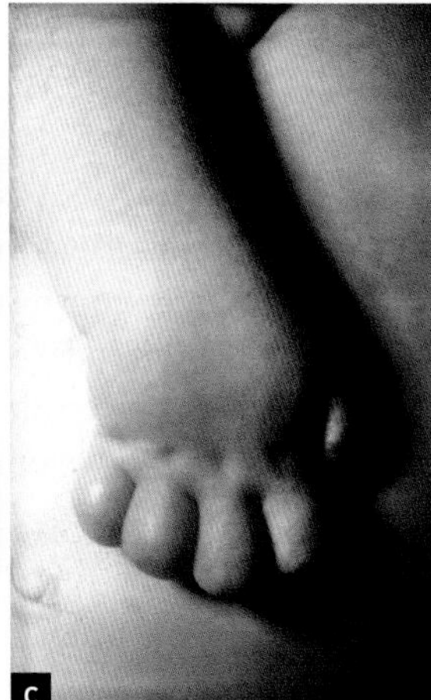

(a) Duchenne–Erb: this infant demonstrates the characteristic posture of the limply adducted and internally rotated arm. (b, c) Infant with Klumpke palsy involving the lower segments of C7 and T1. Note the different posture of the arm compared with the Erb palsy, and the claw-hand deformity

((a) From Brozanski BS. *Zitelli and Davis' atlas of pediatric physical diagnosis*. Philadelphia: Saunders, 2012, with permission; (b, c) courtesy of Dr Michael Painter, Children's Hospital of Pittsburgh.)

FIGURE 38.4

neurone lesion (see Table 38.4 and Fig. 38.4). Brachial plexus lesions occur most commonly during birth (e.g. as a result of shoulder dystocia,[c] which increases the risk 100-fold). Note the size of the hand and arm, the muscle bulk and the presence of joint contractures because injuries can affect normal growth and development of the affected arm.

Respiratory distress could indicate phrenic nerve palsy. Horner syndrome (miosis, partial ptosis, anhidrosis) suggests injury to the T1 spinal root proximal to the point where the sympathetic nerve fibres have separated from the somatic motor nerve fibres. Beware of other abnormalities such as clavicular and humeral fractures, torticollis,[d] cephalohaematoma (see Fig. 38.5) and facial nerve palsy (see Fig. 38.6).

[c] A difficult birth because the width of the shoulders causes obstruction.

[d] Twisting of the head to one side, often as a result of spasm of one sternocleidomastoid muscle.

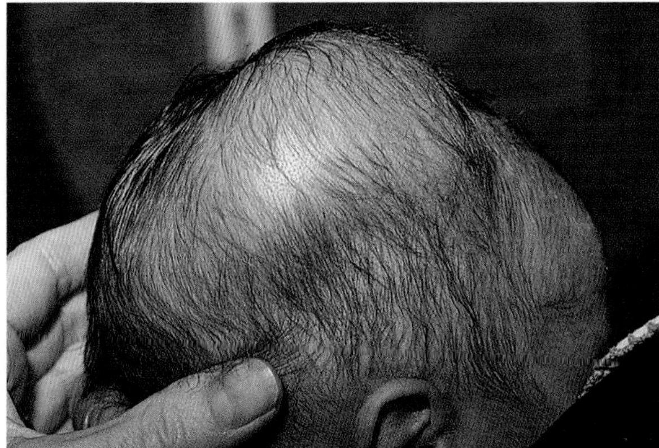

Cephalohaematoma is a subperiosteal haemorrhage and thus limited by the suture lines due to a ruptured vessel within the space between the periosteum and the skull. When finger pressure is applied a bulge forms that disappears once the pressure is released

(From Galbraith SS. In Eichenfield L, Eichenfield L, Frieden I, eds. *Neonatal dermatology*, 2nd edn. Philadelphia: Saunders, 2008.)

FIGURE 38.5

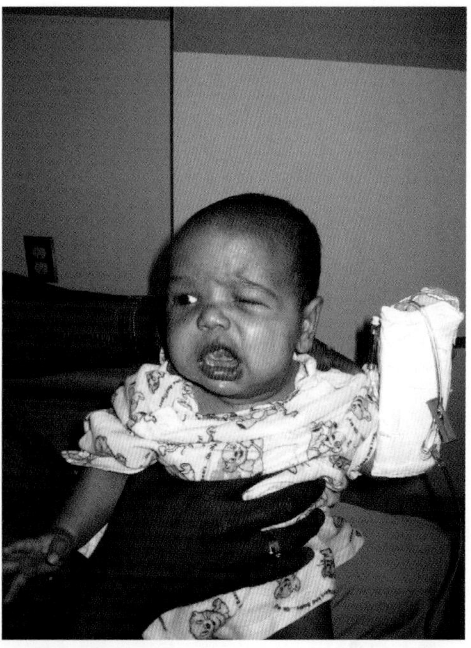

Facial nerve palsy right side

(From Cameron C. *J Cystic Fibrosis* 2006; 6(3):241–243. Figure 1 Photograph of patient on initial admission demonstrating right-sided facial paralysis. ©2006 European Cystic Fibrosis Society.)

FIGURE 38.6

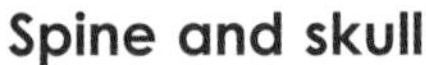

Spine and skull

Inspect the spine carefully for soft-tissue masses and any failure of bony fusion in the posterior midline of the vertebral column (dysraphism), a result of abnormal fusion of the embryonic sacral neural tube. These abnormalities of spinal fusion—lumbosacral meningoceles, myeloceles, myelocystoceles and meningomyeloceles[e] (called spina bifida cystica)—are usually diagnosed before birth by routine fetal ultrasound (see Fig. 38.7). These babies are at risk of infection and should be examined only by clinicians wearing sterile gloves. The associated neurological deficit depends on the localisation of the spinal dysraphic[f] lesion (see Table 38.5).

Hydrocephalus is an increase in the volume of cerebrospinal fluid, usually due to obstruction of drainage pathways; it is a common complication of meningomyelocele (see List 38.2).

The presence of inspiratory stridor, abnormal cry and difficulty with swallowing suggests lower cranial

Localisation of meningomyelocele and neurological deficits

Level of dysraphic spinal lesion	Neurological deficit
Above L3	Combination of upper and lower motor neurone lesions with flaccid (less commonly spastic) paraplegia, areflexia (less commonly hyperreflexia), sensory deficits according to dermatomes affected, bladder and rectal incontinence
L4 and below	Preservation of hip flexors, adductors, extensors
S1 and below	Preservation of feet dorsiflexors, hip extensors, knee flexors
S3 and below	Normal motor function in hip and knee, variable ankle plantar flexor strength, variable bladder and rectal incontinence, saddle anaesthesia

TABLE 38.5

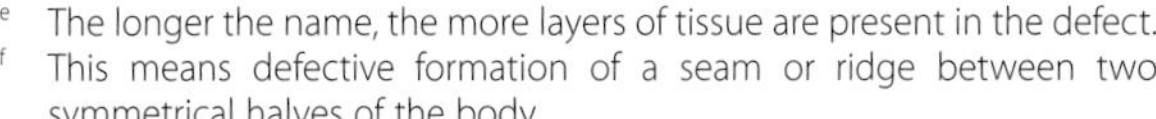

[e] The longer the name, the more layers of tissue are present in the defect.
[f] This means defective formation of a seam or ridge between two symmetrical halves of the body.

Various forms of spina bifida.

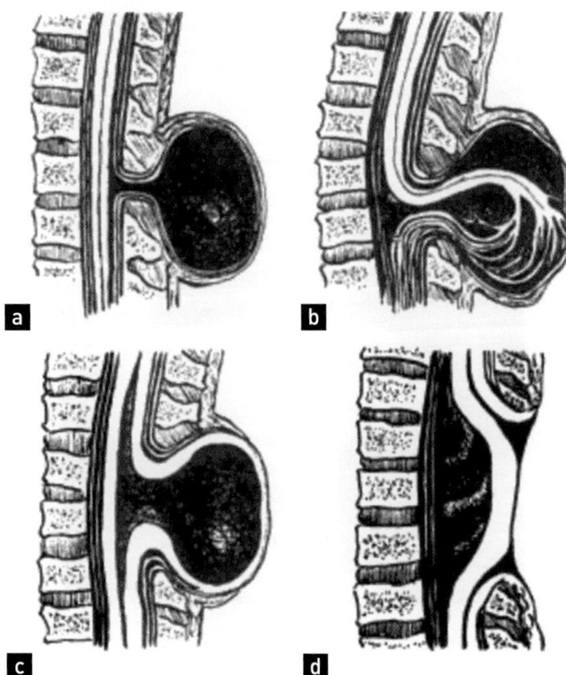

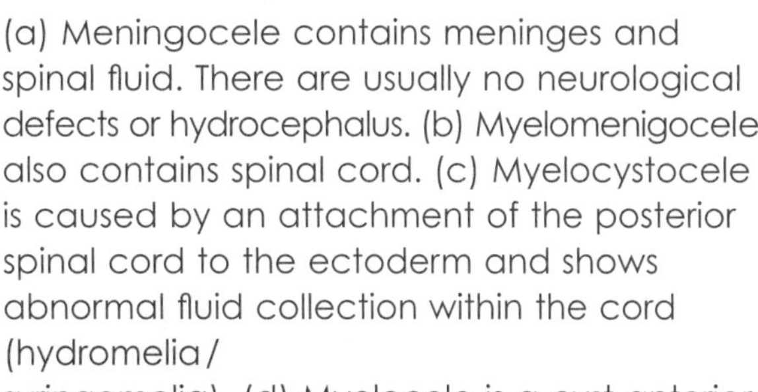

(a) Meningocele contains meninges and spinal fluid. There are usually no neurological defects or hydrocephalus. (b) Myelomenigocele also contains spinal cord. (c) Myelocystocele is caused by an attachment of the posterior spinal cord to the ectoderm and shows abnormal fluid collection within the cord (hydromelia / syringomelia). (d) Myelocele is a cyst anterior to the spinal cord

(From Benda CE. *Developmental disorders of mentation and cerebral palsies*. New York: Grune & Stratton, 1952.)

FIGURE 38.7

SIGNS OF HYDROCEPHALUS

- Increased head circumference
- A large bulging fontanel and wide skull sutures
- Dilated scalp veins
- Loss of upward conjugate gaze with visible sclera between the upper eyelid and iris (setting-sun sign)
- A hyperresonant percussion note of the skullcap (be gentle)

LIST 38.2

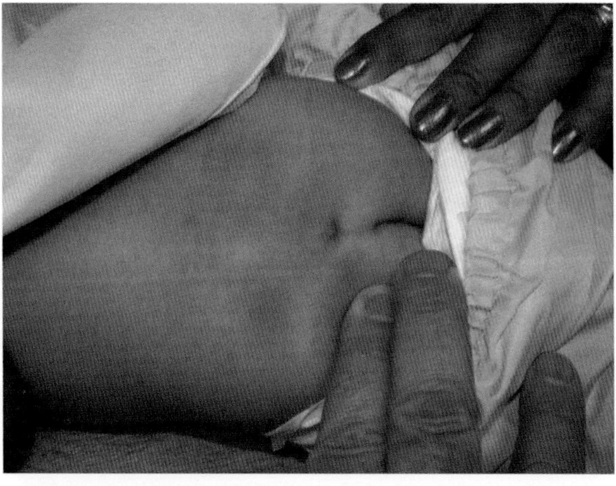

Low sacral dimple

(From Herring JA. *Tachdjian's pediatric orthopaedics: from the Texas Scottish Rite Hospital for Children*. Philadelphia: Saunders, 2008.)

FIGURE 38.8

nerve palsies (bulbar palsy); and apnoeic episodes indicate impaired brainstem function, which is the leading cause of death in these infants.

Spinal and lower extremity deformities and joint contractures are common in patients with spina bifida. If a midline dermal dimple or sinus is present (see Fig. 38.8), measure the depth of the dimple and the distance from the anal verge. An occult spina bifida should be excluded by ultrasound[26] or magnetic resonance imaging (MRI) if the dimple is deeper than 0.5 centimetres, its location is greater than 2.5 centimetres from the anus or a naevus, haemangioma, lipoma or hairy patch is present.[27]

Abnormal limb movements

Jerky limb movements

Sudden brief jerks of the extremities (myoclonus) may be **benign** if they occur only during sleep (non-rapid eye movement [NREM] sleep), are sensitive to stimulation and stop abruptly when the neonate wakes, resolve in the first months of life and are not explained by other disorders. It is important to distinguish benign neonatal sleep myoclonus from other types of jerks that may indicate serious pathologies. Horizontal deviation of the eyes and blinking of the eyelid may indicate seizure activity. In these babies, jerks or abnormal tone of the extremities and orobuccal movements such as grimacing, tongue smacking and extranutritional sucking may be observed (mnemonic: **EEG—Eyes, Extremities, Grimacing**). Dysregulation of the autonomic nervous system with apnoeic spells and increased heart rate in isolation or combination with loss of muscle tone (limbs becoming limp) may be the only sign of neonatal seizures.[16]

Jittery limb movements

Jitters are common in the first days of life and refer to rhythmic tremors of equal amplitude as a presentation of excited neuromuscular activity (jitteriness / tremulousness). They are sensitive to stimulation and can easily be interrupted by gentle flexion or holding of the involved extremities. If persistent or exaggerated they can indicate hypoglycaemia, hypocalcaemia, abstinence syndrome, sepsis and birth asphyxia.

The skin

Inspect the skin from head to toe. A bluish appearance of the hands and feet (acrocyanosis) is common in the first days of life. A number of skin changes without pathological relevance are often present. These include:

- erythema toxicum (see Fig. 38.9(a))
- sebaceous hyperplasia (see Fig. 38.9(b))
- miliae—tiny epidermal cysts, probably the result of blocked pilosebaceous opening (see Fig. 38.9(c and d))
- salmon patches / angel's kiss (naevus simplex; see Fig. 38.9(e))
- hyperpigmentations (congenital dermal melanocytosis; see Fig. 38.9(f)).

However, generalised rashes and blister can be caused by life-threatening disease in neonates.

However, a generalised erythematous rash and fluid-filled small blisters (vesicles) or large blisters (bullae) with exfoliation of the skin on gentle rubbing (Nikolsky's sign—due to toxic epidermal necrolysis) is suggestive of '*Staphylococcus aureus*' infection (called Ritter's disease of the newborn or *Staphylococcus* scalded skin syndrome). Less generalised blisters (bullous impetigo) or erythematous papules (non-bullous impetigo) are more commonly seen and caused by *Staphylococcus* and *Streptococcus* spp. The occurrence of vesicles with surrounding erythema in the face or scalp that develop into pustules filled with purulent or cloudy material in a baby who had a vaginal delivery is indicative of neonatal herpes.

Large pigmented naevi are caused by a benign proliferation of melanocytes but they need to be monitored for changes in size and shape that might indicate the development of malignancy.[28] Port-wine stains (naevus flammeus) are a form of vascular malformation. They are dark-red or purple skin patches with well-defined borders and can be associated with other abnormalities (e.g. Sturge–Weber syndrome).

Haemangiomas of infancy are usually benign and present as a superficial nascent (new) lesion consisting of small dilated blood vessels (capillary telangiectasias) surrounded by a pale halo (see Fig. 38.10(a)), a pale or erythematous macule or a bruise or scratch.[29] Superficial haemangiomas that have progressed from a nascent into a proliferative stage show a strawberry-like appearance with a raised, bright-red and lobulated dermis and may feel warm. A colour change from bright red to grey may indicate shrinkage (involution), which usually starts centrally.[29] A deep haemangioma originating from the subcutis appears as a soft mass with a dusky or bluish colour (see Fig. 38.10(b)) but it can be difficult to distinguish clinically from other vascular birthmarks. Be aware that the presence of haemangiomas on the face or neck is associated with haemangiomas of the airway and that more than five cutaneous haemangiomas anywhere else is associated with visceral haemangiomas.

Visible jaundice develops with a total serum bilirubin of greater than 6 mg / dL or 102.6 mmol / L (1 mg / dL = 17.1 mmol / L). However, it is difficult to estimate the severity of hyperbilirubinaemia by the visual assessment of jaundice.[30] Physiological jaundice is not usually evident in the first 24 hours of life (e.g. less than 6 mg / dL) but peaks at day 3 to day 5 after birth, does not exceed 15 mg / dL and resolves within a week's time in term newborns and within 2 weeks in premature babies. However, some neonates develop excessive hyperbilirubinaemia, which requires careful monitoring and potentially treatment (see List 38.3).

If significant jaundice is present, look for signs of or associated factors that can lead to excessive red blood cell breakdown (haemolysis) such as:

- excessive bruising and cephalohaematoma (e.g. birth trauma)
- splenomegaly (e.g. associated with spherocytosis)
- pallor

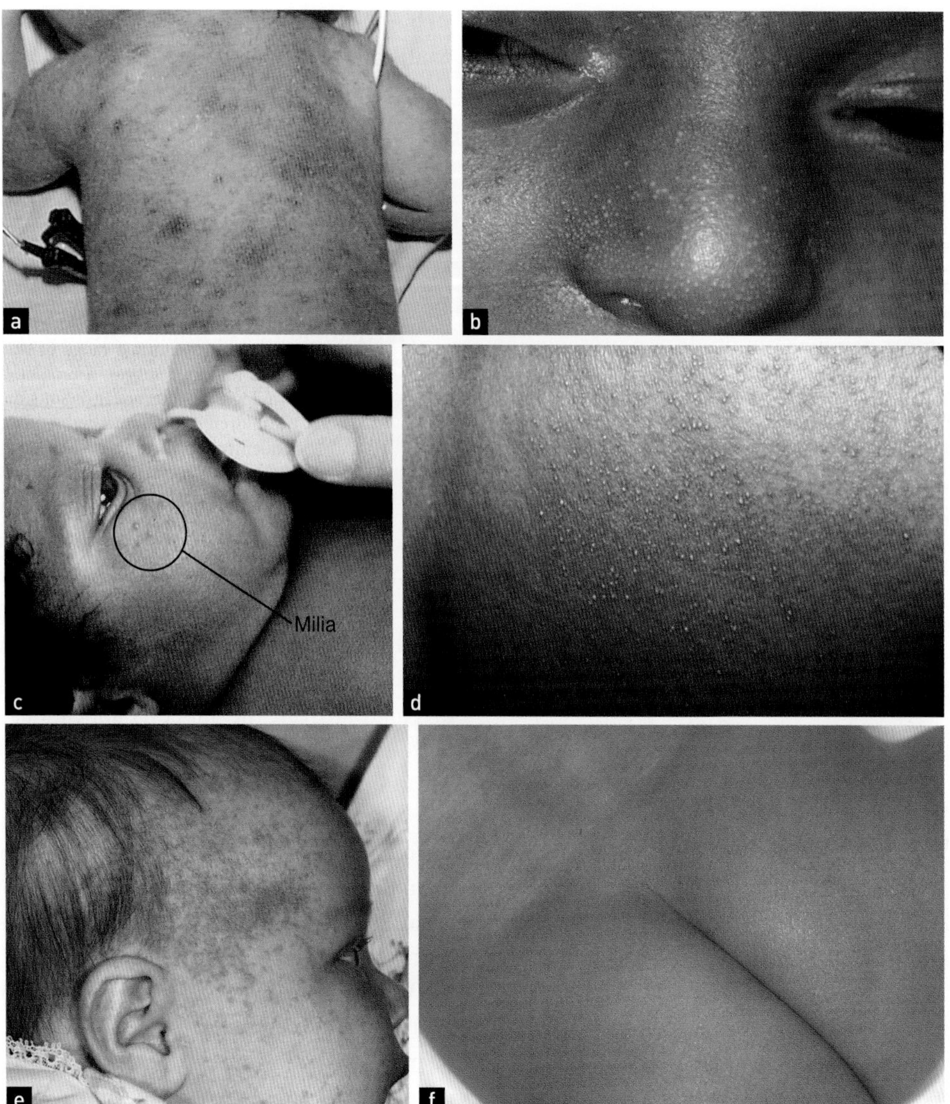

(a) Erythema toxicum; (b) sebaceous hyperplasia; (c, d) miliae; (e) naevus simplex and (f) hyperpigmentations

((a, b and d) from Kliegman RM, Jenson HB, Behrman RE, Stanton BF. *Nelson's textbook of pediatrics*, 18th edn. Philadelphia: Saunders Elsevier, 2007; (c) from Seidel HM, Ball JW, Danis JE, Benedict GW. *Mosby's guide to physical examination*, 6th edn. St Louis, MO: Mosby Elsevier, 2006; (e) from Habif T. *Clinical dermatology*, 4th edn. St Louis, MO: Mosby, 2004; (f) from Lemmi FO, Lemmi CAE. *Physical assessment findings CD-ROM*, Philadelphia: Saunders, 2000.)

FIGURE 38.9

- generalised oedema and signs of heart failure (e.g. severe anaemia as a result of rhesus / ABO incompatibility)
- macrosomia and plethora (e.g. polycythaemia)
- African, African American or Asian descent (e.g. glucose-6-phosphate dehydrogenase deficiency).

Assess for signs of impaired bilirubin elimination, e.g.:

- functional or mechanical bowel obstruction (e.g. increased enterohepatic bilirubin circulation)
- hepatomegaly (e.g. hepatitis, infection)
- pale chalky stools and dark urine staining the nappy (e.g. cholestasis, biliary atresia).

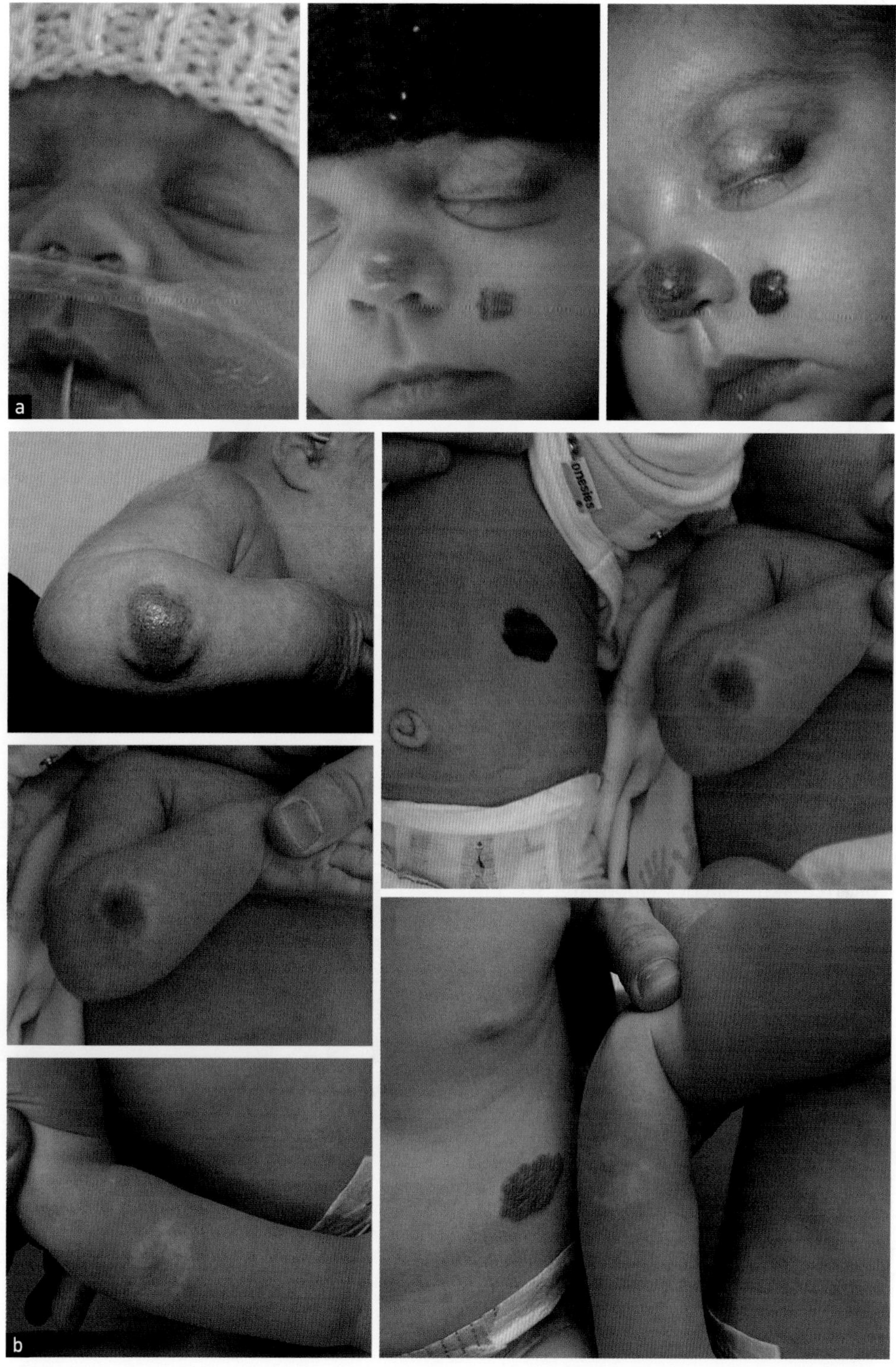

(a) Superficial nascent and (b) deep proliferating haemangioma

(From Drolet BA. Infantile hemangiomas: an emerging health issue linked to an increased rate of low birth weight infants. *J Pediatr* 2008; 153(5):712–715.e1.)

FIGURE 38.10

SIGNS OF EXCESSIVE HYPERBILIRUBINAEMIA*

- Poor feeding
- Lethargy
- Opisthotonus (spasm of the back muscles leads to dramatic arching of the back and extension of the head)
- Irritability
- High-pitched crying
- Apnoea
- Seizures (acute bilirubin encephalopathy)
- Sensorineural hearing loss
- Motor delay
- Extrapyramidal signs
- Gaze palsy
- Dental dysplasia

*Bilirubin deposition in the basal ganglia and its associated neurological signs are called kernicterus.

LIST 38.3

Search for petechiae, which do not empty and disappear when pressed (see Fig. 38.11(a)); if generalised, they may indicate neonatal thrombocytopenia.

Poor perfusion of the peripheries (hypothermia, sepsis, heart failure, hypovolaemia) is suggested by uneven discoloured skin patches (mottling; see Fig. 38.11(b)).

More than six café-au-lait spots, each with a size greater than 5 millimetres, is a diagnostic feature of neurofibromatosis type 1 (see Ch 37).

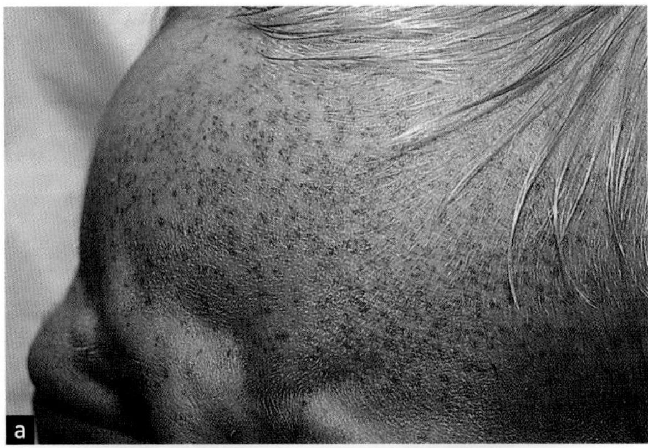

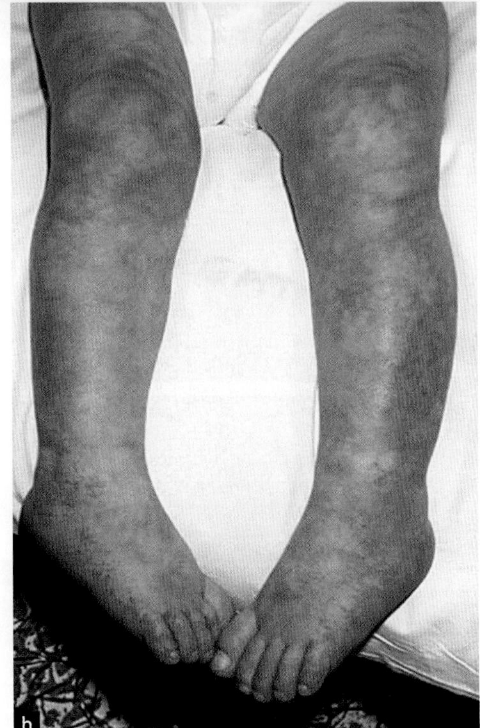

(a) Petechiae and (b) skin mottling

((a) From Weston WL. *Color textbook of pediatric dermatology*, 4th edn. St Louis, MO: Mosby, 2007; (b) from Murphy CC. Late-onset pediatric glaucoma associated with cutis marmorata telangiectatica congenita managed with Molteno implant surgery: case report and review of the literature. Journal of American Association for Pediatric Ophthalmology and Strabismus 2007; 11(5):519–521, with permission.)

FIGURE 38.11

Temperature

A baby who is cold to touch may be very ill. Measure the body temperature in the axilla and if it is abnormal (less than 35.5°C [hypothermia] or more than 37.5°C [hyperthermia]) it is best remeasured in the rectum. Hypothermia and increased body temperature are strong predictors of severe illness in newborn infants.[16,18]

Head

Shape

The head of the newborn is moulded by the baby's intrauterine position and passage through the birth canal. A baby lying in the breech position has its head positioned against the fundus of the uterus, which results in a flatter-appearing top (vertex) and elongation of the occipitofrontal diameter. A baby born head first (cephalic delivery) usually has a shorter biparietal diameter and a more prominent-appearing top. Reassure parents that prominent moulding usually disappears in a couple of days even if bony ridges are palpable owing to a slight overlap of skull bones.

Inspect the head for:

- any signs of swelling and bruising (haematoma)
- lacerations and abrasions (birth injuries)
- asymmetry and protuberances (craniosynostosis, see below)
- abnormal hair growth and pigmentation (see Table 38.6)[31]
- scalp defects (e.g. aplasia cutis)
- caput succedaneum, an area of subcutaneous serosanguineous effusion that is pitting and crosses the cranial sutures, which must be distinguished from
- cephalohaematoma (see Fig. 38.5), a haemorrhage between the periosteum and the skull (which is non-pitting and is limited by the suture lines).

Caput succedaneum resolves within 2 weeks whereas swelling caused by frank haemorrhage may persist for months or even longer if calcification occurs.

Sutures

Feel along the four suture lines for palpable ridges, which may indicate premature fusion of the skull bones (*craniosynostosis*). The metopic suture is the line where the frontal skull bones meet; it extends from the anterior fontanel down the middle of the forehead towards the nose. *Metopic synostosis* results in the development of a triangular-shaped forehead when viewed from above (*trigonocephaly*). The coronal suture marks the point where the frontal and parietal skull bones on each side meet; it extends from ear to ear. Bilateral synostosis leads to a short anterior–posterior and increased transverse head diameter (*brachycephaly*), whereas unilateral synostosis will result in anterior *plagiocephaly*. The sagittal suture line is formed by the two parietal bones; it extends from the anterior to the posterior fontanel. Premature fusion results in a long, narrow head shape and is the most common synostosis (*scaphocephaly*). The lambdoidal suture is the space between the two parietal bones and the single occipital bone and if fused it leads to a trapezoid-shaped head with flattening of the occipital region on one side (posterior *plagiocephaly*). Note, however, that the most common—and self-resolving—presentation, that of posterior plagiocephaly, is caused by positional moulding due to the fetus' position in utero, which may be exacerbated by the infant's preference for placing the head on the same side during sleep. *Oxycephaly* (turricephaly) is the premature fusion of all cranial sutures. Craniosynostoses may be seen in association with Apert, Crouzon, Saethre–Chotzen, Pfeiffer or Carpenter syndrome.

Fontanels

Next, palpate the anterior and posterior fontanels for fullness and size. The anterior fontanel is a diamond-shaped opening of the skull at the point where the frontal and parietal skull bones meet at the junction between the metopic, sagittal and coronal suture lines. The mean area of the anterior fontanel is 220 mm^2 (2.5th to 97.5th centile: 164 to 276 mm^2) in term newborns[32] and is expected to be closed at 18 months of age. The size can be determined by introducing the index finger into each of the four bony corners of the fontanel, marking them with a small circular ink dot immediately distal to the finger, transferring the four dots onto paper by firmly pressing it onto the skin and calculating the area (see Fig. 38.12). The posterior fontanel is triangle shaped, situated at the junction of the sagittal and lambdoidal suture lines and is closed by 3 months of age. **Large or bulging fontanels** may indicate raised intracranial pressure (see List 38.4) whereas an increase in size without fullness is observed in neonates with bony and endocrine abnormalities (see List 38.5).[33] Premature closure of the fontanels may be associated with craniosynostoses (see above). Auscultate for bruits, which can be heard with intracranial aneurysmal malformations (e.g. of the vein of Galen, the great cerebral vein).[34]

Face

Eyes (see Text box 38.2)

Examination of the eyes has the potential to disturb the infant and may best be done last. However, remember that this examination will become virtually impossible if you have made the baby cry.

Conditions that threaten normal sight may require urgent intervention.

Inspect the upper face and orbits for possible dysmorphic features (e.g. short palpebral fissures,

Scalp hair characteristics in neonates and potential clinical significance

Hair abnormality	Potentially associated conditions
Hypopigmentation	
White forelock	Waardenburg syndrome (abnormal iris pigmentation, cochlear deafness) Piebaldism
Silvery metallic sheen	Chediak–Higashi syndrome (immune deficiency, metabolic disease, partial or complete albinism) Prader–Willi syndrome (deletion 15q11-q13) Piebaldism Ectrodactyly–ectodermal dysplasia–cleft (EEC) syndrome Cross (oculocerebral hypopigmentation) syndrome Nutritional deficiency, inborn error of metabolism (phenylketonuria)
Light coloured	Oculocutaneous albinism
Generalised	Chediak–Higashi syndrome
Hypotrichosis / alopecia*	
Localised	Birth trauma, infection, extravasation of intravenous medication Aplasia cutis congenita Naevus
Generalised	Ectodermal dysplasia Ichthyosis Nutritional deficiencies (zinc, vitamins B_6 and B_{12}, biotinidase) Inborn errors of metabolism (homocystinuria, congenital hypothyroidism)
Hypertrichosis**	
Localised	Naevus, encephalocele, meningocele
Generalised	Cornelia de Lange syndrome Coffin–Siris syndrome Hurler syndrome (mucopolysaccharidosis type I) Edwards syndrome (trisomy 18) Fetal hydantoin and alcohol syndrome Congenital hypertrichosis lanuginosa
Abnormal hairline	
Low frontal hairline	Costello syndrome Cornelia de Lange syndrome Coffin–Siris syndrome Fanconi syndrome Fetal hydantoin syndrome Noonan syndrome
Low posterior hairline	Turner syndrome Kabuki syndrome Cornelia de Lange syndrome Fetal hydantoin syndrome

**Too little hair.*
***Too much hair.*

(Furdon SA, Clark DA. Scalp hair characteristics in the newborn infant. *Adv Neonatal Care* [Review] 2003; 3(6):286–296.)

TABLE 38.6

epicanthic folds, flat nasal bridge). Look for ptosis (often due to a third cranial nerve palsy), inability to close the eye (the result of a seventh cranial nerve palsy due to birth trauma) or displacement due to a haemangioma or birth trauma. The size of the eyes may be unequal or enlarged (e.g. *buphthalmos*[g] due to increased intraocular pressure—glaucoma),

g From the Greek words meaning the eye of an ox. Increased intraocular pressure changes the shape of the cornea, enlarging its diameter.

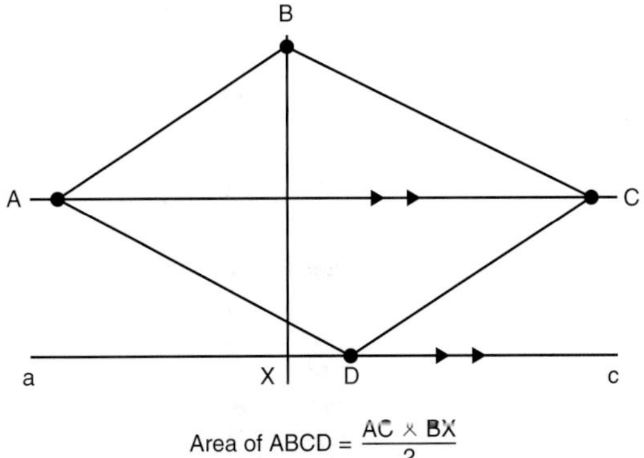

Calculation of anterior fontanel area

(Davies DP, Ansari BM, Cooke TJ. Anterior fontanelle size in the neonate. *Archives of Disease in Childhood* 1975; 50(1):81–3 with permission from BMJ Publishing Group Ltd.)

FIGURE 38.12

CAUSES OF LARGE BULGING FONTANELS

- Hydrocephalus
- Haemorrhage
- Meningitis
- Tumour

LIST 38.4

CAUSES OF LARGE NON-BULGING FONTANELS

- Small for gestational age
- Osteogenesis imperfecta
- Achondroplasia
- Russell–Silver syndrome[34]
- Hypothyroidism
- Hypophosphataemia

LIST 38.5

the sclerae may be blue (premature birth or *osteogenesis imperfecta*) or yellow (jaundice), the conjunctivae injected (glaucoma or subconjunctival haemorrhage; see Fig. 38.13[35]), the irises hypopigmented (oculocutaneous albinism), the cornea cloudy (e.g. metabolic causes, ulcers, transient oedema, trauma tears, dermoids; see Fig. 38.14(a)), the pupils asymmetrical (e.g.

A summary of the neonatal eye examination

Dysmorphic features—epicanthic fold, short palpebral fissures,* flat nasal bridge

Movements—conjugate gaze abnormality; strabismus—consider cranial nerve injury

Ptosis—consider third nerve palsy

Inability to close eye completely—consider seventh nerve palsy

Enlargement of an eye (*buphthalmos*)—glaucoma

Scleral colour—jaundice, osteogenesis imperfecta

Conjunctivae—injected (conjunctivitis, glaucoma, haemorrhage)

Watery eyes—blocked lacrimal duct, conjunctivitis

Irises—hypopigmented (albinism)

Corneas—cloudy (ulcers, oedema, trauma)

Pupils—asymmetrical (amblyopia-blindness, third nerve palsy), irregular (coloboma), opaque (cataract, retinal abnormality)

Abnormal gaze—cranial nerve abnormality

*Palpebra is the Latin word for eyelid.

TEXT BOX 38.2

amblyopia, ocular motor nerve palsy), not round (e.g. coloboma[h]) or opaque (leucocoria due to cataract, retinoblastoma; see Fig. 38.14(b)). Watery eyes may result from nasolacrimal duct stenosis (see Fig. 38.15(a)), which can be associated with cyst formation (dacrocystocele) if the inferior or superior ducts are obstructed. Purulent discharge, however, suggests bacterial infection unless proven otherwise by negative cultures (e.g. *Chlamydia trachomatis* or *Neisseria gonorrhoeae* conjunctivitis).

Observe the baby's vertical and horizontal gaze by moving your face within the baby's visual field. Avoid talking or making noises at the same time. It is common for neonates to lose track intermittently and require readjustment. Look for dysconjugate eye movements

[h] A congenital defect in the iris, retina, choroid and/or optic nerve.

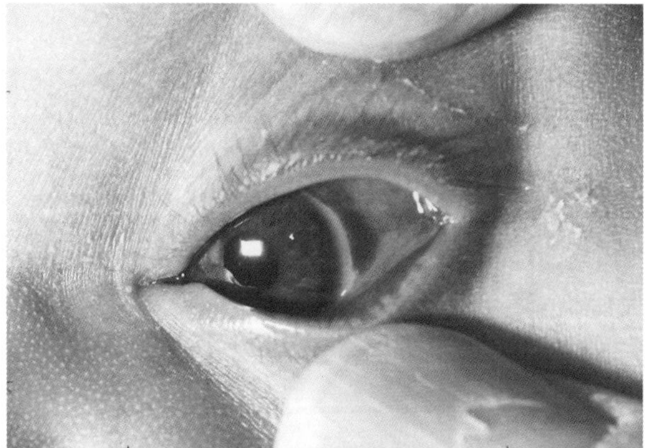

Subconjunctival haemorrhage and petechiae at the forehead commonly as a result from changes in cephalic venous pressure[35]

(From Goldbloom RB. *Pediatric clinical skills*, 4th edn. Philadelphia: Saunders, 2011, pp 38–55.)

FIGURE 38.13

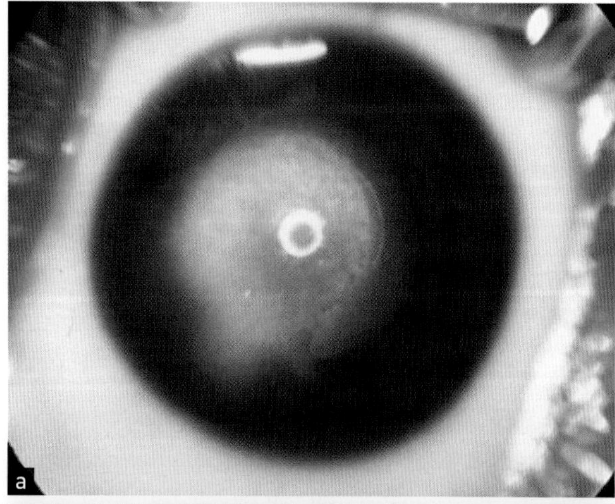

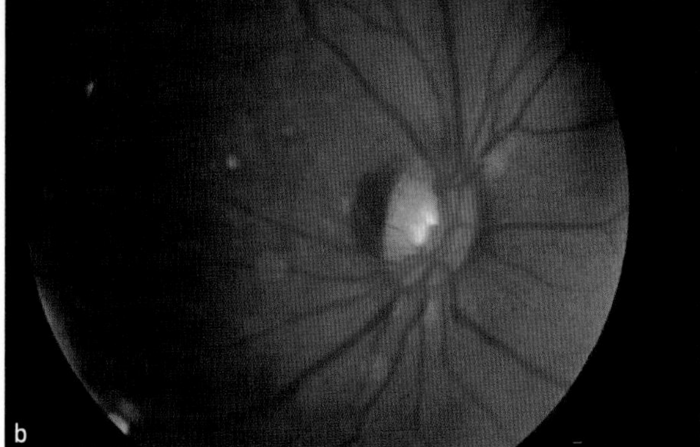

(a) Haziness of the cornea in front of the pupils and involving the iris, versus (b) an opacity behind the pupils

((a) From Krachmer JH, Mannis MJ, Holland EJ. *Cornea*, 3rd edn. Philadelphia: Elsevier Saunders, 2011.)

FIGURE 38.14

(*squint* or *strabismus*[i]) and determine whether these are transiently noticeable (e.g. when falling asleep or waking up) or fixed (e.g. as a result of cranial nerve damage due to birth trauma). A convergent squint can be the result of lateral rectus muscle weakness due to a sixth cranial nerve palsy.

Use an ophthalmoscope to assess pupillary and red reflexes. Darken the room and face the neonate away from any light sources such as windows. Select a small viewing aperture at the front of the ophthalmoscope and dial up the '0' lens with your index finger on the side of the ophthalmoscope (no lens correction). Hold the ophthalmoscope with your right hand vertically in front of your right eye and direct the light beam laterally towards the baby's right and left eye from a distance of approximately 15 centimetres. **P**upils should be **e**qual and **r**eactive to **l**ight (**PEARL**). The red reflex is a light reflection from the retina and a lack of the reflex is suggestive of lens opacities (e.g. cataract), retinal abnormalities such as haemorrhage or detachment, or retinoblastoma. On closer inspection, the retina should appear yellow-white, grey or red depending on pigmentation.

Ears

Look for periauricular pits and skin tags, which are common findings. The presence of these increases the risk of hearing impairment five-fold. Hearing loss can be detected by hearing screening (e.g. transient-evoked otoacoustic emissions or auditory brainstem response audiometry).[36]

Note the position of the ear. Approximately 30% of the auricle (pinna) should be positioned above an

[i] These words mean the same thing. When one eye looks at an object the other may look too far inwards (convergent strabismus), too far outwards (divergent strabismus) or too far up or down (vertical strabismus).

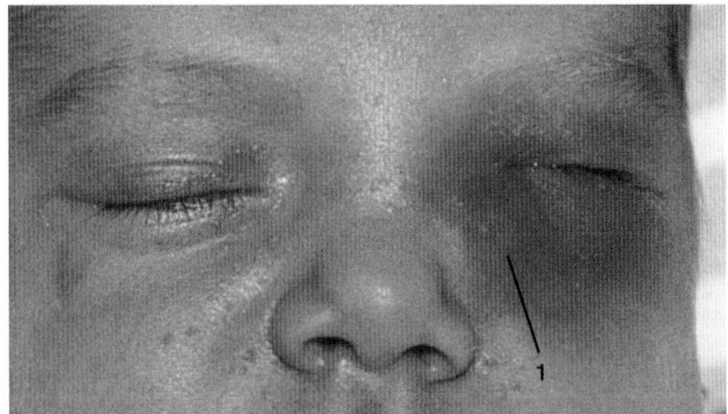

Acute dacryocystitis in a 4-week-old child with redness and swelling of left upper and lower lids and a prominent nasolacrimal sac

(From Krachmer JH, Mannis MJ, Holland EJ. *Cornea*, 3rd edn. Philadelphia: Elsevier Saunders, 2011.)

FIGURE 38.15

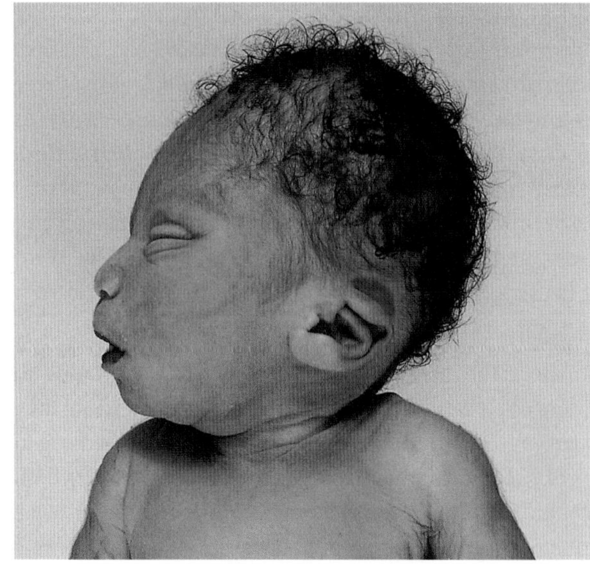

Low-set and hypoplastic left ear

(From Corrin B. *Pathology of the lungs*. Philadelphia: Elsevier Saunders, 2011 (courtesy of the late Dr AH Cameron, Birmingham, UK).)

FIGURE 38.16

imaginary line drawn from the inner and outer canthus[j] to the occipital bone. The ear is clearly low set (see Fig. 38.16) if the upper margin of the ear helix is below the eye level and this may be associated with chromosomal anomalies.

Inspection of the tympanic membranes with an otoscope is not performed routinely because the ear canals may be obscured by vernix[k] or blood. Applying a positive pressure using a pneumatic otoscope prevents the collapse of the cartilaginous auricular meatus for better visualisation of the tympanic membrane, which is greyer, thicker and more vascular in newborns than in older children.[37] Middle ear effusions are commonly seen but resolve in the first 3 days of life in most neonates.[38]

Nose

Inspect the external nose for any deformity and asymmetry of the nasal bridge and nares, which can affect nasal airway patency. Nasal flaring may indicate respiratory distress. Infants are preferential nose breathers and bilateral nasal airway patency should therefore be verified, particularly in those babies with signs of respiratory distress or apnoeic spells. The presence of cyanosis exacerbated by feeding and relieved by crying suggests nasal obstruction, which may be due to:

- choanal[l] atresia—posterior nasal obstruction
- piriform aperture[m] stenosis—anterior obstruction
- dacryocystoceles[n] with intranasal extension.

Inspect both nasal passages by inserting the tip of the otoscope a few millimetres into the anterior nasal apertures to assess for nasal septum deviation and uncommon masses (e.g. encephalocele, dermoid cysts, haemangiomas).

Several functional tests have been described. For example, look for movement of thin cotton fibres, or for condensation on metal or a mirror held beneath each nostril. Alternatively, close the baby's mouth and one nasal aperture with your left thumb and index finger and auscultate for airflow sounds with a stethoscope held beneath the other nostril (and vice versa).[39] If in any doubt, check patency by gently trying to pass a nasogastric feeding tube (e.g. 6 French,

[j] The angle formed by the junction of the eyelids, also called the palpebral angle.

[k] This greasy deposit covers a baby's skin at birth. It consists of skin scales and fine hairs. The full name is vernix caseosa and comes from the Latin words for varnish and cheese.

[l] Choana means funnel and these are the funnel-shaped openings between the nose and the nasopharynx.

[m] Piriform means pear shaped; this is the bony opening of the nose.

[n] This is a protrusion of the lacrimal sac.

2 millimetres) through each nasal aperture into the hypopharynx. However, partial obstruction (e.g. piriform aperture stenosis) cannot be excluded with these manoeuvres. Non-structural abnormalities such as mucosal oedema may also cause nasal obstruction. Clear nasal discharge is commonly caused by a virus-induced upper respiratory tract infection (and very rarely by a cranial cerebrospinal fluid leak), whereas purulent discharge may indicate a bacterial aetiology.

Mouth

Inspect the mandibles from the front and sides to identify lower facial asymmetry and abnormal jaw size. A Pierre Robin[o] sequence is suggested by a proportionally small mandible (*micrognathia*), which includes posterior displacement of the tongue into the pharynx (*glossoptosis*) and airway obstruction. It may be associated with a cleft palate.[40]

If you have made the baby cry, look for the symmetrical opening of the mouth and for apparently unrestricted side and forward mobility. This excludes temporomandibular joint fixation (ankylosis).[41]

Note the presence of lip cyanosis and a cleft lip or any other dysmorphic features (e.g. small upper lip and smooth philtrum in fetal alcohol spectrum disorder).

Inspect the oral cavity for cleft palate and a bifid uvula, which may occasionally indicate a submucous cleft. Cleft lip and palate interfere with swallowing and feeding, whereas the clinical relevance of a submucous cleft may surface only later in life with symptoms of velopharyngeal[p] insufficiency (nasal regurgitation, recurrent ear infections, hypernasality of speech). Exclusion of a cleft palate requires palpation of the hard and soft palate with the index finger and while wearing an examination glove, in addition to direct visualisation of the palate with a torch, with the aid of a spatula, to avoid missing a submucous cleft. Prevent full closure of the mouth during the examination of the palate as strong sucking by the neonate otherwise precludes assessment of the soft palate.

Small white cysts at the junction between the soft and hard palates or the gum (Epstein's pearls; see Fig. 38.17(a)) are common and harmless if they do not interfere with function (e.g. feeding). Natal (present at birth) or neonatal (erupting in the first month of life) teeth, mostly lower central incisors, are often loose and show enamel hypoplasia, making extraction the treatment of choice.[42] Assess the size of the tongue (e.g. *aglossia* or *microglossia*, which is associated with micrognathia; and *macroglossia*, which is associated with Beckwith–Wiedemann, Down syndrome or hypothyroidism). Look at its position (e.g. for glossoptosis) and mobility (e.g. tongue tie [lingual frenulum[q]]; see Fig. 38.17(b)).[43] The need for treatment of ankyloglossia can be assessed using standardised score sheets. Look beneath the tongue for sublingual (central) cyanosis.

Neck

Examine the neck for symmetry and abnormal skinfolds. **Loose nuchal[r] skin** can be seen in several conditions (e.g. intrauterine lymphoedema, Down syndrome, Noonan's syndrome and Turner syndrome; see Fig. 38.18).

Look at the sternocleidomastoid muscles for unilateral shortening or swelling to rule out congenital torticollis. In this condition the head tilts towards the affected side while the chin points to the opposite side. Turn the baby's head gently from side to side as far as the neck will allow. The full range of movement is restricted when torticollis is present.

Look for cervical masses (e.g. cystic hygromas,[s] thyroglossal cysts, epidermoid cysts), which present with painless, soft or semifirm swellings. In newborn infants, cystic hygromas are most commonly found in the posterior cervical space on one side and vary in size. Large ones may cause compromise to the airway and extend into the mediastinum or face.[44] Thyroglossal cysts are most commonly localised in the midline at or below the level of the hyoid bone and move upwards with tongue protrusion.[45] Epidermoid cysts are found at the floor of the mouth and superior to the hyoid bone. Isolated palpable cervical lymph nodes (up to 12 millimetres in diameter) are common in healthy newborns but warrant documentation and follow-up.[46]

A short and asymmetrical neck may indicate maldeveloped cervical vertebrae (Klippel–Feil syndrome).

[o] This sequence includes micrognathia, cleft palate, glossoptosis and sometimes glaucoma and retinal detachment.

[p] A velum is a sail or curtain in Latin and refers here to the posterior part of the soft palate.

[q] The Latin word for a bridle.

[r] The *nucha* is the nape of the neck.

[s] This is a cystic cavity arising from distended lymphatics.

Oral examination in the neonate.

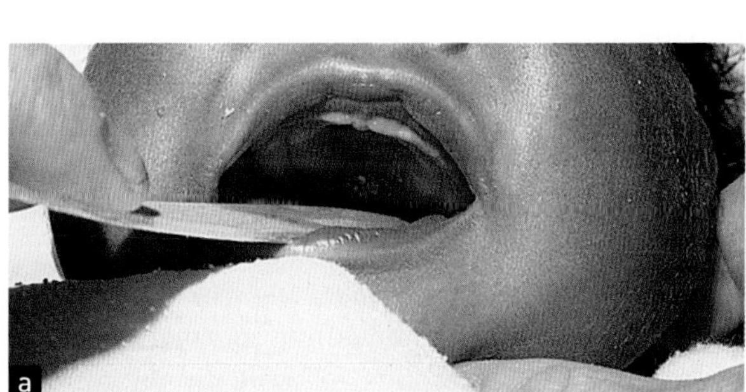

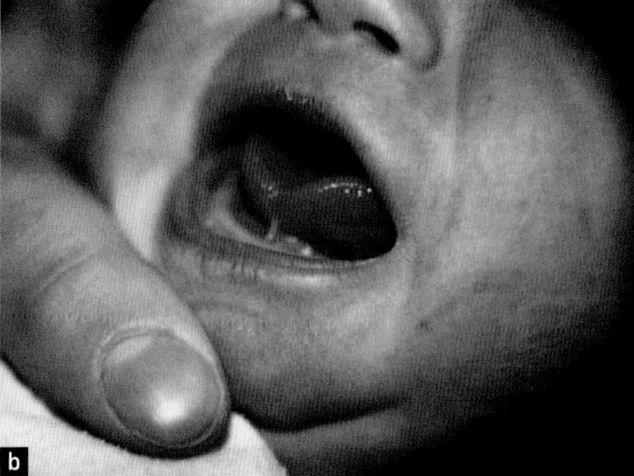

(a) Epstein's pearls of the hard palate. (b) An infant with ankyloglossia (tongue-tie). Note the short frenulum, which extends to the tip of the tongue. Ankyloglossia interferes with protrusion of the tongue and may make breastfeeding difficult

((a) From Metry DW. *Neonatal dermatology*. Philadelphia: Saunders, 2008, with permission. (b) Courtesy of Dr Evelyn Jain, Lakeview Breastfeeding Clinic, Calgary, Alberta, Canada; from: Moore KL. *The developing human*. Philadelphia: Saunders, 2013.)

FIGURE 38.17

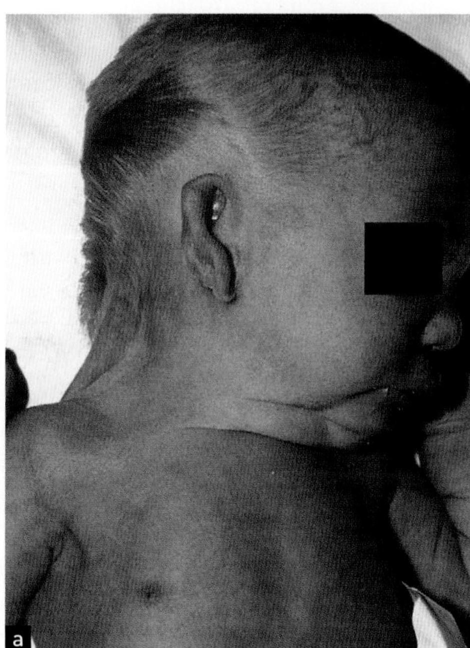

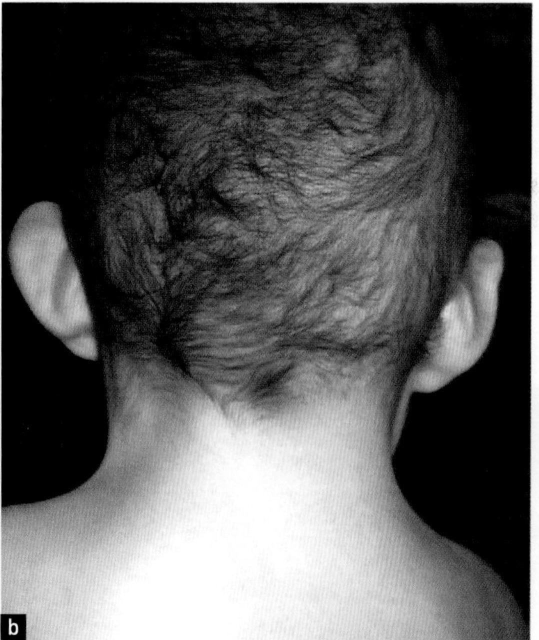

Clinical photographs show several physical manifestations associated with Turner syndrome. (a) In this newborn a webbed neck with low hairline, shield chest with widespread nipples, abnormal ears, and micrognathia are seen. (b) The low-set posterior hairline can be better appreciated in this older child who also has protruding ears. The newborn shown in (a) also had prominent lymphoedema of the hands and feet

(From Zitelli BJ, McIntire SC, Nowalk AJ. *Atlas of pediatric physical diagnosis*, 6th edn. Philadelphia: Saunders, 2012 (Figure 1.25 a and b).)

FIGURE 38.18

Chest and cardiovascular system

Approximately half of the evidence-based clinical signs best identifying severe illness in newborn infants can be detected during a chest examination.[16] Note that the sequence of 'look, listen and feel' will change in an opportunistic fashion during the examination. If you have made the baby cry, auscultation may be impossible.

Inspect the chest for symmetrical expansion and any deformities. These may be acquired (fracture or pneumothorax) or congenital (pectus or dystrophy). A depressed sternum (pectus excavatum—funnel chest; see Fig. 38.19) is the most commonly observed congenital deformity.[47] A protuberance of the sternum (pectus carinatum—pigeon chest) may be symmetrical or affect only one side of the chest wall, which results in asymmetry with sternal rotation and depression of the contralateral site of the chest wall. A narrow chest due to the intrauterine failure of chest wall growth (e.g. Jeune syndrome [asphyxiating thoracic dystrophy], Poland syndrome [hypoplasia of the chest wall variably involving soft tissues, muscles and ribs], Ellis–van Creveld syndrome [chondroectodermal dysplasia]) may be associated with bilateral lung hypoplasia. Unilateral lung hypoplasia is commonly observed with a left-sided diaphragmatic hernia.

Count the respiratory rate over one full minute (normal is 40–60 breaths per minute) by assessing both chest movements and breath sounds. Fast breathing (tachypnoea) predicts severe illness moderately well.[16]

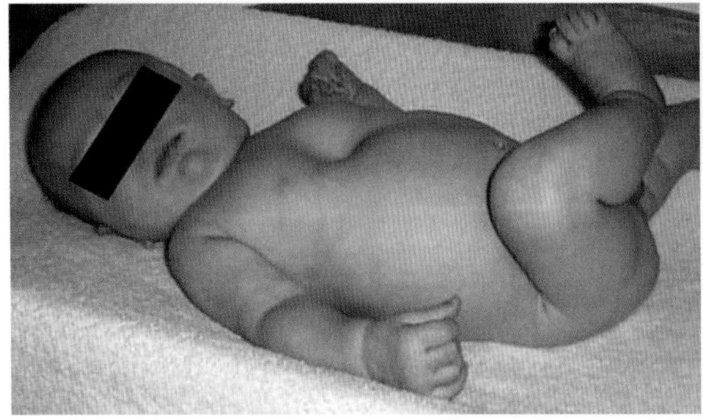

Pectus excavatum

(From Hebra A. *Semin Thorac Cardiovasc Surg* 2009; 21(1):76–84.)

FIGURE 38.19

Assess for intermittent upper airway obstruction (e.g. Pierre Robin sequence, choanal atresia, tracheo- or laryngomalacia). These babies cannot move air sufficiently despite normal or increased respiratory efforts. Asymmetry in chest movements suggests that phrenic nerve palsy has caused unilateral paralysis of the diaphragm. If you have made the baby cry, use the opportunity to note the presence of abnormal crying (e.g. weak or hoarse). Paradoxical inward movements of the chest and outward movements of the abdomen during inspiration are normal in newborns, particularly in sleep when chest compliance increases.

Episodes of periodic breathing (normal breathing for as long as 20 seconds followed by an apnoeic period of less than 10 seconds) that occur at least three times in succession[48] are normal in newborn infants. However, **apnoeas** defined as cessations of airflow for longer than 20 seconds (or associated with oxygen desaturation or bradycardia)[49] in a term neonate are commonly a manifestation of serious potentially life-threatening illnesses requiring urgent evaluation and intervention.[50]

Look carefully for other signs of respiratory distress such as nasal flaring, intercostal and subcostal chest recessions, tracheal tug and grunting. Central cyanosis occurs when the amount of deoxygenated haemoglobin is greater than 3 g / dL or so.[51] The aetiology may be a right-to-left shunt due to pulmonary or intracardiac conditions.

Central cyanosis is associated with low partial arterial oxygen pressure (P_aO_2) and a variable degree of reduction in the percentage of haemoglobin saturated with oxygen (S_aO_2), which depends on the total haemoglobin concentration.[51] For example, a severely anaemic neonate with a total haemoglobin of 8 g / dL will appear cyanosed only if the S_aO_2 is less than 63%, whereas a polycythaemic infant with a total haemoglobin of 25 g / dL will appear cyanosed with a S_aO_2 of 88%.[51] It is important to remember that peripheral cyanosis (acrocyanosis) in the first days of life is common and usually without any pathological relevance.

Chest

Test the capillary refill time by pressing your index finger onto the neonate's chest for 2 seconds. This inhibits skin perfusion and leaves a pale area, which should regain its colour (refill) within 2 seconds. A prolonged capillary refill indicates poor peripheral

CAUSES OF INCREASED CAPILLARY REFILL TIME

- Low body temperature
- Cardiac failure (consider congenital heart disease)
- Infection (pneumonia, meningitis, urinary tract infection, omphalitis)
- Anaemia (haemolysis or bleeding)
- Dehydration (feeding difficulties or vomiting)

LIST 38.6

Situs explained

Situs	Commonly associated abnormalities
Levocardia + situs inversus abdominalis	Complex congenital heart disease
Dextrocardia + situs inversus abdominalis	Primary ciliary dyskinesis
Dextrocardia + abdominal situs solitus	Atrial or ventricular septal defects

TABLE 38.7

perfusion (see List 38.6). Feel the brachial and femoral pulses on all four extremities. These will be diminished if the baby has heart failure and bounding if he or she has a patent ductus arteriosus. Coarctation of the aorta (without cardiac failure) results in weak or absent femoral pulses only.

Heart

Assess the location, size and quality of the impulse of the heart apex beat, which should be located in the fourth intercostal space approximately on the left midclavicular line in the case of the normal arrangement of the heart (left-sided, levocardia).[52] An increased size may indicate ventricular dilation, and a forceful beat ventricular hypertrophy.

Note that when the heart is on the correct side (levocardia) but the abdominal organs are inverted (situs inversus abdominalis; see Table 38.7) there is commonly congenital heart disease.[53,54] In contrast, a cardiac apex located on the right side (dextrocardia) in association with situs inversus abdominalis (situs inversus totalis) usually occurs without structural heart defects but can be associated with primary ciliary dyskinesia leading to bronchiectasis and chronic sinusitis in later life (Kartagener syndrome).[55] Dextrocardia in combination with normal arrangement of the abdominal organs (abdominal situs solitus[t]) is commonly associated with left-to-right shunts at the atrial or ventricular level.[53] Dextroposition of the heart is acquired (e.g. left diaphragmatic hernia, pneumothorax, congenital lung emphysema, congenital cystic adenomatoid malformation), in which case breath sounds on the left side are often reduced or absent.

Approximately 1% of newborns have a murmur and about half of them have structural heart defects even if they are asymptomatic.[56] A murmur may not be heard at birth and may develop after a couple of days. Conversely, it may disappear in the first hours of life (e.g. a patent ductus arteriosus) or in the first months of life (e.g. a muscular ventricular septum defect) even though the structural abnormality remains. Start by feeling for a vibration under your hand (a palpable thrill is consistent with a murmur of grade 4 or more) held onto the left upper sternal edge (pulmonary stenosis) and left lower sternal border (ventricular septal defect). A left parasternal impulse or lift may be felt with right ventricular hypertrophy (e.g. tetralogy of Fallot).

While auscultating decide whether the cardiac rhythm is regular or irregular. Count the heart rate over 15 seconds. Normal is between 120 and 160 beats per minute in an active neonate.

Proceed to auscultation of heart sounds using the diaphragm at first and then the bell of the stethoscope. At least four praecordial areas should be auscultated: the apical or mitral area (fourth intercostal space between the midclavicular and anterior axillary lines), the tricuspid area (left lower sternal border in the fourth intercostal space), the pulmonary area (left upper sternal border; second intercostal space) and the aortic area (right upper sternal border; second intercostal space).

Listen for any murmurs and if present aim at assessing the mnemonic **CARDIO**:

Character of the sound

Area of the sound where they are best heard

Radiation of the sound into other areas

[t] Solitus means accustomed or usual in Latin.

Degree or **I**ntensity of the loudness of the sound
Occurrence of the sound in the cardiac cycle.

Table 38.8 summarises potential auscultation notes for some common congenital structural heart defects.[57] Clearly, assessment of heart murmurs in infants for the purpose of identifying the underpinning structural abnormality is challenging (e.g. due to the faster heart and respiratory rate and lack of cooperation as compared with older children). Thus, the absence of a murmur in a neonate does not necessarily exclude serious cardiac disease. The sensitivity of the examination for the detection of congenital heart disease can be markedly increased when combined with measurement of peripheral cutaneous oxygen saturation (S_pO_2) employing pulse oximetry.[58]

If central cyanosis is present (see Table 38.9) or there is any doubt about its presence, perform a preductal (right arm) and postductal (either foot) S_pO_2 measurement employing pulse oximetry. These should both be 95% or above[59] but may be lower (91–96%) at altitudes greater than 2000 metres.[60]

Auscultation findings in common congenital heart diseases[58]

Cause	CARDIO	
Ventricular septal defect (3:1000 persistent [mostly membranous defect]; 50:1000 spontaneously closing [mostly muscular defect])	C	High frequency if very restrictive/small Low frequency (harsh) if moderately restrictive/large
	A	Left lower sternal border
	R	Back
	D	Systole at least grade 2 (faint but immediately audible) or greater (3 moderately loud, 4 loud with thrill, 5 audible with rim of stethoscope, 6 audible with stethoscope raised off the chest) Diastole grade 1 to 2 (out of 4)
	I	
	O	Early systolic if restrictive (small) Pansystolic murmur (moderately large) Mid-diastolic flow mitral murmur/rumble if very large
Isolated patent ductus arteriosus (1:2000 to 1:5000)	C	Machinery
	A	Left upper sternal border
	R	Suprasternal notch, left infraclavicular region +/– thrill
	D	Variable (systole grade 1 to 6)
	I	
	O	Pansystolic tricuspid valve regurgitation murmur Diastolic decrescendo pulmonic regurgitation murmur +/– systolic aortic ejection murmur; S_2 may not be audible ('buried' in the murmur)
Atrium septum defect (1:1000)	C	Harsh
	A	Systolic murmur: left upper sternal border +/– palpable click Diastolic murmur: left lower sternal border
	R	Back
	D	Systole grade 2, diastole grade 1 to 2
	I	
	O	Crescendo–decrescendo pulmonic ejection murmur Early-diastolic tricuspid flow murmur if large Loud, wide split and fixed S_2
Tetralogy of Fallot (3:10,000)	C	Harsh
	A	Left upper sternal border
	R	Lung fields, back
	D	Variable
	I	
	O	Crescendo–decrescendo pulmonic ejection murmur, single S_2

(Based on Keane JF, Lock JE, Fyler DC, Nadas AS. *Nadas' pediatric cardiology*. 2nd edn. Philadelphia: Saunders, 2006.)

TABLE 38.8

Causes of right-to-left shunt leading to central cyanosis in the first weeks of life	
Intrapulmonary (2 Ps)	Persistent pulmonary hypertension of the neonate Pulmonary arteriovenous malformations
Intracardiac (5 Ts and others)	Transposition of the great arteries Tetralogy of Fallot Total anomalous pulmonary venous return Truncus arteriosus Tricuspid atresia Ebstein's anomaly (abnormal tricuspid valve) Pulmonary atresia Hypoplastic left heart Atrioventricular canal defect

TABLE 38.9

Reduced postductal S_pO_2 indicates right-to-left shunting through a patent ductus arteriosus, which may be caused by duct-dependent congenital heart disease. This means the patent ductus is required to maintain circulation. Causes include tricuspid atresia and transposition of the great arteries. It can also be caused by duct-independent congenital heart disease such as a tetralogy of Fallot.

Blood pressure is not routinely measured in healthy neonates, but non-invasive oscillometric measurements should be performed in ill infants. However, the accuracy of this method fails in very premature hypotensive and critically ill babies and invasive measurement via an arterial catheter may thus be required.[61]

Lungs

Continue the chest examination with auscultation of the lung sounds, which are bronchovesicular (medium pitch and volume, equally in expiration and inspiration) unlike the vesicular (low pitch and soft, dominant in inspiration) sounds heard in adults.[37] Listen for reduced breath sounds, which may be due to:

- collapse (atelectasis)
- fluid collection (effusion)
- intra-alveolar fluid collection (consolidation)
- diaphragmatic hernia
- pneumothorax in pleural space
- emphysema
- obstruction.

Listen also for bronchial breath sounds, which are high-pitched, loud and dominant in expiration. They are normally present when auscultation is performed over the trachea but when heard elsewhere indicate consolidation or interstitial lung disease.

Prolonged breath sounds are a sign of airway obstruction. Added breath sounds include **stridor**, which is a harsh continuous sound often audible without the stethoscope. Stridor may be heard during inspiration if an obstruction is localised outside of the chest wall. Causes include:

- laryngomalacia[u]
- infection
- gastro-oesophageal reflux
- subglottic stenosis due to a web, cyst or haemangioma
- vocal cord paralysis
- enlarged thyroid.

Stridor that occurs during expiration may be due to intrathoracic obstruction. Causes include:

- tracheomalacia
- bronchomalacia

due, for instance, to a vascular ring.

Stridor that occurs in both expiration and inspiration may be a result of severe obstruction or obstruction at multiple sites.

Grunting is produced at the start of expiration when air is forced against a closed glottis. This is in an attempt to prevent small airway collapse during expiration by generating a positive airway pressure and is not pathognomonic for a specific condition. It may indicate (like tachypnoea, apnoeas and cyanosis) respiratory distress, which has an extremely wide range of differential diagnoses in neonates (see Table 38.10).

Wheeze is more high-pitched and musical sounding and is usually heard during expiration only. However, wheeze may also occur during inspiration (it is then called biphasic) if airway obstruction is very severe.

[u] Softening and destruction of the cartilage of the trachea.

Conditions manifesting with respiratory distress in neonates[37]		
Respiratory	Parenchymal	Respiratory distress syndrome, transient tachypnoea, pneumonia, aspiration syndrome, persistent or primary pulmonary hypertension, pulmonary oedema / haemorrhage, lung hypoplasia, lobar emphysema, interstitial lung disease
	Extraparenchymal	Nasal, laryngeal, tracheal or bronchial obstruction, pneumothorax, haemothorax, chylothorax, pleural effusion
Cardiovascular	Structural	Congenital heart disease, cardiomyopathy, large aneurysm, haemangioma, vascular malformation
	Non-structural	Septicaemia, hypovolaemia, arrhythmia, anaemia, polycythaemia, methaemoglobinaemia
Neurological	Central / cranial	Asphyxia, pain, seizure, hydrocephalus, infection (meningitis, encephalitis), haemorrhage, aneurysmal malformation, cerebrovascular accident (stroke), drugs, maternal sedation
	Peripheral	Diaphragmatic and vocal cord paralysis, neonatal myasthenia gravis, spinal muscular atrophy, drugs
Abdominal		Diaphragmatic hernia, necrotising enterocolitis, large tumours, pneumoperitoneum
Metabolic		Hypo / hyperthermia, hypoglycaemia, metabolic alkaloses (e.g. hyperammonaemia), organic aciduria, hypocalcaemia

(Based on Fletcher MA. *Physical diagnosis in neonatology*. Philadelphia: Lippincott-Raven, 1998.)

TABLE 38.10

Crackles are non-musical interrupted lung sounds of short duration that may occur at any time during inspiration or expiration. Crackles may be high-pitched (fine) or of variable pitch (coarse). They are sometimes unwisely referred to as râles or crepitations. Inspiratory crackles are produced by the abrupt opening of closed airways.[62] Thus crackles during early inspiration may be assumed to originate from the abrupt opening of larger airways, while those generated during late inspiration may stem from terminal bronchioli or alveoli (e.g. as a result of bronchiolitis or pneumonia).[63]

Percussion is not part of the routine examination in neonates but may potentially be helpful in a few circumstances (e.g. unilateral pneumothorax versus effusion).

Gastrointestinal and urogenital systems

Remove the nappy (if not done beforehand) and inspect it for the presence of meconium (first stool), which should be passed in the first 48 hours in healthy term newborns.[64]

Inspect the abdomen for vertical bulging (diastasis recti;[v] see Fig. 38.20) or general distension, which may indicate bowel obstruction. Functional causes of bowel obstruction include:

- Hirschsprung's disease
- hypoganglionosis
- neuronal intestinal dysplasia type B
- megacystis–microcolon–intestinal hypoperistalsis syndrome.

Mechanical causes include:

- duodenal atresia
- anal atresia
- meconium plug syndrome
- meconium ileus as a result of cystic fibrosis.[65]

You may be fortunate enough to see the baby vomiting. If not, ask to see any vomitus, which may have been kept by the helpful staff or parents. Bilious vomiting, in particular, raises the suspicion of the presence of gastrointestinal obstruction. However, bile is not seen if an obstruction is proximal to the ampulla of Vater[w] (causes include oesophageal atresia and proximal duodenal atresia). Early vomiting associated with respiratory distress is highly suggestive of oesophageal

[v] A weakness of the rectus sheath.

[w] The joint opening of the pancreatic and common bile duct into the distal part of the duodenum.

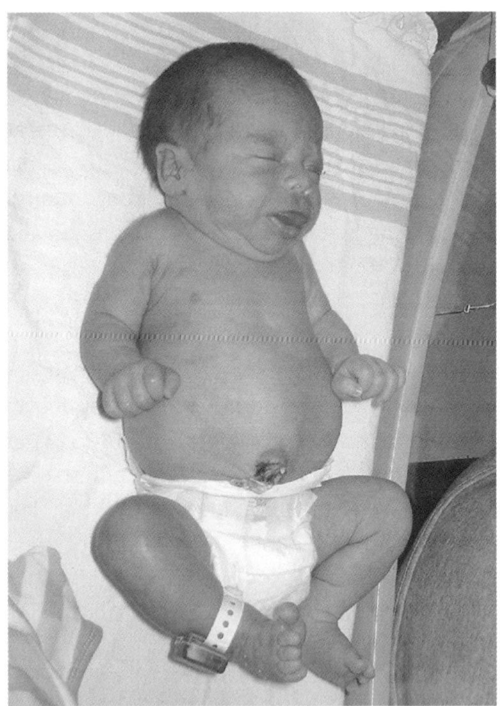

A premature newborn with Beckwith–Wiedemann syndrome, macroglossia, and rectus diastasis

(From Gleason CA, Devaskar S. *Avery's diseases of the newborn*, 9th edn. Philadelphia: Elsevier, 2012.)

FIGURE 38.20

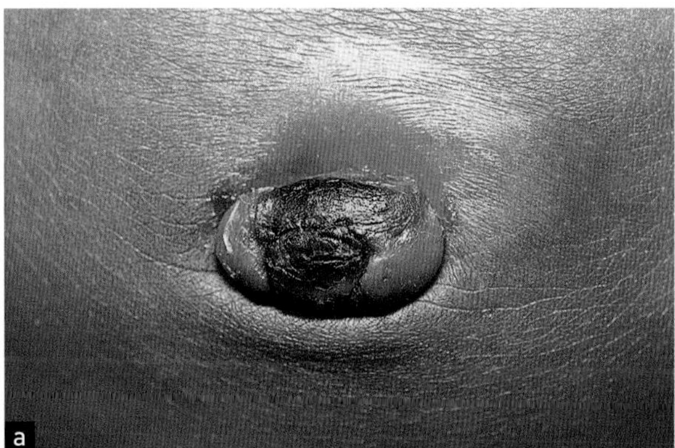

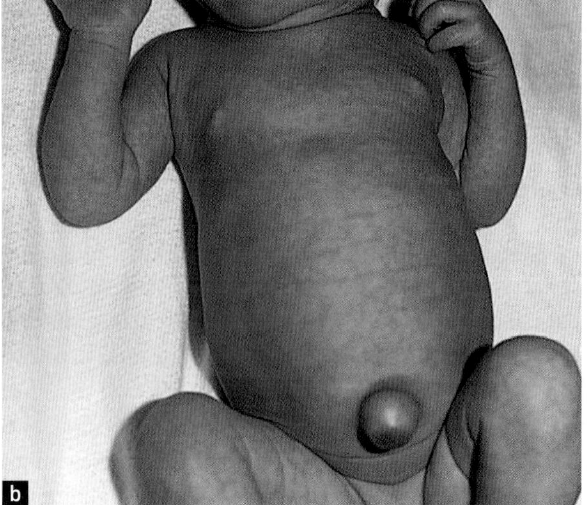

(a) Omphalitis and (b) umbilical hernia

(From (a) Püttgen KB, *Pediatric dermatology*: Expert Consult—Online and Print, Elsevier, 2013; Chapter 2, 14–67. (b) Seidel HM, Ball JW, Dains JE et al. *Mosby's guide to physical examination*, 7th edn. St Louis, MO: Mosby, 2011, pp 482–534.)

FIGURE 38.21

atresia, which is commonly associated with a tracheo-oesophageal fistula (TOF). This results in aspiration of gastric contents into the lungs.

Identify the umbilical vein (one) and the umbilical arteries (two) and look for signs of infection (omphalitis; see Fig. 38.21(a)) or an umbilical hernia (see Fig. 38.21(b)). Inspect the inguinal areas for swelling, which may indicate an inguinal hernia or the presence of an inguinal ovary or testis. Look for a concave or scaphoid contour of the abdomen, which is seen when its contents have moved into the chest as a result of a diaphragmatic hernia.

Look carefully for the presence and position of the anus, as the presence of faeces does not exclude anal atresia.

Palpate the abdomen gently for masses, which may be a result of organomegaly or tumours. Palpate the liver, which can be felt up to 2 centimetres below the rib cage on the right side, while the tip of the spleen may be felt below the left rib cage in healthy newborns with situs solitus abdominalis. Feel for abdominal masses and the bladder. The upper edge of a full bladder can be verified with percussion and should be below the umbilicus; otherwise, further investigations for causes leading to urinary retention (e.g. urethral valves, drugs, dysraphic spinal lesion) and appropriate intervention are urgently warranted. Inspect the back for spinal dysraphism (spina bifida).

Percuss the abdomen. Masses and fluid have a dull percussion note, whereas an obstructed abdomen will generally be resonant.

Next listen for bowel sounds. They should be easily heard. They may be increased if there is mechanical bowel obstruction or heard clearly in the chest if the baby has a diaphragmatic hernia. Auscultate for renal bruits.

Inguinal region and genitals

If an inguinal hernia has been seen on inspection an attempt should be made to see whether it is reducible, using gentle pressure in the direction of the inguinal canal. However, if the hernia is non-reducible or appears to be painful, incarceration of herniated bowel, ovary or testis should be considered (a surgical emergency). Advise parents to be very vigilant for reducibility and pain if a hernia is detected.

If the scrotum is empty and an inguinal or suprascrotal testis (size 1.0–1.5 centimetres) can be palpated, try carefully to manipulate the testis into the scrotum. A retractable testis that remains in the scrotum for some time is a normal finding. A testis that immediately returns into the original position is an undescended testis, which requires further management to prevent infertility and increased risk for malignancy. If a testis is impalpable that may be because it is located in the abdomen (undescended), too small to be found by you (atrophic) or absent (e.g. in combination with ambiguous genitalia, see below).

Scrotum and penis

Examine the scrotum. Discoloration of the scrotum may occur as a result of ischaemia due to testicular torsion, which is another surgical emergency. A large painless fluctuant scrotum can be assessed with a torch (see Fig. 18.11 on p 315) to demonstrate translucency of light due to fluid accumulation (hydrocele). This occurs in 2%–5% of baby boys. It often resolves spontaneously in the first year of life but may require correction if persistent.

Examine the penis. A length of less than 2.5 centimetres is abnormal. Do not withdraw the foreskin (prepuce) for routine inspection of the urethral meatus because adherence to the glans penis is normal in infants. However, an abnormal opening of the prepuce on the ventral side of the penis is often associated with malposition of the urethral meatus (hypospadias). The urethral meatus should also be inspected if there is bending of the penis (chordee) or the neonate does not pass urine. A urethral meatus that opens at the dorsum of the penis in association with a marked chordee is a severe but rare penile abnormality that requires urgent assessment of associated renal tract abnormalities (by ultrasound).

Female genitalia

Inspect the female genitalia for the presence of normal labia majora, which should not be fused but cover the labia minora in term newborns. The clitoris is found at the upper border of the labia minora and the urethra is visible below, with the hymen below that. Inspect for any skin tags or mucoid cysts. Effects of maternal hormones regularly cause mucoid vaginal discharge, occasionally mixed with blood, which is normal in the first days of life.

Ambiguous genitalia

Ambiguous genitalia are a medical emergency. Congenital adrenal hyperplasia (CAH) secondary to 21-hydroxylase deficiency (less commonly 11-hydroxylase, 3β-hydroxysteroid dehydrogenase) causes overvirilisation (labial fusion, clitoral enlargement, joint vagina and urethra [urogenital sinus]) leading to masculinised external genitalia in female (karyotype 46, XX) neonates. Babies with 21-hydroxylase deficiency are at risk of life-threatening salt wasting.

Neonates with syndromes such as Smith–Lemli–Opitz (microcephaly, syndactyly, cleft palate, hypospadias, growth retardation) and **VACTERL** (**v**ertebral abnormalities, **a**nal atresia, **c**ardiac abnormalities, **T**OF, oesophageal atresia, **r**enal abnormalities, **l**imb defects) may show variable degrees of genital ambiguity.

Musculoskeletal system

Limbs

Examine the upper and lower limbs for symmetry, in particular symmetry of the leg creases (asymmetry is a sign of congenital hip dysplasia; see Fig. 38.22), muscle bulk, range of motion and strength. Look for spontaneous symmetrical movements and consider nerve damage or long-bone fractures sustained during

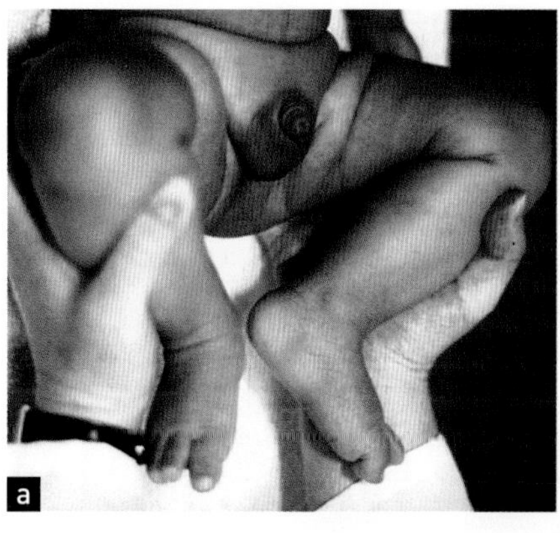

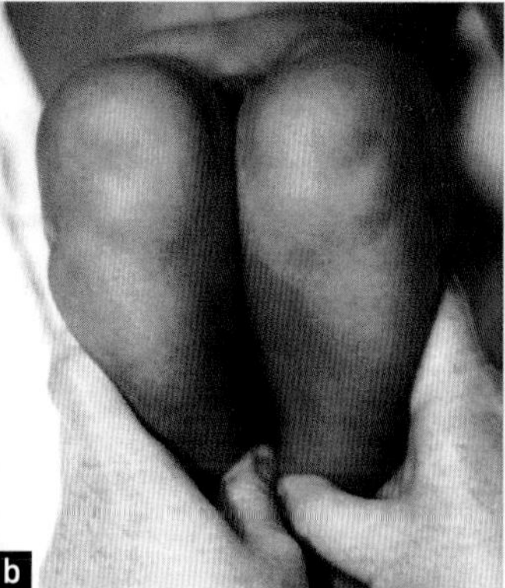

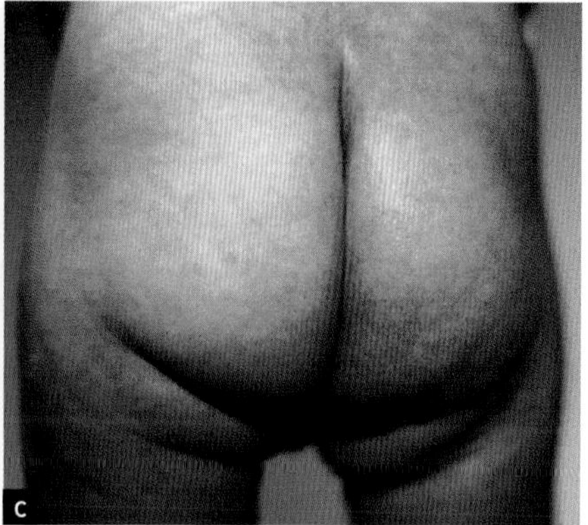

Developmental dysplasia of the hip in an older infant with rigid spine myopathy. Aberrantly increased muscular forces resulted in postnatal hip dislocation, evident as (a) tight hips with limited abduction, (b) upper leg length discrepancy with uneven knee height and (c) asymmetric thigh creases

(From Graham JM. *Smith's recognizable patterns of human deformation*. Philadelphia: Elsevier, 2007, pp 69–76.)

FIGURE 38.22

the birth process (clavicle and humeral fractures are the most common). Compared with term infants, premature infants are at higher risk of birth-associated fractures, particularly multiple fractures.[66]

Upper limbs

Examine the hands and forearms for dysmorphic features. Causes of anomalies can be genetic (e.g. Diamond–Blackfan anaemia), environmental (amniotic bands, congenital infection) or unknown. Around half of all cases with multiple anomalies will be due to a known syndrome and more than a hundred recognised syndromes are described with hand anomalies (see Table 38.11, Fig. 38.23).[67,68] The term *malformation* is preferred if the cause of the anomaly is unknown.

When examining the hands, remember to examine each hand separately and then both hands together to compare them, particularly when checking for size disparity (e.g. hemihyperplasia). On the dorsal surface, examine the skin, joints and nails before turning the hands over to examine the palms, taking particular care to check the palmar creases. Gently move the wrist and finger joints through their respective ranges of motion, looking for flexibility, asymmetry and any unusual positions.

Lower limbs

As with the hands, systematically examine the skin, joints and nails of the feet before moving on to the soles of each foot. Examine for symmetry and any unusual positioning or skinfolds, and gently move each joint through its respective ranges of motion. Common newborn foot abnormalities include:

- metatarsus adductus
- clubfoot deformity
- calcaneovalgus (flexible flatfoot)
- congenital vertical talus (rigid flatfoot)
- multiple digital deformities (polydactyly, syndactyly)
- overlapping toes
- amniotic bands.[69]

It is particularly important in children with congenital foot deformities that careful and repeated hip examinations are performed, as developmental dysplasia of the hip or acetabular dysplasia is commonly seen in these patients.

Metatarsus adductus (MTA) is a transverse plane deformity in the tarsometatarsal joints, in which the metatarsals are deviated medially (see Fig. 38.24(a) and (b)). It is particularly seen in breech

Proposed classification of upper limb malformations[67] and frequencies[68]

Type	Malformations
Type I: Failure of formation: Transverse arrest Longitudinal arrest	Amputations at any level from shoulder to phalanx (7%) Preaxial: varying degrees of hypoplasia of the thumb (4%) or radius (1%) Central: divided into typical and atypical types of cleft hand Postaxial: varying degrees of ulnar hypoplasia to hypothenar hypoplasia Intercalated longitudinal arrest: various types of phocomelia* (<1%)
Type II: Failure of differentiation: Soft tissue Skeletal Tumourous conditions	Syndactyly (18%; see Fig. 38.23(a)), trigger thumb, Poland syndrome (2%), camptodactyly** (7%; see Fig. 38.23(b)) Radioulnar synostosis (1%), carpal coalitions Include all vascular and neurological malformations
Type III: Duplication	Applies to whole limb, mirror hand, polydactyly (15%; see Fig. 38.23(c) and (d))
Type IV: Overgrowth	Hemihypertrophy and macrodactyly (1%)
Type V: Undergrowth	Brachydactyly (5%), radial hypoplasia (<1%), brachysyndactyly
Type VI: Constriction band syndromes	Involves amputation at any level (2%) with or without distal lymphoedema
Type VII: Generalised anomalies and syndromes	Clinodactyly*** (6%; see Fig. 38.23(e))

**This is abnormal development of the arms or legs but with hands and feet still present.*
***Fixed flexion at one or both phalangeal joints.*
****Abnormal bending of the fingers or toes.*

(Canale ST, Beaty JH, Campbell WC. *Campbell's operative orthopaedics*, 12th edn. St Louis, MO: Elsevier/Mosby, 2013; and Flatt AE. *The care of congenital hand anomalies*, 2nd edn. St Louis, MO: Quality Medical, 1994.)

TABLE 38.11

presentations and in oligohydramnios babies. In the mild form, the forefoot can be passively abducted to the midline and the condition resolves without treatment. A quick test for MTA is to place the heel

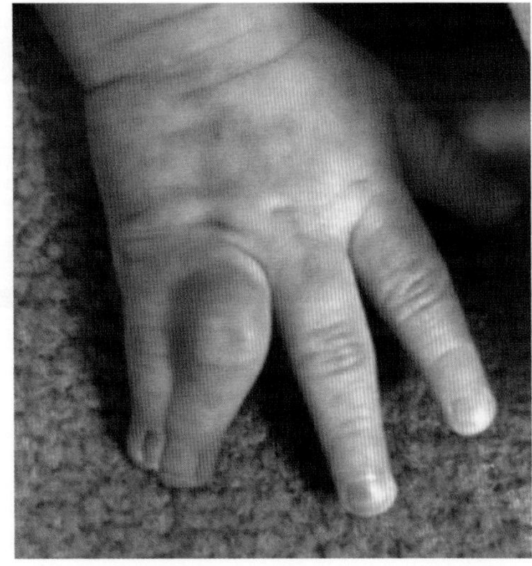

Clinical photograph of complex syndactyly. Note both the flexion posture of the ring finger and the synonychia between the ring and little fingers

(From Charles A, Goldfarb MD, Jennifer A, Steffen BS, Christopher M, Stutz MD. Complex syndactyly: aesthetic and objective outcomes. *J Hand Surg* 2012; 37(10) 2068–2073, Copyright ©2012 American Society for Surgery of the Hand.)

FIGURE 38.23

of the neonate's foot between your index and middle fingers and to observe the lateral aspect of the foot from the plantar side for medial or lateral deviation from your middle finger. Medial deviation indicates MTA.[69]

Clubfoot (talipes equinovarus) (see Fig. 38.24(c)) is another relatively common condition. The four basic components can be remembered by the mnemonic CAVE:

C avus
A dduction
V arus[x]
E quinus.[y]

This varies in severity from mild positional clubfoot (passively correctable) to severe clubfoot with extreme,

[x] Varus is displacement or angulation towards the midline of the body; valgus is the opposite.
[y] In severe cases the foot looks like that of a horse.

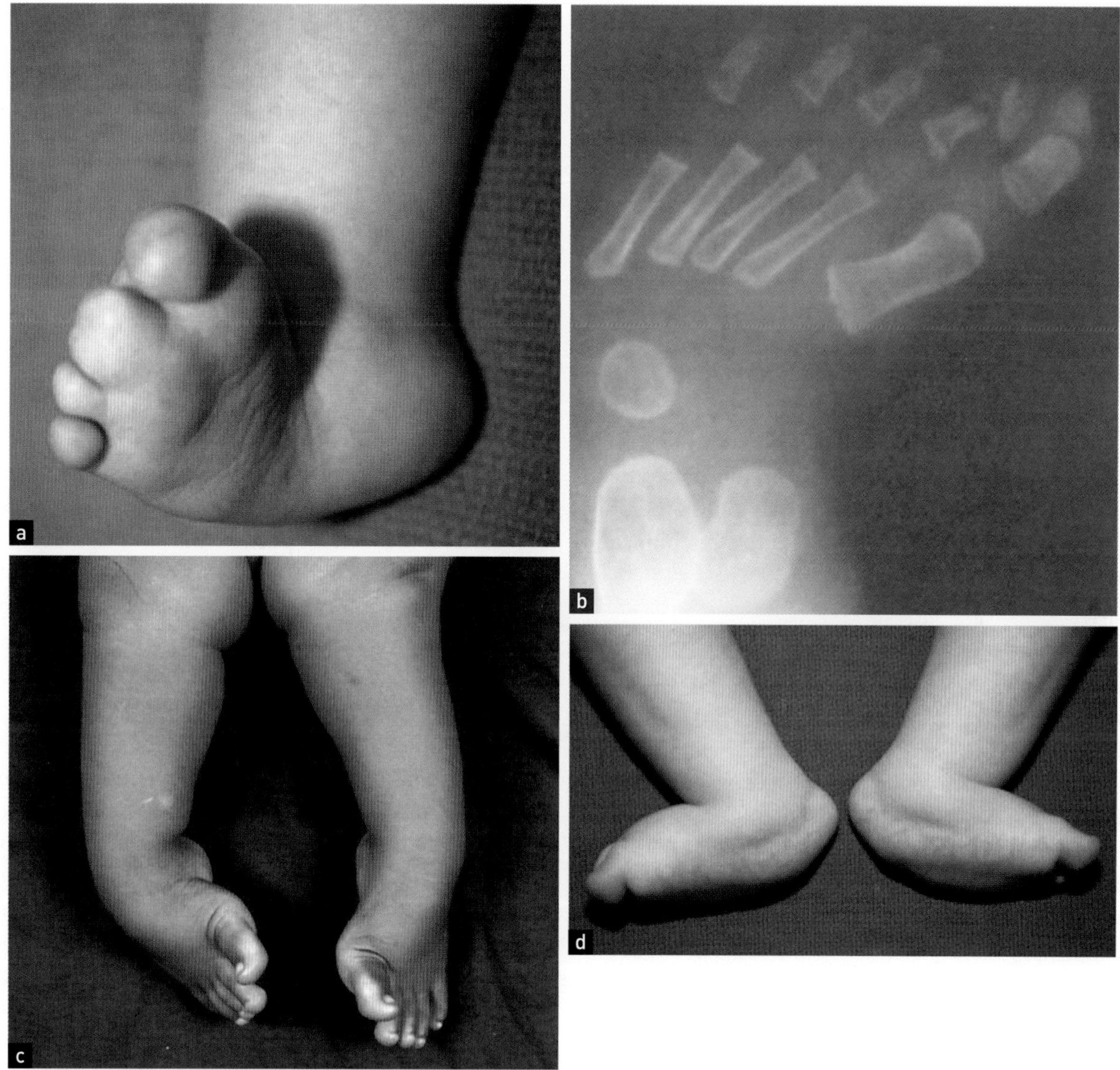

(a) and (b) Metatarsus adductus (severe); (c) talipes equinovarus; and (d) congenital vertical talus

((a), (b) and (d) from Canale ST, Beaty J. *Campbell's operative orthopaedics*, 12th edn. St Louis, MO: Mosby, 2012; (c) from Kliegman RM, Stanton BMD. *Nelson textbook of pediatrics*, 19th edn. Philadelphia: Saunders, 2011.)

FIGURE 38.24

rigid hindfoot equinus. On examination, the foot appears small, with a flexible, soft heel that is internally rotated so as to make the soles of the feet face each other. All patients exhibit calf atrophy, and internal tibial torsion and shortening of the ipsilateral extremity may be seen.

Calcaneovalgus foot is seen in up to 30%–50% of newborns secondary to in utero positioning. The newborn typically presents with a dorsiflexed and everted foot; the dorsum may occasionally be in contact with the anterolateral surface of the lower leg. If there is a full passive range of motion present at birth, then no active treatment is required, but gentle stretching may be required if there is restriction of movement. In severe cases, casting may be considered.

Rocker-bottom foot (congenital vertical talus) is a rare foot deformity where the midfoot is dorsally dislocated on the hindfoot (see Fig. 38.24(d)). Although approximately 60% of cases are idiopathic, up to 40% are associated with an underlying neuromuscular condition or syndrome.[69] On examination, it is noted that the plantar surface of the foot is convex, with a prominent talar head along the medial border of the midfoot. The fore part of the foot is dorsiflexed and abducted relative to the hindfoot, and the hindfoot is in equinus and valgus. Examine closely for any coexisting neurological or musculoskeletal abnormalities (e.g. arthrogryposis and meningomyelocele). This does not respond to stretching, and usually requires surgery.

Hips

The hip examination is of critical importance to check for **developmental dysplasia of the hip (DDH)**. It has been estimated that approximately 15% of DDH is not detectable at birth, even by experienced examiners or ultrasonographers.[70] Careful repeated examination of the infant in the first year of life by a skilled practitioner is crucial. Be aware of the increased risk of DDH seen in breech deliveries, girls and babies who have a positive family history of this condition. The rationale and importance of repeated examination needs to be explained to parents prior to the examination. Examination of the hips is often best left until the end of the neonatal examination, as it can be distressing to the child (and parents!).[z]

After inspecting the lower limbs, perform the Ortolani and Barlow tests (see below). Ensure that the baby is relaxed and undressed and lying supine. Examine each hip individually, with your free hand stabilising the contralateral side of the pelvis. Very little force is required for each of these manoeuvres. Forceful and repeated examinations can damage the femoral head. A high-pitched 'click' may be heard during these manoeuvres. This is often musculoskeletal or ligamentous in origin and is usually of no clinical significance. If the examination is equivocal, or the baby is at increased risk of DDH, then sonography at 6 weeks is recommended.

Ortolani test: this is performed to elicit the sensation of the dislocated hip being reduced. The hip is flexed to 90° with the knee resting in the palm of your hand. Place your index and middle fingers along the greater trochanter and your thumb on the inner thigh. Hold the leg in a neutral position. Gently abduct the hip while lifting the leg anteriorly. A positive Ortolani sign is when a 'clunk' is felt as the dislocated femoral head reduces into the acetabulum.

Barlow provocation test: this is performed to detect the unstable hip dislocating from the acetabulum. It is performed with your hands in the same positions as for the Ortolani test, with the hips flexed to 90°. The leg is adducted while posteriorly directed pressure is placed on the knee. A positive Barlow's sign occurs when a palpable 'clunk' or sensation of movement is felt as the femoral head exits the acetabulum posteriorly.

Central and peripheral nervous systems

Examine for tone and positioning taking into account the gestational age of the neonate. The normal term infant will usually position him- or herself with the hips abducted and slightly flexed, knees flexed, upper limbs adducted with flexion at the elbows and hands softly clenched (the well-known 'fetal position'). The hypotonic infant (and the preterm infant) often adopts a 'frog-like' position with abducted hips and extended elbows (see Fig. 38.25). Very premature infants (less than 30 weeks) will have very minimal flexor tone, and this will develop first in the lower limbs and then in the upper limbs (between 34 and 36 weeks' corrected age).[aa]

Another quick check for tone is to suspend the baby in a ventral position, lying supported over your hand and forearm (see Fig. 38.26). There should be some resistance to gravity in the normal baby, whereas the hypotonic baby will flop like a rag-doll. Bear in mind that following a feed even a normal term infant may appear slightly hypotonic, and repeat examination is suggested.

[z] In fact, most parts of the neonatal examination seem best left to the end.

[aa] For babies up to at least 2 years of age, subtract the number of weeks the baby was premature from its age (and for longer in the extremely premature infant).

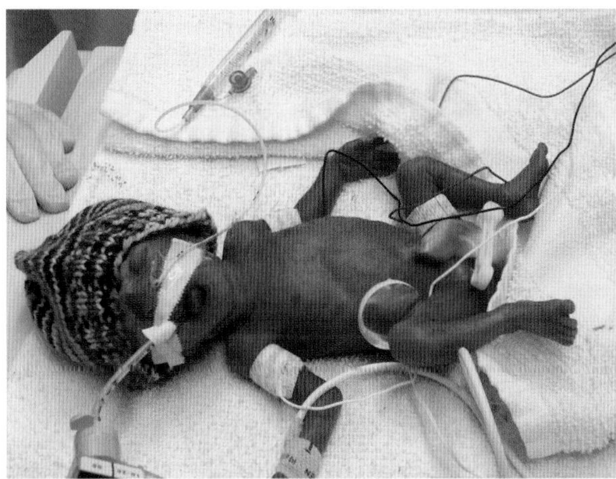

The 'frog-like' position in the extreme premature infant

FIGURE 38.25

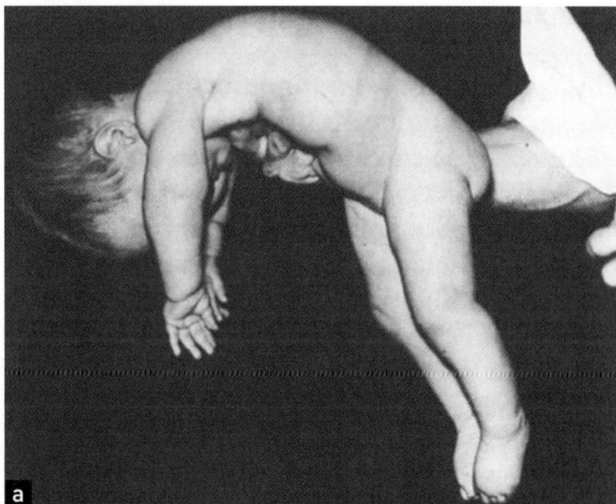

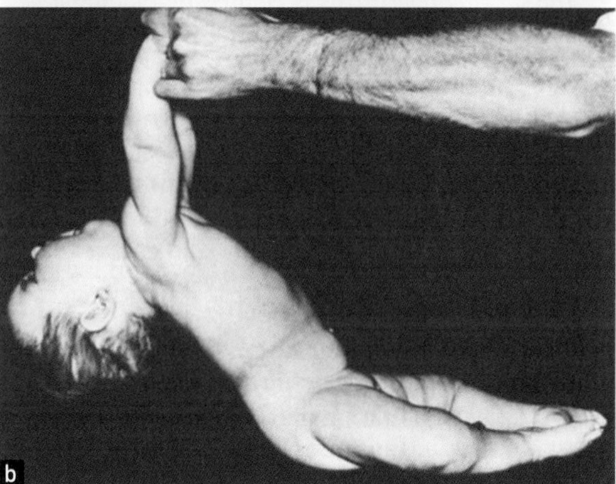

Type 1 spinal muscular atrophy (Werdnig–Hoffmann disease). Clinical manifestations of weakness of limb and axial musculature in a 6-week-old infant with severe weakness and hypotonia from birth. Note the marked weakness of (a) the limbs and trunk on ventral suspension and (b) of neck on pull to sit

(From Volpe J. *Neurology of the newborn*, 5th edn. Philadelphia: Saunders, 2008, Figure 18.2, p 771.)

FIGURE 38.26

Developmental reflexes

Examination of the developmental (or primitive) reflexes can be disturbing for the baby and should join the queue at the end of the neonatal examination. The most commonly elicited reflex in newborns is the Moro reflex, but it is useful to check others including grasp, tonic neck and the Galant reflex. Again, explain the examination in detail to the parents and perform the various manoeuvres while they are present if possible. It is a great opportunity for parents to experience their baby's developmental maturity and responsiveness even if these reflexes are mediated at the brainstem or spinal cord level.

The following reflexes are usually all present in the normal term infant.[71]

- *The Moro reflex:* this can be elicited by suddenly allowing the infant to fall back from a semierect position to supine with the head supported in your hand (carefully, and preferably over a soft surface, just in case). The infant will abduct and extend the arms and open the hands, and then flex them. This is seen in newborns from about 32 weeks' gestation and usually disappears between 3 and 6 months of age. Warn the parents that this manoeuvre may be accompanied by an audible cry. Absence of this reflex usually signifies dysfunction of the central nervous system and is an ominous sign that mandates investigation. Unilateral absence may indicate brachial plexus palsy or fractures.
- *The stepping reflex:* this can be elicited by holding the infant vertically with the feet on a flat surface. The infant will then alternatively flex and extend the legs initiating a slow stepping

action. This is seen from about 32 weeks' gestation and disappears by around 1–2 months of age. The significance of this reflex is not entirely clear.[72]

- *The Galant reflex:* this is elicited by stroking gently down either side of the spine from the thorax to the sacrum while the baby is held in ventral suspension. The infant's trunk and hips will move towards the side of the stimulus. This gives some indication of segmental integrity from T2 to S1.[73] This reflex is usually present by 32 weeks' gestation and disappears by around 2–4 months of age.
- *The sucking reflex:* this is elicited by placing a gloved finger in the infant's mouth to evaluate the coordination and strength of the suck. A firm grip should be felt on the finger and a strong seal formed by the newborn's lips. This usually appears by 28 weeks' gestation and disappears by around 3–4 months of age.
- *The rooting reflex:* this is elicited by stroking along the infant's cheek towards the corner of the mouth. The head will turn towards the stimulus and the mouth will open. This is usually present by 34 weeks' gestation and disappears by around 3–4 months of age.
- *The grasp reflex/palmar grasp:* this is elicited by placing your index finger into the infant's palm. When you attempt to withdraw your finger, the infant should tighten his or her grasp—so much so that the term infant can be lifted off the bed for a few seconds. This reflex is usually present by 26 weeks' gestation, although fetal palmar reflex grasping of the umbilical cord is often seen on routine ultrasound examination from around 16 weeks' gestation.[74] The reflex usually disappears by around 3 months of age. The absence of this reflex usually reflects peripheral or spinal cord involvement, particularly if it is asymmetrical.[74]
- *The plantar grasp:* this is elicited by pressing your thumb against the sole of the infant's foot, just behind the toes. The infant should flex and adduct the toes. Alternatively, the infant can be held vertically and the feet stimulated by floor contact. Again, the toes should flex and adduct. This reflex is usually present by 30 weeks' gestation and disappears between 10 and 15 months of age. A reduced or negative plantar grasp reflex during early infancy can be a sensitive indicator of later development of spasticity.[74]
- *The asymmetric tonic neck reflex (ATNR):* this is elicited by turning the infant's head to the side. There should be extension of the upper extremity on the side to which the head and neck are turned and flexion of the contralateral upper extremity (the fencing posture). The lower extremity responds similarly, but is much less striking. This reflex is usually present by 35 weeks' gestation and disappears by around 6 months of age.[72] When this is seen as a resting posture, it is never normal.

Gestational age

The gestational age can be determined by fetal ultrasound, maternal menstrual cycle and postnatal neuromuscular and physical maturation. Although not performed routinely,[75] if there are doubts about the exact gestational age (e.g. late recognition of pregnancy), use the New Ballard Score (NBS)[75] for postnatal estimation of gestational age in neonates up to 1 week old.[76]

T&O'C ESSENTIALS

1. *Babies cannot cooperate with the examiner and their examination must be performed as the opportunity occurs.*
2. *The parents must be involved at all stages and nothing should be done without their being informed.*
3. *Parts of the examination may be performed while the mother nurses the baby.*
4. *Do not let the baby get cold or fall off the examination table.*
5. *Taking serial measurements and charting these results are essential for monitoring a baby's progress.*

Continued

T&O'C ESSENTIALS *continued*

6. *Always remember to look for asymmetry—a vital guide to abnormality.*
7. *Certain congenital abnormalities must always be looked for (e.g. hip dysplasia, spina bifida).*
8. *A below-normal temperature is a significant sign of acute illness.*
9. *If the baby's parent says that the baby is sick, take this very seriously.*

OSCE REVISION TOPICS – **THE NEONATAL HISTORY AND EXAMINATION**

Use these topics, which commonly occur in the OSCE, to help with revision.

1. Take a history of the pregnancy from these new parents and any risk factors for their baby in their own history. (p 719)
2. Talk to this mother about the delivery of her baby. (p 720)
3. Chart this baby's size and weight and discuss the results. (p 724)
4. This neonate has some dysmorphic features. Please examine him. (pp 723, 741, 744, 753)
5. Examine this baby's primitive reflexes. (p 757)
6. Examine this baby's chest. She has had some problems with her breathing. (p 746)
7. This baby has a murmur. Please examine her. (p 747)
8. This baby's family think his feet look abnormal. Please examine him. (p 753)

References

1. Morris T. *Cultural aspects of birthing*, 2011. Sydney: NSW Government.
2. Weintrob N, Karp M, Hod M. Short- and long-range complications in offspring of diabetic mothers. *J Diabetes Complications* 1996; 10(5):294–301.
3. Fitzpatrick DL, Russell MA. Diagnosis and management of thyroid disease in pregnancy. *Obstet Gynecol Clin North Am* 2010; 37(2):173–193.
4. Smyth A, Oliveira GHM, Lahr BD et al. A systematic review and meta-analysis of pregnancy outcomes in patients with systemic lupus erythematosus and lupus nephritis. *Clin J Am Soc Nephrol* 2010; 5(11):2060–2068.
5. Namazy JA, Murphy VE, Powell H et al. Effects of asthma severity, exacerbations and oral corticosteroids on perinatal outcomes. *Eur Respir J* 2013; 41(5):1082–1090.
6. Lenke RR, Levy HL. Maternal phenylketonuria and hyperphenylalaninemia. An international survey of the outcome of untreated and treated pregnancies. *N Engl J Med* 1980; 303(21):1202–1208.
7. Hernandez-Diaz S, Smith CR, Shen A et al. Comparative safety of antiepileptic drugs during pregnancy. *Neurology* 2012; 78(21):1692–1699.
8. Jefferies AL. Selective serotonin reuptake inhibitors in pregnancy and infant outcomes. *Paediatr Child Health* 2011; 16(9):562–563.
9. Gilbert GL. 1: Infections in pregnant women. *Med J Aust* 2002; 176(5):229–236.
10. Cutland CL, Schrag SJ, Zell ER et al. Maternal HIV infection and vertical transmission of pathogenic bacteria. *Pediatrics* 2012; 130(3):e581–e590.
11. Montoya JG, Rosso F. Diagnosis and management of toxoplasmosis. *Clin Perinatol* 2005; 32(3):705–726.
12. Janakiraman V. Listeriosis in pregnancy: diagnosis, treatment, and prevention. *Rev Obstet Gynecol* 2008; 1(4):179–185.
13. Cherpes TL, Matthews DB, Maryak SA. Neonatal herpes simplex virus infection. *Clin Obstet Gynecol* 2012; 55(4):938–944.
14. Wong S, Ordean A, Kahan M. Substance use in pregnancy. *J Obstet Gynaecol Can* 2011; 33(4):367–384.
15. Apgar V. A proposal for a new method of evaluation of the newborn infant. *Curr Res Anesth Analg* 1953; 32(4):260–267.
16. Opiyo N, English M. What clinical signs best identify severe illness in young infants aged 0–59 days in developing countries? A systematic review. *Arch Dis Child* 2011; 96(11):1052–1059.
17. Bang AT, Bang RA, Reddy MH et al. Simple clinical criteria to identify sepsis or pneumonia in neonates in the community needing treatment or referral. *Pediatr Infect Dis J* 2005; 24(4):335–341.
18. Young Infants Clinical Signs Study Group. Clinical signs that predict severe illness in children under age 2 months: a multicentre study. *Lancet* 2008; 371(9607):135–142.
19. Robinson JN, Abuhamad AN. Abdominal wall and umbilical cord anomalies. *Clin Perinatol* 2000; 27(4):947–978, ix.
20. National Health Service. Newborn and infant physical examination screening: standards. 2008, updated April 2016. www.gov.uk/government/publications/newborn-and-infant-physical-examination-screening-standards.
21. Polin RA, Denson S, Brady MT. Strategies for prevention of health care-associated infections in the NICU. *Pediatrics* 2012; 129(4):e1085–e1093.
22. Babson SG, Benda GI. Growth graphs for the clinical assessment of infants of varying gestational age. *J Pediatr* 1976; 89(5):814–820.
23. Lubchenco LO, Hansman C, Boyd E. Intrauterine growth in length and head circumference as estimated from live births at gestational ages from 26 to 42 weeks. *Pediatrics* 1966; 37(3):403–408.
24. Dancis J, O'Connell JR, Holt LE. A grid for recording the weight of premature infants. *J Pediatr* 1948; 33(11):570–572.
25. Myrelid A, Gustafsson J, Ollars B, Annerén G. Growth charts for Down's syndrome from birth to 18 years of age. *Arch Dis Child* 2002; 87(2):97–103.
26. American Institute of Ultrasound in Medicine; American College of Radiology; Society for Pediatric Radiology; Society of Radiologists in Ultrasound. AIUM practice guideline for the performance of an ultrasound examination of the neonatal spine. *J Ultrasound Med* 2012; 31(1):155–164.
27. Kriss VM, Desai NS. Occult spinal dysraphism in neonates: assessment of high-risk cutaneous stigmata on sonography. *Am J Roentgenol* 1998; 171(6):1687–1692.
28. Moss C. Genetic skin disorders. *Semin Neonatol* 2000; 5(4):311–320.
29. Bruckner AL, Frieden IJ. Hemangiomas of infancy. *J Am Acad Dermatol* 2003; 48(4):477–493; quiz 494–496.
30. Kaplan M, Hammarman C. Neonatal hyperbilirubinaemia. In Polin RA, Yoder MC (eds) *Workbook in Practical Neonatology*, 4th edn, Ch 5. Philadelphia: Saunders, 2007.

31. Furdon SA, Clark DA. Scalp hair characteristics in the newborn infant. *Adv Neonatal Care* 2003; 3(6):286–296.
32. Davies DP, Ansari BM, Cooke TJ. Anterior fontanelle size in the neonate. *Arch Dis Child* 1975; 50(1):81–83.
33. Popich GA, Smith DW. Fontanels: range of normal size. *J Pediatr* 1972; 80(5):749–752.
34. Chen MY, Liu HM, Weng WC et al. Neonate with severe heart failure related to vein of Galen malformation. *Pediatr Neonatol* 2010; 51(4):245–248.
35. Brown RL. Samba San: the Japanese midwife. *Midwives Chron* 1970; 83(993):344–345.
36. Roth DA, Hildesheimer M, Bardenstein S et al. Preauricular skin tags and ear pits are associated with permanent hearing impairment in newborns. *Pediatrics* 2008; 122(4):e884–e890.
37. Fletcher MA. *Physical diagnosis in neonatology*. Philadelphia: Lippincott-Raven, 1998.
38. Roberts DG, Johnson CE, Carlin SA et al. Resolution of middle ear effusion in newborns. *Arch Pediatr Adolesc Med* 1995; 149(8):873–877.
39. Capasso A, Capasso L, Raimondi F et al. A nontraumatic and inexpensive clinical maneuver to check nasal patency at birth. *Pediatrics* 2001; 107(1):214.
40. Singh DJ, Bartlett SP. Congenital mandibular hypoplasia: analysis and classification. *J Craniofac Surg* 2005; 16(2):291–300.
41. Nwoku AL, Kekere-Ekun TA. Congenital ankylosis of the mandible. Report of a case noted at birth. *J Maxillofac Surg* 1986; 14(3):150–152.
42. Baumgart M, Lussi A. Natal and neonatal teeth. *Schweiz Monatsschr Zahnmed* 2006; 116(9):894–909.
43. Ballard JL, Auer CE, Khoury JC. Ankyloglossia: assessment, incidence, and effect of frenuloplasty on the breastfeeding dyad. *Pediatrics* 2002; 110(5):e63.
44. Koeller KK, Alamo L, Adair CF, Smirniotopoulos JG. Congenital cystic masses of the neck: radiologic–pathologic correlation. *Radiographics* 1999; 19(1):121–146; quiz 152–153.
45. Park YW. Evaluation of neck masses in children. *Am Fam Physician* 1995; 51(8):1904–1912.
46. Bamji M, Stone RK, Kaul A et al. Palpable lymph nodes in healthy newborns and infants. *Pediatrics* 1986; 78(4):573–575.
47. Haller JA, Kramer SS, Lietman SA. Use of CT scans in selection of patients for pectus excavatum surgery: a preliminary report. *J Pediatr Surg* 1987; 22(10):904–906.
48. Kelly DH, Shannon DC. Periodic breathing in infants with near-miss sudden infant death syndrome. *Pediatrics* 1979; 63(3):355–360.
49. Committee on Fetus and Newborn. American Academy of Pediatrics. Apnea, sudden infant death syndrome, and home monitoring. *Pediatrics* 2003; 111(4 Pt 1):914–917.
50. Duke T, Oa O, Mokela D et al. The management of sick young infants at primary health centres in a rural developing country. *Arch Dis Child* 2005; 90(2):200–205.
51. Sasidharan P. An approach to diagnosis and management of cyanosis and tachypnea in term infants. *Pediatr Clin North Am* 2004; 51(4):999–1021, ix.
52. Antia AU, Maxwell SR, Gough A, Ayeni O. Position of the apex beat in childhood. *Arch Dis Child* 1978; 53(7):585–589.
53. Perloff JK. *The clinical recognition of congenital heart disease*. Philadelphia: Saunders, 2003.
54. Gindes L, Hegesh J, Barkai G et al. Isolated levocardia: prenatal diagnosis, clinical importance, and literature review. *J Ultrasound Med* 2007; 26(3):361–365.
55. Le Mauviel L. Primary ciliary dyskinesia. *West J Med* 1991; 155(3):280–283.
56. Ainsworth S, Wyllie JP, Wren C. Prevalence and clinical significance of cardiac murmurs in neonates. *Arch Dis Child Fetal Neonatal Ed* 1999; 80(1):F43–F45.
57. Keane JF, Lock JE, Fyler DC, Nadas AS. *Nadas' pediatric cardiology*. Philadelphia: Saunders, 2006.
58. Bakr AF, Habib HS. Combining pulse oximetry and clinical examination in screening for congenital heart disease. *Pediatr Cardiol* 2005; 26(6):832–835.
59. de-Wahl Granelli A, Wennergren M, Sandberg K et al. Impact of pulse oximetry screening on the detection of duct dependent congenital heart disease: a Swedish prospective screening study in 39,821 newborns. *BMJ* 2009; 338:a3037.
60. Ravert P, Detwiler TL, Dickinson JK. Mean oxygen saturation in well neonates at altitudes between 4498 and 8150 feet. *Adv Neonatal Care* 2011; 11(6):412–417.
61. Takci S, Yigit S, Korkmaz A, Yurdakök M. Comparison between oscillometric and invasive blood pressure measurements in critically ill premature infants. *Acta Paediatr* 2012; 101(2):132–135.
62. Forgacs P. Crackles and wheezes. *Lancet* 1967; 2(7508):203–205.
63. Nath AR, Capel LH. Inspiratory crackles and mechanical events of breathing. *Thorax* 1974; 29(6):695–698.
64. Clark DA. Times of first void and first stool in 500 newborns. *Pediatrics* 1977; 60(4):457–459.
65. Loening-Baucke V, Kimura K. Failure to pass meconium: diagnosing neonatal intestinal obstruction. *Am Fam Physician* 1999; 60(7):2043–2050.
66. Wei C, Stevens J, Harrison S et al. Fractures in a tertiary neonatal intensive care unit in Wales. *Acta Paediatr* 2012; 101(6):587–590.
67. Canale ST, Beaty JH. *Campbell's operative orthopaedics: hand surgery*. St Louis, MO: Mosby, 2012.
68. Flatt AE. *The care of congenital hand anomalies*, 2nd edn. St Louis, MO: Quality Medical Pub, 1994.
69. Gore AI, Spencer JP. The newborn foot. *Am Fam Physician* 2004; 69(4):865–872.
70. Cady RB. Developmental dysplasia of the hip: definition, recognition, and prevention of late sequelae. *Pediatr Ann* 2006; 35(2):92–101.
71. Zafeiriou DI. Primitive reflexes and postural reactions in the neurodevelopmental examination. *Pediatric Neurology* 2004; 31(1):1–8.
72. Volpe JJ, Inder T, Darras B et al. *Neurology of the newborn*, 6th edn. Philadelphia, Elsevier, 2017.
73. Harris W. *Examination paediatrics*, 5th edn. Sydney: Elsevier Australia, 2017.
74. Futagi Y, Toribe Y, Suzuki Y. The grasp reflex and moro reflex in infants: hierarchy of primitive reflex responses. *Int J Pediatr* 2012; 2012:191562.
75. Ballard JL, Khoury JC, Wedig K et al. New Ballard Score, expanded to include extremely premature infants. *J Pediatr* 1991; 119(3):417–423.
76. Sasidharan K, Dutta S, Narang A. Validity of New Ballard Score until 7th day of postnatal life in moderately preterm neonates. *Arch Dis Child Fetal Neonatal Ed* 2009; 94(1):F39–F44.

SECTION 11

Women's health history and examination

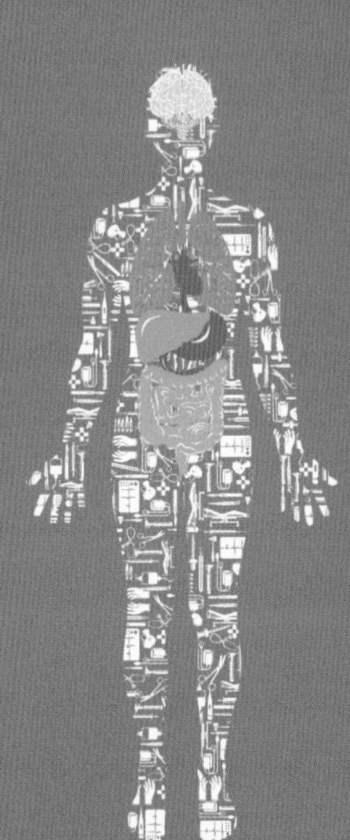

CHAPTER 39

The obstetric history and examination

Wendy Carseldine and Ian Symonds

Life is always a rich and steady time when you are waiting for something to happen or to hatch.

E B WHITE, Charlotte's Web

THE OBSTETRIC HISTORY

Obstetrics is the branch of medicine concerned with pregnancy and childbirth. It is derived from the Latin *obstetrix*, which literally means midwife: 'mid' meaning 'with' (Old English, still seen in 'mit' in German) and 'wife' meaning 'the woman'. The obstetric system is mostly concerned with normal processes, rather than a disease state. There are also two patients, and not one. Both of these factors differentiate it from other branches of medicine. It is important to understand the symptoms and signs of a normal pregnancy so as to understand what is pathological.[1–5]

EARLY PREGNANCY SYMPTOMS

(See Questions box 39.1.)

Amenorrhoea

Amenorrhoea is the absence of a menstrual period in a woman of reproductive age. In a woman presenting with amenorrhoea, pregnancy must be assumed until proven otherwise. A urinary or serum hCG level will confirm the presence of a pregnancy. The dating of pregnancy is done using the last external physical sign prior to pregnancy, which is the first day of the **last menstrual period** (LMP). This assumes that the patient's cycle length is 28 days and that ovulation thus occurs on day 14 (as ovulation occurs 14 days prior to the onset of menses). The estimated date of confinement (EDC), or due date, is calculated at 280 days, or 40 weeks from the LMP. When the cycle length varies

QUESTIONS TO ASK A WOMAN WHO MAY BE PREGNANT

1. When was the first day of your last menstrual period?
2. Was it normal in volume and length? (A light bleed may occur at the time of implantation and be confused with a period.)
3. Are your periods usually regular? What is the usual number of days from the first day of one period to the first day of the next period?
4. Are you currently sexually active?
5. Have you had previous pregnancies?
6. Have you had difficulty becoming pregnant or have you been using fertility treatment?
7. Have you been using any form of contraception? What have you used?
8. Have you performed a urine pregnancy test or had a blood test to confirm the pregnancy?
9. Have you had breast tenderness?
10. Have you been troubled by nausea?
11. How do you feel about the possibility of pregnancy?

QUESTIONS BOX 39.1

from 28 days, but remains regular, the EDC can be calculated accordingly. When the cycle length is irregular, the woman does not remember her LMP, she is breastfeeding or has ceased hormonal contraception within 3 months of the pregnancy, the date of the pregnancy should be confirmed with a pelvic ultrasound examination.

Another method of calculation of EDC is Naegele's rule. This is done by counting back 3 calendar months from the LMP and adding 7 days. For example, if the LMP is 15 May then the EDC will be 22 February. This rule also assumes a 28-day cycle.

Breast changes

Although not diagnostic of pregnancy, breast tenderness and paraesthesia are common symptoms in the first weeks of pregnancy. As the pregnancy progresses the breasts enlarge and the subcutaneous veins become more prominent. The nipple area enlarges and the pigment darkens. Later in the pregnancy the nipple may produce colostrum, a thick yellow fluid.

Nausea and vomiting

The majority of women experience nausea in pregnancy and approximately half will experience vomiting. It is correlated with the rise of hCG levels and is usually present from 6–16 weeks' gestation. When a woman presents with very early or intractable vomiting, it is important to investigate with an ultrasound to rule out multiple pregnancy or gestational trophoblastic disease. In some cases it can lead to hyperemesis gravidarum[a] (see below).

MINOR SYMPTOMS IN PREGNANCY

Pregnancy is traditionally divided into three trimesters. The first trimester and its complications are considered 'gynaecological' by convention and are covered in Chapter 40, 'The gynaecological history and examination and basic investigations'. The following symptoms may occur at any stage of the pregnancy, but are more common in the second and third trimesters. (See List 39.1.)

[a] 'Gravidus' means 'burdened' in Latin.

MINOR SYMPTOMS IN PREGNANCY

- Nausea and vomiting
- Heartburn and acid regurgitation
- Constipation
- Back pain
- Pubic symphysis pain
- Vaginal discharge
- Pruritus
- Neuropathies
- Tiredness
- Breathlessness
- Palpitations
- Ankle oedema

LIST 39.1

Nausea and vomiting

Nausea and vomiting occurs commonly in pregnancy and is normally transient resolving by 16 weeks gestation although it can continue through the entire pregnancy. Where the vomiting is intractable and associated with weight loss and ketonuria, it is described as hyperemesis gravidarum and may be associated with increased hCG levels such as in multiple gestation and molar pregnancy. Hyperthyroidism should be excluded on initial investigations and treatment is guided by symptoms. Hyperemesis gravidarum can occur as early as 5 weeks gestation, although it can continue through the entire pregnancy.

Heartburn and acid regurgitation

Increased progesterone levels in pregnancy cause decreased gastrointestinal motility and slower gastric emptying. Levels of gastric acid secretion reduce; however, the oesophageal pressure is also reduced, leading to acid regurgitation.

Constipation

Constipation is a very common symptom in pregnancy, which is likely also to be associated with the effect of the progesterone. This is often worsened by iron supplementation. Haemorrhoids are a common side effect of the constipation, which usually resolve postnatally.

Back pain

As the uterine size increases, there is increasing lordosis in the lumbar spine and a relaxation of the musculature, contributing to back pain. As the fetal head descends into the pelvis, the pain may also occur in the vagina and buttocks and radiate into the upper legs.

Pubic symphysis pain

This is point tenderness over the pubic symphysis, which is usually exacerbated with movement. This is a result of ligament laxity as well as increasing uterine pressure. The pain can be relieved by rest, pelvic support belts, warm water immersion and simple analgesia.

Vaginal discharge

In the early stages of pregnancy the cervical mucus is thick, obstructs the cervical canal and creates a barrier to protect the uterine contents. During the early stages of labour, this mucous plug is expelled and is colloquially called 'the show'. Overall, there is an increase in vaginal discharge throughout pregnancy. It is usually thick and white, resulting from the increased lactic acid production from the glycogen in the epithelium of the vagina. Candidal vaginal infection is also common and if the discharge has more of a 'cottage cheese' appearance associated with itch then a culture should be performed and the infection treated with topical anti-yeast cream.

Pruritus

Itch is a common complaint in pregnancy. There are a number of pregnancy-related conditions that manifest with pruritus, including *intrahepatic cholestasis of pregnancy* with the itch often worse in the palms of the hands and soles of the feet. This is associated with abnormal liver function tests and an increased risk of fetal death in utero. Evaluation and treatment should be prompt and delivery should be considered from 37 weeks' gestation. *Pruritic urticarial papules and plaques of pregnancy (PUPPS)* is the most common dermatosis of pregnancy, which usually resolves soon after delivery and has no significant increase in fetal morbidity. The itch is likely to be on the abdomen, thighs, arms and buttocks.

Neuropathies

The most common neuropathy in pregnancy is carpal tunnel syndrome. This is often present in the third trimester, associated with increasing oedema and subsequent compression of the median nerve. Bell's palsy (unilateral lower motor neurone lesion of the facial nerve) has an increased incidence during pregnancy and the puerperium.[b] Compression and damage of the lumbar and sacral nerves are also associated with pregnancy and delivery.

Tiredness

This is most common in the first and third trimesters, affecting almost all pregnant women at some stage during their pregnancy. As the uterus enlarges, women feel uncomfortable and have increasing urinary frequency, causing sleep to become difficult.

Breathlessness

Dyspnoea is reported in up to 70% of pregnant patients. Most of this is physiological. Asthma exacerbations must be excluded in women in whom it is pre-existing.

Palpitations

Heart rate increases in pregnancy in response to the increasing blood volume and cardiac output requirements. There is poor correlation between symptoms and pathological arrhythmias; however, if the palpitations are persistent, they should be investigated with an ECG, Holter monitor and evaluation of full blood count, electrolytes and thyroid function.

MAJOR SYMPTOMS IN PREGNANCY

The major symptoms in pregnancy are summarised in List 39.2.

Change in fetal movements

Fetal movements are a good indication of fetal wellbeing. They are usually first appreciated at 17–22 weeks' gestation (the 'quickening') and continue until delivery. Towards the end of the third trimester the movements are often not as vigorous, but should be as frequent. If

[b] The Latin word for 'childbirth'.

MAJOR SYMPTOMS IN PREGNANCY

- Change in fetal movements
- Vaginal bleeding
- Rupture of membranes
- Abdominal pain
- Headache
- Non-dependent oedema

LIST 39.2

the fetal movements are decreased, fetal evaluation with electronic heart rate monitoring and ultrasound should be undertaken and, once full term is reached, delivery should be considered. All women should receive antenatal education regarding monitoring of fetal movements.

Vaginal bleeding

Vaginal bleeding in pregnancy is never normal, but it is relatively common. In early pregnancy it may be associated with miscarriage or ectopic pregnancy or occur as a result of a subchorionic haematoma. In the second and third trimesters, vaginal bleeding may herald more sinister pathology. The three diagnoses that should be excluded include **placental abruption** (separation of the placenta from the uterine wall), **placenta praevia** (when the placenta is near or covering the cervical os) and **vasa praevia** (vessels containing fetal blood crossing the cervical os). Non-pregnancy-related causes are also possible including trauma, malignancy and cervical polyp.

Assessment should include a full history, abdominal and vaginal examinations (once the location of the placenta is known), ultrasound and bloods, including full blood count groups and hold and Kleihauer (a test to assess the amount of fetal haemoglobin). Prompt resuscitation of the mother is required if there is significant haemorrhage.

Rupture of membranes

When the 'waters break', or rupture of the membranes (amnion and chorion) occurs, the colour of the liquor should be assessed. The liquor should be clear (not cloudy) and pale yellow in colour. Light bloodstaining may cause the fluid to become pink and is also acceptable. Cloudy, offensive, brown or green liquor should be addressed quickly. In the setting of ruptured membranes prior to 37 weeks' gestation, infection is often the cause and should be treated. At term, if the woman is group B *Streptococcus* (GBS) negative and otherwise uncomplicated, then a period of expectant management is usually allowed. If GBS is present, then antibiotic cover and consideration for induction of labour is recommended.

Abdominal pain

Throughout pregnancy, the uterine muscle contracts and relaxes. When this is a painless process, it is termed a Braxton–Hicks contraction. Once these become painful and regular, they are termed contractions. The nature of contractions is that they are intermittent and associated with uterine firmness, with the pain being in the abdomen and mid–lower back.

Constant or instantly severe abdominal pain in pregnancy should receive prompt assessment. Placental abruption, which may be concealed or associated with vaginal bleeding, can cause constant, severe pain. There is usually also frequent uterine activity with no period of relaxation. The other, potentially catastrophic causes of abdominal pain include uterine rupture, which is usually associated with previous uterine surgery or prolonged, obstructed labour. In all cases the mother and the fetus should be examined. Non-obstetric causes of abdominal pain include ruptured viscera and hepatic capsule oedema as well as causes seen outside of pregnancy.

Headache

Headache in pregnancy deserves special consideration as it may be the symptom of more ominous pathology such as cerebral irritation or haemorrhagic stroke associated with hypertensive disorders of pregnancy such as pre-eclampsia. Migraine can also manifest in pregnancy and should be treated initially with simple analgesia and hydration.

Oedema

Pedal and hand oedema in the third trimester is almost universal and transient in nature. More significant oedema that occurs over the course of a few days or affects the face should trigger evaluation of the blood pressure and urinalysis to exclude pre-eclampsia.

HISTORY

(See Questions box 39.2.)

QUESTIONS TO ASK WHEN PREGNANCY HAS BEEN CONFIRMED

Obstetric history

1. Have you been pregnant before? If so, how many times?
2. Have you had any miscarriages, ectopic pregnancies or terminations of pregnancy?
3. Did you go into labour prematurely? Did you have any problems with the delivery?
4. Were the babies delivered vaginally or by caesarean section?
5. Did you have any problem with high blood pressure or diabetes during your previous pregnancies?
6. Did you have problems with depression after the delivery?

Medical history

7. Do you currently have or have a history of any of the following?
    - Diabetes
    - Heart disease (especially congenital or valvular) or high blood pressure
    - Epilepsy
    - Kidney, thyroid, liver disease
    - Connective tissue disorders
    - Clotting or bleeding disorders
    - Chronic viral infection (hepatitis B or C, HIV)
    - Sexually transmitted diseases
8. Positive cervical screening test (HPV) and ask When was your last test?
9. Have you had any operations before? If so, were there any complications?
10. Do you suffer from anxiety, depression or other psychiatric illnesses?

Medications

11. Have you been taking any of the following?
    - Anticonvulsants
    - ACE inhibitors
    - Cytotoxic drugs
    - Statins
    - Anticoagulants
12. Have you been taking folic acid or a pregnancy multivitamin?
13. Do you have any allergies?

Family history

14. Do you have a family history of any genetic disorders?
15. Does anyone in your family suffer from blood clots?
16. Are there any other medical disorders that run in the family?

Social questions

17. Are you a smoker?
18. Do you drink alcohol? How many days a week do you drink and how much each day?
19. Do you take any recreational drugs? Which ones?
20. Are you working or studying? What type of work do you do?
21. How do you feel you will manage during the pregnancy and once the baby is born?
22. Do you have a partner? Are they supportive? Do you feel safe at home?
23. What supports do you have at home?

QUESTIONS BOX 39.2

Current pregnancy history

Firstly, the EDC should be confirmed and agreed upon with the woman. The antenatal screening tests should be checked: blood group and antibodies, rubella, syphilis, hepatitis B, hepatitis C, HIV serology, midstream urine culture and full blood count. If anaemia is present, serum ferritin and thalassaemia screening should also be performed. Glucose tolerance testing should be undertaken at around 28 weeks, with an earlier test at 16–20 weeks' gestation if the woman is high risk for gestational diabetes (see List 39.3). Group B *Streptococcus* (GBS) should be screened for after 36 weeks.

First-trimester screening for aneuploidy and pregnancy complications (see List 39.4) and second-trimester morphological ultrasound examination results should be reviewed. The morphology, or fetal anomaly ultrasound, includes placental location and cervical length assessment to screen for placenta praevia and cervical shortening respectively. Cervical length is most accurately measured by transvaginal ultrasound. A shortened cervix is a risk factor for preterm delivery and treatment should be considered.

Reviewing the antenatal record also gives an overview of the examination findings over previous visits. Trends in blood pressure and fundal height over time give an indication of whether the pregnancy is progressing normally.

RISK FACTORS FOR HYPERGLYCAEMIA IN PREGNANCY

- Previous hyperglycaemia in pregnancy.
- Previously elevated blood glucose level.
- Maternal age ≥40 years.
- Ethnicity: Asian, Indian subcontinent, Aboriginal, Torres Strait Islander, Pacific Islander, Māori, Middle Eastern, non-white African.
- Family history of diabetes mellitus (first-degree relative with diabetes or a sister with hyperglycaemia in pregnancy).
- Prepregnancy BMI >30 kg/m^2
- Previous macrosomia (baby with birth weight >4500 g or >90th centile).
- Polycystic ovarian syndrome.
- Medications: corticosteroids, antipsychotics.

(From https://www.adips.org.)

LIST 39.3

Past obstetric history

A detailed history of each prior pregnancy, regardless of outcome, should be obtained. Recurrent miscarriage (three or more first-trimester miscarriages or any second-trimester miscarriage), preterm birth or adverse pregnancy outcome warrants investigation for underlying cause.

Past intrapartum and postnatal events such as preterm delivery, caesarean section, postpartum haemorrhage, shoulder dystocia and third/fourth-degree perineal tears should be noted and an appropriate screening, prevention and/or management plan formulated.

Past gynaecological history

The antenatal period is an appropriate opportunity for a full maternal health check. This includes cervical screening history; whether it is up to date and normal. If there have been previous abnormal results, were they treated and how many times? If there has been more than one treatment for cervical abnormalities, or a cone biopsy, the woman should be considered for transvaginal ultrasound cervical length screening from 14 weeks' gestation. Find out whether the patient has received human papillomavirus (HPV) vaccination.

It is important to ask about a history of sexually transmitted infections, especially *Chlamydia trachomatis*, *Neisseria gonorrhoeae* and herpes simplex virus (HSV), syphilis (*Treponema pallidum*) and human immunodeficiency virus (HIV) as these can be screened for and treated as they can potentially affect the fetus and newborn.

Past medical history

This should include all pre-existing medical conditions. Importantly, women should be questioned regarding a history of cardiac, respiratory, renal, endocrine and neurological disease. Commonly overlooked chronic conditions such as rheumatic fever and cardiac valve replacement, epilepsy, asthma, hypertension, diabetes, thromboembolic events or depression should be specifically asked about. Previous surgeries, particularly abdominal or pelvic procedures, should be noted and

FIRST-TRIMESTER SCREENING OPTIONS

- **Combined first-trimester screening** (cFTS) is also known as nuchal translucency screening. This method is performed at 11–14 weeks and screens for trisomies 21,18 and 13 using maternal demographics and history, serum biochemistry (free bHCG, Papp-A, PlGF and alpha-fetoprotein) and ultrasound markers (nuchal translucency, nasal bone, ductus venosus and tricuspid flows). This screening has a detection rate of 90%–95% with a false positive rate of 5%.
- **Non-invasive prenatal screening** (NIPS) is also known as non-invasive prenatal testing (NIPT) or cell-free fetal DNA testing (cfDNA). This examines the cell-free DNA released from the placenta which is in the maternal circulation and can be performed from 10 weeks' gestation. Screening is available for all trisomies and sex chromosome as well as subchromosome changes. For trisomy 21 the test has a detection rate of >99% with a false-positive rate of <1%.
- **Screening for pregnancy complications including preterm pre-eclampsia** can also be performed in the first trimester. For pre-eclampsia this combines maternal demographics and history, serum biochemistry (PlGF, sFLT-1, Papp-A), mean arterial blood pressure and uterine artery Doppler. For pre-eclampsia prior to 37 weeks' gestation, the detection rate is approximately 75%. Screenings for other adverse outcomes including miscarriage, stillbirth, intrauterine growth restriction, macrosomia and preterm birth are possible; however, these are currently less well validated and remain the subject of ongoing research.
- **Early fetalanatomy or morphology assessment** is performedeither at the time of cFTS or at 11–14 weeks in addition to NIPS. Most major structural fetal abnormalities can be detected at this stage byultrasound.
- **Invasive diagnostic testing** is with either chorionic villous sampling (CVS) or amniocentesis for genetic testing. CVS is performed from 11 weeks onwards by either a transabdominal or a transcervical route to sample the placental villi. Amniocentesis can safely be performed once the amnion and chorion have fused, which usually occurs after 15 weeks. A needle is passed into the amniotic sac and a sample of 20–30 mL of amniotic fluid is taken. Both procedures are performed under ultrasound guidance and have a small risk of pregnancy loss.

(From https://fetalmedicine.org.)

LIST 39.4

operative notes obtained in the event that a caesarean section is required so that intraoperative complications can be predicted.

It is routine for a screening tool for depression, for example the Edinburgh Depression Scale, to be administered at least once during the antenatal period. This is usually performed at the booking visit by the midwife. Antenatal depression is one of the strongest predictors of postnatal depression.

Treatment history

The treatment history is very important, especially in regard to the fetus. All medications have a pregnancy category rating (List 39.5).[6] All medications rated other than category A should be risk-assessed against the benefits and, if appropriate, changed after consultation with the patient. All women should be advised to take 0.5 mg of folic acid per day for 3 months prior to pregnancy and through the first trimester to reduce the risk of fetal neural tube defects. High-dose folic acid (5 mg / day) is recommended for high-risk groups of women—for example, type 1 diabetes, women on antiepileptic medication, those with a body mass index (BMI) >35 and those with a previous history of a fetus with a neural tube defect. Vitamin A supplements should be avoided in pregnancy. Vitamin D supplementation should be considered after screening for deficiency, especially in high-risk groups, such as those with limited sunlight exposure or dark skin or who are obese. Calcium supplementation should be considered in women who are calcium deficient.

PREGNANCY DRUG CATEGORY RATINGS

Category A

Drugs that have been taken by a large number of pregnant women and women of childbearing age without any proven increase in the frequency of malformations or other direct or indirect harmful effects on the fetus having been observed.

Category B1

Drugs that have been taken by only a limited number of pregnant women and women of childbearing age, without an increase in the frequency of malformation or other direct or indirect harmful effects on the human fetus having been observed. Studies in animals have not shown evidence of an increased occurrence of fetal damage.

Category B2

Drugs that have been taken by only a limited number of pregnant women and women of childbearing age, without an increase in the frequency of malformation or other direct or indirect harmful effects on the human fetus having been observed. Studies in animals are inadequate or may be lacking, but available data show no evidence of an increased occurrence of fetal damage.

Category B3

Drugs that have been taken by only a limited number of pregnant women and women of childbearing age, without an increase in the frequency of malformation or other direct or indirect harmful effects on the human fetus having been observed. Studies in animals have shown evidence of an increased occurrence of fetal damage, the significance of which is considered uncertain in humans.

Category C

Drugs that, owing to their pharmacological effects, have caused or may be suspected of causing harmful effects on the human fetus or neonate without causing malformations. These effects may be reversible. Accompanying texts should be consulted for further details.

Category D

Drugs that have caused, are suspected to have caused or may be expected to cause an increased incidence of human fetal malformations or irreversible damage. These drugs may also have adverse pharmacological effects. Accompanying texts should be consulted for further details.

Category X

Drugs that have such a high risk of causing permanent damage to the fetus that they should not be used in pregnancy or when there is a possibility of pregnancy.

From Australian categorisation system for prescribing medicines in pregnancy, 2011, Therapeutic Goods Administration, used by permission of the Australian Government https://www.tga.gov.au/australian-categorisation-system-prescribing-medicines-pregnancy

LIST 39.5

Social history

Due to the harmful effects of both cigarette smoking and alcohol on the health of the fetus, both should be explored. Quit-smoking advice and referral should be made during the initial consultation as well as at each subsequent interaction. Quitting smoking decreases the risks of placental abruption, preterm delivery and fetal abnormalities. Although fetal alcohol syndrome is rare, women should be advised that there is no safe level of alcohol consumption in pregnancy.

Some workplaces have inherent risks for pregnant women, and these should be discussed. Specifically, contact with infectious diseases, radiation and potential abdominal trauma should be avoided. Many workplaces will also require a medical certificate if the woman wishes to work after 34 weeks' gestation. With the increasing weight, tiredness and general discomfort of advanced pregnancy, some work and exercise may not be possible. Appropriate advice regarding exercise, weight gain and manual work can be given on an individualised basis. In general terms, women with a normal prepregnancy BMI should gain 10–15 kg throughout the entire pregnancy. This should be more if the woman is underweight and less if overweight or obese.

FACTORS INDICATING A RISK OF INHERITED GENETIC DISEASE IN THE FETUS

- Previous child affected
- Either parent with a known genetic defect
- Affected relative
- Family history of sex-linked disease (e.g. Duchenne's muscular dystrophy)
- Ethnicity (e.g. beta-thalassaemia in families of Mediterranean or Middle Eastern origin)
- Consanguinity

LIST 39.6

Food hygiene should be discussed during pregnancy in order to avoid both food poisoning and food-associated infectious diseases such as *Toxoplasmosis* (unwashed salads and fruit), *Listeria* (soft cheeses, uncooked meat, unpasteurised milk, pâté) and *Salmonella* (raw eggs, uncooked meat).

Pregnancy is a time of increased risk of domestic violence for some women. All women should be formally screened for domestic violence without their partner present at the earliest opportunity in the pregnancy, with additional discussion if domestic violence is disclosed or suspected from signs of trauma on physical examination at any stage during the pregnancy.

Family history

A family history of inherited disorders is important, especially if screening or diagnostic tests may be used in decision making for the patient (see List 39.6).

EXAMINATION ANATOMY

The **uterus** is centrally located in the pelvis and throughout the pregnancy grows directly superiorly. The gravid uterus is usually palpable abdominally (above the pubic symphysis) by 12–14 weeks' gestation, depending on the adiposity of the patient.

EXAMINATION

A suggested method for the examination is given in Text box 39.1.

The antenatal obstetric examination: a suggested method

This examination is a targeted examination designed to screen for abnormalities in both the mother and the fetus in the progression of the pregnancy. As with all other systems, it starts with an examination of general appearance. Special interest is taken in respiratory distress, increased oedema and pallor.

Position the patient initially in a sitting position with the feet supported on the floor. Measure the blood pressure in the right arm.

Reposition the patient to a semirecumbent position. Measure the symphyseal–fundal height and perform Leopold manoeuvres. Auscultate the fetal heart rate for at least 15 seconds.

If the history or examination is suggestive of hypertension or pre-eclampsia, then reflexes, clonus and oedema should be assessed in this position prior to assisting the woman to sit again.

Genital examination should be performed with a chaperone, after informed consent, only when indicated. Perform a urinalysis.

Further investigation by electronic fetal heart rate monitoring and ultrasound should be considered if there are any concerns for fetal wellbeing.

TEXT BOX 39.1

Positioning the patient

The blood pressure should be taken with the woman sitting with her feet on the floor. It should initially be measured on both arms and if it is equal should be measured on the right arm at subsequent visits.

Supine hypotension can complicate the examination once the pregnancy reaches the third trimester. For abdominal palpation, the woman should not lie flat if uncomfortable, but be at approximately 30°, with a pillow or bed head tilt. If the patient must lie flat, she should be placed with a slight left lateral tilt, using a pillow under the right hip / flank, to avoid venocaval compression.

General appearance

The woman should have her height and weight measured at her booking visit, and BMI calculated. The weight should be measured at subsequent visits in underweight, overweight and obese patients to monitor weight changes in pregnancy and guide treatment. Referral to a dietitian early in the pregnancy may be beneficial for these women. Those women with increased BMI should also be referred to anaesthetic services antenatally for assessment should the need arise for regional analgesia in labour or caesarean section.

All women should be examined for pallor and jaundice. Anaemia due to iron deficiency is common in pregnancy. Anaemia due to vitamin B_{12} or folate deficiency or thalassaemia can occur, but is less common. Jaundice may result from viral hepatitis, gallstones, drug-induced or pregnancy-related causes such as AFLP (acute fatty liver of pregnancy), obstetric cholestasis, pre-eclampsia or HELLP (**H**aemolysis, **E**levated **L**iver enzymes, **L**ow **P**latelets) syndrome.

Observations

Blood pressure should be measured at each antenatal visit or presentation. Physiological changes in the cardiovascular system of peripheral vasodilation and increased cardiac output give rise to profound haemodynamic changes during pregnancy. During the first and second trimester, the blood pressure usually falls for both systole and diastole. Diastolic blood pressure may be unrecordable owing to the decreased peripheral resistance of the maternal circulation. The blood pressure then returns to prepregnancy values in the third trimester.

The heart rate usually increases 10–20 beats per minute above baseline rate, although a persisting heart rate of over 100 b.p.m. should always be investigated for a cause.

The hands

Carpal tunnel syndrome is common in pregnancy, as discussed above. The tingling, numbness and pain can be recreated by pressing on the anterior aspect of the wrist. Anaemia can cause palmar crease pallor.

The face

Periorbital and generalised facial oedema can be a sign of pre-eclampsia. This can be difficult to determine if you have not examined the patient previously. Often when questioned the patient or her partner will volunteer a recent history of facial swelling.

The neck and chest

The pregnant woman's neck is commonly oedematous, which can make anaesthetic intubation problematic. The normal breast hypertrophy also makes ventilation under anaesthetic difficult. These anatomical changes are just two of the reasons a regional anaesthetic is preferred in the pregnant woman.

Initial antenatal visit examination should include examination of the thyroid for goitre or nodules. A routine breast examination can be performed; as well as screening for breast masses, the breasts can be assessed for nipple inversion, asymmetry or previous surgery. All of these factors may influence breastfeeding and an antenatal lactation consultation may be of benefit. Women should be encouraged to perform their own breast checks routinely and can be educated on the procedure at this time.

The abdomen: mother and fetal findings

The symphyseal–fundal height (SFH) is measured from the fundus of the uterus in the midline, to the symphysis pubis with a non-elastic measuring tape (Fig. 39.1). By 20 weeks the fundus of the uterus should be at the level of the umbilicus. After this, the SFH in centimetres should equate to the number of weeks' gestation of the pregnancy, with an allowable margin of up to 3 cm. It should be recorded at each visit and the trend can be observed over time. There can be discrepancy in the measurements if: the EDC is incorrectly calculated, the woman is overweight / obese, uterine fibroids are present, there is a multiple pregnancy, and there are abnormalities in either fetal growth or liquor volume. If there is any clinical concern over the SFH measurement, the woman should be referred for an ultrasound assessment.

Leopold manoeuvres (Fig. 39.2) can be used to palpate the gravid uterus in the second and third trimester to assess fetal lie, presentation, position and engagement into the maternal pelvis. Fetal lie is the relation of the fetal long axis to the maternal long axis, and is described as longitudinal, transverse or oblique. Fetal presentation describes the fetal part that is foremost within the maternal pelvis, or closest to it. Presentations include cephalic (head presenting) and breech (sacrum, knees or feet presenting). Malpresentations such as shoulder, brow, face or umbilical cord are also possible

Measurement of SFH.

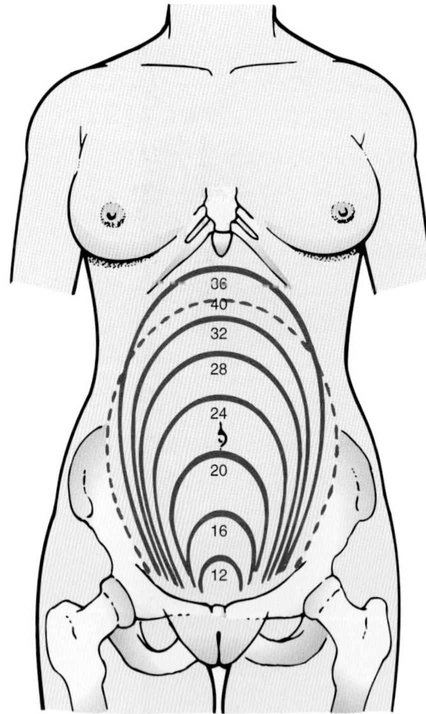

Changes in fundal height with pregnancy. Weeks 10 to 12: uterus within pelvis; fetal heartbeat can be detected with Doppler. Week 12: uterus palpable just above symphysis pubis. Week 16: uterus palpable halfway between symphysis and umbilicus; ballottement of fetus is possible by abdominal and vaginal examination. Week 20: uterine fundus at lower border of umbilicus; fetal heartbeat can be auscultated with a fetoscope. Weeks 24 to 26: uterus changes from globular to ovoid shape; fetus palpable. Week 28: uterus approximately halfway between umbilicus and xiphoid; fetus easily palpable. Week 34: uterine fundus just below xiphoid. Week 40: fundal height drops as fetus begins to engage in pelvis

(From Seidel HM, Ball JW, Dains JE et al. *Mosby's guide to physical examination*, 7th edn. St Louis, MO: Mosby, 2011, Ch 18, pp 535–599.)

FIGURE 39.1

(Fig. 39.3). If the presenting part is unable to be identified, an ultrasound should be performed to confirm the presentation, especially after 36 weeks' gestation. Fetal position refers to the relation of fetal part to the right or left side. Most commonly, if the fetus is in a cephalic presentation the fetal occiput is described as being anterior (OA), posterior (OP) or transverse (ROT or LOT) (Fig. 39.4). Engagement is measured abdominally as the proportion of the fetal head that has descended into the maternal pelvis. It is expressed in fifths, and can be described as fifths palpable abdominally or as fifths in the pelvis. The fetal head may engage prior to labour or after the start of labour, especially in multiparous women.

Once the uterus has been palpated and the fetal orientation identified, the fetal heart rate should be auscultated. This is usually done over the anterior-most shoulder with either a Pinard stethoscope or an electronic Doppler fetal heart rate monitor. The heart rate should be between 110 and 160 b.p.m. in the third trimester. A faster heart rate may be heard if the fetus is active and auscultation should continue until it returns below 160 b.p.m. If a slower heart rate is auscultated, comparison should be made with the maternal heart rate to ensure it is not the maternal rate being detected. If it is not, the woman should be positioned into a left lateral position. If there is no recovery of the fetal heart rate over the following 30 seconds, immediate assistance should be sought.

During labour the fetal heart rate can be assessed either by intermittent auscultation or by continuous electronic fetal heart rate monitoring. The method will be determined by the risk factors present in the patient. Local electronic fetal heart rate assessment tools should be consulted. An example of these can be found at www.ranzcog.edu.au or www.rcog.org.uk.

The genitals

Examination of the external genitalia may reveal vaginal discharge or vulval lesions such as HSV. If the symptoms suggest further examination is warranted, this usually begins with a speculum examination (see Ch 40). The labia majora and minora are carefully parted and the speculum (usually a Graves speculum) is passed with gentle downward pressure along the posterior vaginal wall. Once the speculum has been inserted as far as it will easily go, the speculum can be opened until the cervix can be directly visualised. The cervix is usually

Leopold manoeuvres.

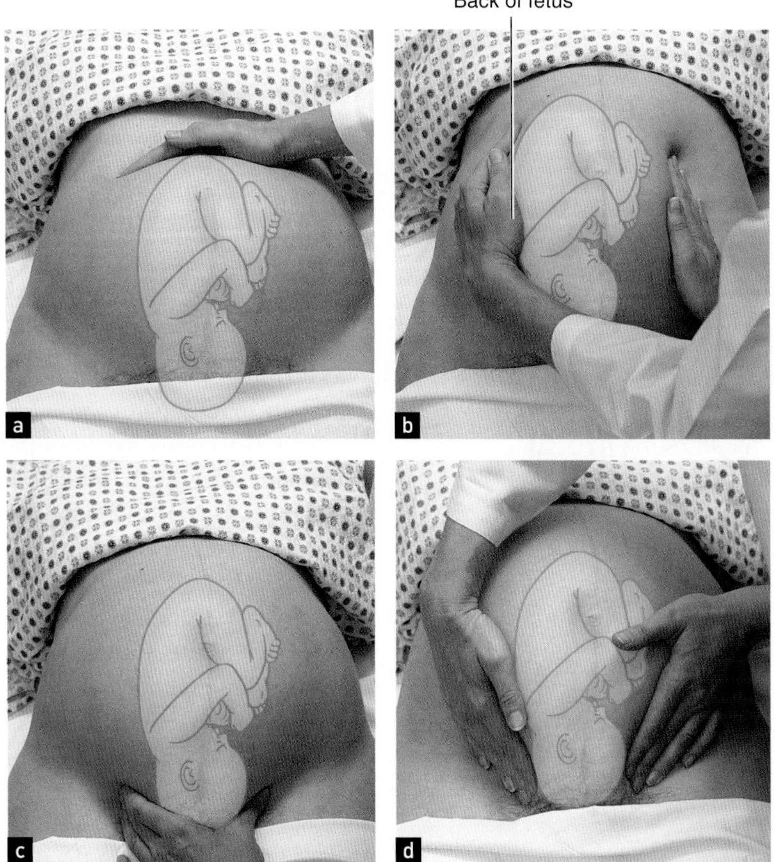

(a) First manoeuvre: place hand(s) over fundus and identify the fetal part. (b) Second manoeuvre: use the palmar surface of one hand to locate the back of the fetus; use the other hand to feel the irregularities, such as hands and feet. (c) Third manoeuvre: use thumb and third finger to grasp presenting part over the symphysis pubis. (d) Fourth manoeuvre: use both hands to outline the fetal head; with a head presenting deep in the pelvis, only a small portion may be felt

(From Seidel HM, Ball JW, Dains JE et al. *Mosby's guide to physical examination*, 7th edn. St Louis, MO: Mosby, 2011, Ch 18, pp 535–599.)

FIGURE 39.2

in the posterior aspect of the upper vagina, but may be more anterior or deviated laterally. The vaginal walls should be inspected during insertion of the speculum for lesions, discharge or bleeding areas.

Once the cervix is in view, it should be inspected for lesions, ectropion appearance and for any fluid coming through the os. This may be blood, liquor, pus or normal cervical discharge. Asking the patient to perform the Valsalva manoeuvre may elicit pooling of the liquor if the diagnosis of ruptured membranes is uncertain.

Vaginal examination is usually performed with the index and middle finger of the dominant hand of the examiner inserted gently into the vagina to assess the cervix. Examination of the cervix in pregnancy has five main features, which should each be assessed. In the antenatal period, this examination has a scoring system called the Bishop score (Table 39.1), where the

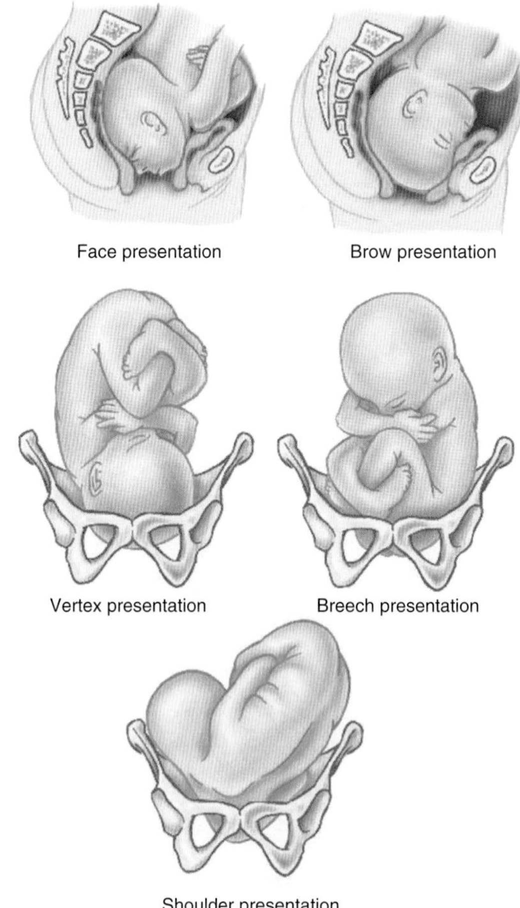

Fetal presentations and positions in labour

(Modified from Norwitz ER, Robinson J, Repke JT. The initiation and management of labor. In Seifer DB, Samuels P, Kniss D, eds. *The physiologic basis of gynecology and obstetrics*. Philadelphia: Lippincott Williams & Wilkins, 2001; Gabbe SG, Niebyl JR, Simpson JL et al. *Obstetrics: normal and problem pregnancies*, 6th edn. Ch 13, pp 267–286. Philadelphia: Elsevier Saunders. © Elsevier, 2012.)

FIGURE 39.3

cervix can be objectively described, usually when making decisions for the best method of induction of labour. The first feature is **cervical dilation**, which is measured in centimetres. This is how open the cervix is at the level of the internal os when the examination starts, not after manipulation. During the first stage of labour the cervix dilates to 'full' dilation at 10 cm, when the start of the second stage of labour begins. The second feature is **cervical length (effacement)**, which starts at 3–4 cm dilation and effaces to become 'paper' thin. The third feature is **consistency**, which is described as soft, medium or firm. The prelabour cervix is firm, similar in consistency to the tip of the nose, and gradually softens as labour progresses. The fourth feature is the **cervical position**, which describes whether the cervix has started to move from the initial 'posterior' position, through to 'mid' position or has progressed to an 'anterior' position. The final feature is **station** of the presenting part. This is measured in centimetres above or below the ischial spines, which are located at approximately 5 and 7 o'clock in the upper vagina. During labour the vaginal examination should also include assessment of fetal head position, application to the cervix, caput and moulding.

Bishop score

Cervical feature	Bishop score			
	0	1	2	3
Dilation	<1 cm	1–2 cm	3–4 cm	>4 cm
Length	4 cm	2–4 cm	1–2 cm	<1 cm
Consistency	Firm	Medium	Soft	
Position	Posterior	Central	Anterior	
Station	3	2	1, 0	>+1

(Goh J, Flynn M. *Examination obstetrics and gynaecology*, 3rd edn. Sydney: Elsevier Australia, 2011, Table 42.1.)

TABLE 39.1

The lower limbs

The lower limbs should be examined with the patient lying. Initial inspection should assess for oedema; often the patient should be asked to clarify whether the level of oedema is usual or increased. If oedema is present, the level of pitting should be checked from the ankle upwards on both sides. The calves and ankles can be palpated for tenderness consistent with deep vein thrombosis.

If hypertension is present, neurological signs are easily elicited in the lower limbs. Patella reflexes in pregnancy are usually normal to brisk and a tendon hammer is rarely required. Clonus is best assessed in the ankle joint by moving the foot in a quick upward motion to flex the joint. One or two beats are acceptable in pregnancy. Increased reflexes and/or clonus may reflect neurological irritation in the setting of pre-eclampsia and should be addressed in a timely fashion.

Fetal head positions.

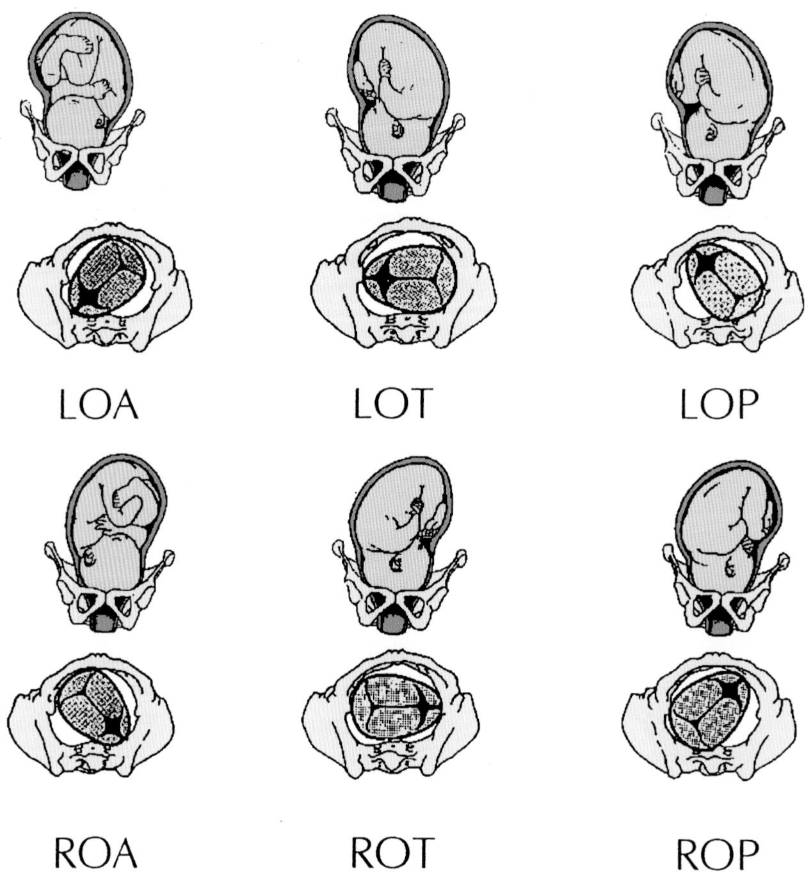

LOA=left occiput anterior; LOT=left occiput transverse; LOP=left occiput posterior; ROA=right occiput anterior; ROT=right occiput transverse; ROP=right occiput posterior

(From *Dorland's medical dictionary for health consumers*. Philadelphia: © 2007 Saunders.)

FIGURE 39.4

Urinalysis

A midstream urine specimen should be collected at the first antenatal visit to exclude infection. At subsequent visits dipstick urinalysis should be performed if infection is suspected or there are signs / symptoms of pre-eclampsia to check for the presence of proteinuria.

Obstetric ultrasound: a systematic approach

First-trimester obstetric ultrasound can be used for dating of the pregnancy as described previously. At 10–14 weeks' gestation the first-trimester screening for aneuploidy and pregnancy complications should be offered (see List 39.4).

At 18–20 weeks' gestation a full morphological assessment of the fetus is performed, including head, face, chest, heart, abdomen, limbs and spine being visualised. The placental location is also observed at this examination, with a further ultrasound to be performed at about 34 weeks if it is low-lying, which is classified as within 20 mm of the internal os. If any abnormality is seen, then tertiary referral is usually ought for advice and management.

Further ultrasound assessment may be required to estimate the growth velocity of the fetus. The

T&O'C ESSENTIALS

1. *Vaginal bleeding in pregnancy is never normal. Both pregnancy- and non-pregnancy-related causes should be explored.*
2. *Medical disorders can both affect pregnancy and be affected by pregnancy.*
3. *If a medication is being used (or being considered for use) in pregnancy or breastfeeding, always check the pregnancy category rating.*
4. *Supine positioning in pregnancy causes vena caval compression; use the left lateral or semirecumbent position to avoid hypotension and hypoperfusion of the uterus.*
5. *Fetal lie, presentation, position and engagement can be obtained from abdominal palpation.*
6. *Assessment of cervical dilation, effacement, position, consistency and fetal station is acquired by vaginal examination.*

OSCE REVISION TOPICS – THE OBSTETRIC HISTORY AND EXAMINATION

1. A multiparous woman presents for her routine antenatal visit at 37 weeks' gestation. Please explain how you would perform a routine examination. (pp 771–6)
2. A woman presents with severe nausea and vomiting at 8 weeks' gestation. Please describe your investigations and initial management. (p 764)
3. A primiparous woman presents to the delivery suite at 36 weeks' gestation with a severe frontal headache and a blood pressure of 170/110. Please take a history of the presenting illness. (pp 766–71)
4. At 41 weeks' gestation, a multiparous woman presents for cervical assessment for induction of labour. What are the five features assessed for the Bishop score? (p 775)
5. This 34-year-old woman presents at 38 weeks with spontaneous rupture of membranes. Please take a history and explain how you would perform the appropriate examination. (pp 766, 773–5)

measurements used include head circumference, biparietal diameter, abdominal circumference and femur length. These are used to calculate an estimation of the fetal weight. Liquor volume is assessed by single deepest pool or amniotic fluid index (the sum of the pools in the four quadrants of the uterus). The placental location is again observed. Assessment of fetal wellbeing can also be performed using blood flow Doppler in the umbilical artery, middle cerebral artery and ductus venosus vessels.

References

1. Cunningham FG, Leveno KJ, Bloom SL et al. *Williams obstetrics*, 23rd edn. Sydney: McGraw Hill Medical, 2010.
2. Goh J, Flynn M. *Examination obstetrics and gynaecology*, 3rd edn. Sydney: Elsevier Australia, 2011.
3. Luesley DM, Baker PN. *Obstetrics and gynaecology: an evidence-based text for MRCOG*, 2nd edn. London: Hodder Arnold, 2010.
4. Nelson-Piercy C. *Handbook of obstetric medicine*, 4th edn. London: Informa Healthcare, 2010.
5. Sarris I, Bewley S, Agnihotri S. *Training in obstetrics and gynaecology: the essential curriculum*. London: Oxford University Press, 2009.
6. Therapeutic Goods Administration. The Australian categorisation system for prescribing medicines in pregnancy. www.tga.gov.au/hp/medicines-pregnancy.htm.

CHAPTER 40

The gynaecological history and examination

Wendy Carseldine and Ian Symonds

The good physician treats the disease; the great physician treats the patient who has the disease.

SIR WILLIAM OSLER (1849–1919)

Gynaecology is the field of medicine that includes disorders of the female genital tract and reproductive system. It also includes complications of early pregnancy such as miscarriage and ectopic pregnancy.

HISTORY

As with all areas of medicine a precise and comprehensive history is the most important component in making an accurate gynaecological diagnosis. The basic structure of the gynaecological history is similar to that for other systems, but with more emphasis on the patient's menstrual, sexual and past reproductive history. It is important to note the patient's age as this will influence the likely diagnosis for a number of presenting problems. Occupation may be relevant both to the level of understanding that can be assumed and to the effect of different gynaecological problems on the patient's life. Pay attention to LGBTI patients; refer to Chapter 2.

A method for the gynaecological history and examination is given in Text box 40.1.

Presenting symptoms

Ask the patient to describe the nature of her problem. Where there are multiple symptoms these may not be related to the same pathology and it is useful to address each of these in turn with appropriate open and closed questioning. Ascertain the timescale of the problem and, where appropriate, the circumstances surrounding the onset of symptoms and their relationship to the menstrual cycle. It is also important to discover the degree of disability experienced for any given symptom.

More detailed questions will depend on the nature of the presenting complaint. List 40.1 outlines some of the more common presenting symptoms encountered in the outpatient clinic. Further details for some of these are discussed below.

COMMON PRESENTING SYMPTOMS IN GYNAECOLOGY

- Disorders of menstruation
- Heavy menstrual bleeding
- Intermenstrual bleeding
- Oligomenorrhoea / amenorrhoea
- Postmenopausal bleeding
- Premenstrual syndrome
- Disorders of sexual function
- Dyspareunia
- Loss of libido
- Vaginismus
- Infertility
- Pain and / or bleeding in early pregnancy
- Pelvic / lower abdominal pain: acute and chronic
- Perimenopausal symptoms
- Symptoms of uterovaginal prolapse
- Urinary incontinence
- Urinary urgency / frequency
- Voiding difficulties
- Vaginal discharge and genital tract infection
- Vulval pain / pruritus

LIST 40.1

The gynaecological history and examination: a suggested method

1. **History**
- Presenting symptoms
  - Onset and duration of main complaint
  - Associated symptoms, relationship to menstrual cycle
  - Previous treatment and response
  - Specific closed questions
- Previous gynaecological history
  - Previous investigations or treatment
  - Contraceptive history
  - Sexual history
  - Cervical screening test
  - Menstrual history (menarche, last menstrual period, cycle)
- Previous pregnancies
  - How many (gravidity)
  - Outcome (parity)
  - Surgical deliveries
  - Birth weight and health of previous babies
- Past surgical and medical history
  - Previous abdominal surgery
  - Major cardiovascular/respiratory disease
  - Endocrine disease
  - Thromboembolic disease
  - Breast disease
- Drug history and allergies
- Social and family history
  - Home circumstances
  - Support
  - Smoking
  - Family history

2. **Examination**
- General examination
  - General condition, weight, height
  - Pulse, blood pressure
  - Anaemia
  - Goitre
  - Breast examination (if indicated)
  - Secondary sex characteristics, body hair, acne
- Abdominal examination
  - Inspection: distension, scars
  - Palpation: masses, organomegaly, tenderness, peritonism, nodes, hernial orifices
  - Percussion: ascites
- Pelvic examination
  - Explanation, comfort, privacy, chaperone
  - Inspection of external genitalia
  - Speculum examination
  - Bimanual examination
- Rectal examination, if indicated

TEXT BOX 40.1

Menstrual history

A full menstrual history should be taken from all women of reproductive age, starting with the first day of the last menstrual period.

The length of the menstrual cycle is the time between the first day of one period and the first day of the following period. While there is usually an interval of between 26 and 32 days, occasionally the duration of the cycle may be as short as 21 days or as long as 42 days without necessarily indicating any underlying abnormality.

Normal menstruation lasts from 4 to 7 days, and normal blood loss varies between 30 and 80 mL. A change in pattern is often more noticeable and significant than the actual duration and volume of loss. Self-reported assessment of the amount of bleeding is subjective, with up to 50% of women who report excessive bleeding actually having a measured blood loss of less than 80 mL. Excessively prolonged or heavy regular periods are sometimes referred to as **menorrhagia**, but the term **heavy menstrual bleeding (HMB)** is now generally used to describe all excessive menstrual blood loss regardless of the regularity of the cycle (see below).

The cessation of periods for at least 12 months at the end of menstrual life is known as the **menopause**. Bleeding that occurs after this is described as **postmenopausal bleeding**. A history of irregular vaginal bleeding or blood loss that occurs after coitus or between periods should be noted.

Heavy menstrual bleeding

HMB is defined as menstrual loss of more than 80 mL per month or 'excessive menstrual loss leading to

CAUSES OF HEAVY MENSTRUAL BLEEDING

Structural

- Uterine leiomyomata (fibroids)
- Adenomyosis
- Endometrial polyps
- Endometrial hyperplasia
- Endometrial cancer

Non-structural

- Disorders of ovulation (polycystic ovary syndrome, perimenopause, puberty)
- Clotting disorders
- Iatrogenic (intrauterine contraceptive device)
- Dysfunctional bleeding (see below)
- Hypothyroidism

LIST 40.2

interference with the physical, emotional, social and material quality of life in a woman and which occurs alone or in combination with other symptoms'.[1] It affects about 10% of women. In most cases the cause is an imbalance in the mechanisms that regulate clotting at the endometrial level without any obvious structural pathology. However, it may be associated with a number of benign pathologies and, occasionally, with malignancy (see List 40.2).

Diagnosis

In practice, the diagnosis of HMB is made on the basis of symptoms, not measured blood loss. Symptoms of clotting, flooding (soiling of clothing), the use of a large amount of sanitary protection, bleeding lasting more than 7 days and treatment for anaemia are likely to indicate HMB. A change in the pattern of bleeding is more likely to be associated with a structural lesion. Malignancy is rare in women under the age of 40. A history of polycystic ovary syndrome (PCOS), diabetes, hypertension and obesity are associated with an increased risk of endometrial hyperplasia and malignancy.

All women with HMB should have a general examination for signs of anaemia and thyroid disease and a pelvic examination including cervical screening. The finding of a pelvic mass is most likely to be associated with a diagnosis of fibroids but can indicate malignancy.

A full blood count (FBC) should be requested for all patients with HMB. Additional investigation is mainly directed at excluding malignancy and usually includes a pelvic ultrasound scan. Endoscopic examination of the endometrial cavity (hysteroscopy) with endometrial biopsy is indicated when:

- there is a history of irregular or intermenstrual bleeding
- risk factors for endometrial cancer are present
- pelvic examination is abnormal
- there is no response to first-line treatment.

Young women under the age of 25 should have a partial coagulation screen to exclude Von Willebrand's disease.

Bleeding in early pregnancy

Any women of reproductive age presenting with abnormal vaginal bleeding should have the possibility of pregnancy considered. If a pregnancy test is positive, the cause of the bleeding can usually be determined by a combination of vaginal examination and ultrasound (see Table 40.1). The most common cause of bleeding in early pregnancy (before 20 weeks) is miscarriage, or threatened miscarriage, although hydatidiform and ectopic pregnancy may also present with bleeding. Miscarriage is the spontaneous termination of pregnancy prior to 20 weeks' gestation; it affects about 15–20% of pregnancies. It is important to remember that bleeding in pregnancy can result from the same lower genital tract lesions as in non-pregnant women.

Amenorrhoea and oligomenorrhoea

The onset of the first period, the **menarche**, commonly occurs at 12 years of age and can be considered to be abnormally early at 7 years. **Primary amenorrhoea** is the absence of menarche. The age at which the diagnosis is made depends on the presence or absence of other features of puberty. In the absence of other signs of puberty this is 14 years, but where there are other pubertal changes it is 16.

Secondary amenorrhoea is defined as the cessation of menses for 6 months or more in a woman who has previously menstruated. **Oligomenorrhoea** is the occurrence of five or fewer periods over 12 months. In practice, the distinction between the two can be somewhat arbitrary as they share many of the same causes.

Diagnosis of bleeding in early pregnancy

Symptoms and examination	Ultrasound	Diagnosis
Light vaginal bleeding with minimal pain; closed cervix	Viable intrauterine pregnancy	Threatened miscarriage
Heavy vaginal bleeding with cramping lower abdominal pain; open cervix	Products of conception in uterus with or without fetal heartbeat	Inevitable miscarriage
Heavy vaginal bleeding with cramping; open cervix, possibly with tissue	Products of conception in uterus, usually without fetal heartbeat	Incomplete miscarriage
Painless light bleeding or no symptoms; closed cervix	No fetal pole or fetal heartbeat in gestation sac >25 mm diameter	Missed miscarriage
Minimal bleeding after history of heavier bleeding and cramps; closed cervix	Empty uterus	Complete miscarriage (also consider ectopic pregnancy and very early viable pregnancy)
Mild-to-moderate bleeding; uterus large for dates, exaggerated pregnancy symptoms (e.g. hyperemesis)	Snowstorm appearance with or without gestation sac	Molar pregnancy
Light vaginal bleeding with unilateral abdominal pain; closed cervix; cervical excitation	No intrauterine pregnancy when hCG >1500; free fluid outside the uterus and/or an adnexal mass	Ectopic pregnancy

hCG=human chorionic gonadotrophin.

TABLE 40.1

Diagnosis

Amenorrhoea can be physiological or pathological (see List 40.3), with the most common causes being pregnancy, menopause and lactation. The possibility of pregnancy should be excluded in any woman of reproductive age by undertaking a urinary pregnancy test. Ask about recent emotional stress, changes in weight, menopausal symptoms and current medication. Relevant findings on examination are a low or high body mass index, hirsutism (PCOS), galactorrhoea and bitemporal hemianopia (pituitary tumours).

In cases of primary amenorrhoea look for features of secondary sex characteristics development, signs of imperforate hymen (P) and features of Turner syndrome (short stature, wide carrying angle and widely spaced nipples).

The differential diagnosis is established by measurement of follicle-stimulating hormone (FSH), luteinising hormone (LH) and prolactin, and thyroid function tests. A pelvic ultrasound can provide additional evidence of polycystic ovary syndrome (POCS), ovarian tumours and abnormalities of the lower genital tract. In women with primary amenorrhoea, a karyotype should also be obtained.

Dysmenorrhoea

Dysmenorrhoea, or painful menstruation, is the most common of all gynaecological symptoms.

Primary dysmenorrhoea occurs in the absence of any significant pelvic pathology. It usually develops within the first 2 years of the menarche. The pain is typically described as central and cramping. Symptoms can be severely incapacitating, causing major disruption of social activities. The onset of symptoms is usually associated with the onset of menstrual blood loss but may begin on the day preceding menstruation. The pain occurs only in ovulatory cycles and often disappears or improves after the birth of the first child. Dysmenorrhoea may be associated with vomiting and diarrhoea. Pelvic examination reveals no abnormality of the pelvic organs.

Secondary or **acquired dysmenorrhoea** is more likely to be caused by organic pelvic pathology and usually has its onset many years after the menarche. Commonly associated pathologies include endometriosis (see Fig. 40.1), adenomyosis, pelvic infections and intrauterine lesions such as submucous fibroid polyps.

CAUSES OF AMENORRHOEA

Primary

- Constitutional
- Anatomical
  - Imperforate hymen
  - Transverse vaginal septum
  - Müllerian agenesis: Mayer–Rokitansky–Küster–Hauser syndrome
- Hypergonadotrophic hypogonadic
  - Androgen insensitivity (XY)
  - Turner syndrome
  - Gonadal dysgenesis
- Hypogonadotrophic hypogonadic
  - CNS lesions (tumours, infection, trauma)
  - Kallmann's syndrome

Secondary

- Physiological causes
  - Pregnancy
  - Lactation
  - Menopause
- Pathological causes
- Hypothalamic disorders
  - Excessive weight loss or exercise
  - Stress
  - Chronic kidney disease
- Pituitary disorders
  - Prolactin-secreting tumours of the anterior pituitary (micro- or macroadenoma)
  - Postpartum necrosis (Sheehan's syndrome)
  - Antidopaminergic drugs
- Ovarian disorders
  - Premature ovarian failure
  - Autoimmune disease
  - Surgical removal of the ovaries
  - Oestrogen- or testosterone-secreting ovarian neoplasms
- Polycystic ovary syndrome
- Failure of uterine response
  - Surgical removal of the uterus
  - Asherman syndrome
  - Cryptomenorrhoea
  - Cervical stenosis, as a result of surgical trauma or infection

LIST 40.3

Investigations

A careful history is of great importance in this condition. Pelvic examination should be performed and, if this is abnormal, a pelvic ultrasound scan arranged. Laparoscopy is the gold standard investigation for the diagnosis of conditions such as endometriosis. It is performed in cases with primary dysmenorrhoea only if the condition is particularly resistant to therapy.

Acute abdominal pain

In women with a negative pregnancy test and acute pelvic pain, gynaecological disorders include pelvic inflammatory disease (PID), functional ovarian cysts, ovarian or peritoneal endometriosis and ovarian torsion. The most common gastrointestinal causes that can present with acute pelvic pain include appendicitis, acute sigmoid diverticulitis and Crohn's disease. In your assessment it is important to exclude those diagnoses that require urgent intervention: PID, ovarian torsion, ectopic pregnancy and appendicitis.

The history should include the onset site and the nature of the pain, the date of the last menstrual period and the presence of associated symptoms. On examination, identify the site of maximal tenderness and the presence of rebound tenderness and guarding. It is vital to always exclude pregnancy, particularly ectopic pregnancy.

Ovarian torsion usually occurs in the presence of an enlarged ovary. Women with torsion present with sudden onset of sharp, unilateral pelvic pain that is often accompanied by nausea and vomiting. The sonographic findings are variable. The ovary is enlarged and can be seen in an abnormal location above or behind the uterus. The absence of blood flow is an important sign, and a lack of venous wave form on Doppler ultrasound has a high positive predictive value.

Endometriotic patches on the surface of the ovary.

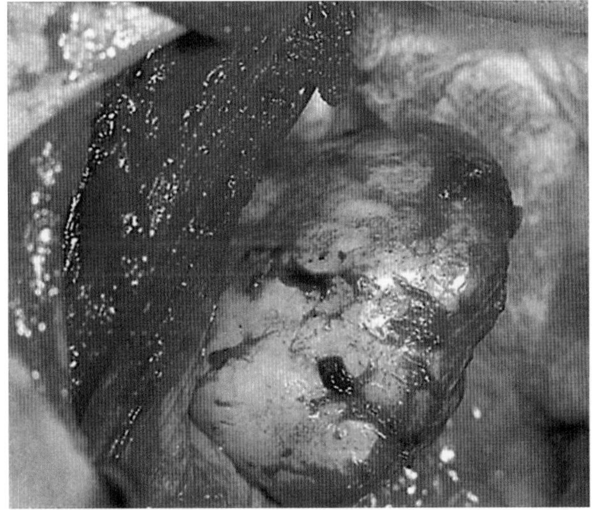

(From Symonds EM, Symonds IM. *Essential obstetrics and gynaecology*, 4th edn. Edinburgh: Churchill Livingstone, 2004.)

FIGURE 40.1

However, the presence of arterial and venous flow does not exclude torsion and any cases where it is suspected clinically require laparoscopy to visualise the adnexa (ovaries and fallopian tubes). If the torsion is reversed early in the process, the ovary may be saved.

Approximately 1% of pregnancies are ectopic (occur outside the uterus) but the individual risk depends on the past history (see Table 40.2). Ectopic pregnancy presents classically with sudden onset of unilateral pain and irregular vaginal bleeding after a period of amenorrhoea. The presence of shoulder tip pain (due to diaphragmatic irritation) and peritonism are suggestive of rupture with intraperitoneal bleeding. In practice, it is rare for all three symptoms to be present and chronic presentation with atypical pain and bleeding are more common. Clinical examination findings include cervical excitation (increased pain on movement of the cervix during pelvic examination), adnexal pain and swelling with or without signs of hypovolaemic shock. The diagnosis is usually made by measurement of human chorionic gonadotrophin (hCG) levels and pelvic ultrasound and confirmed at laparoscopy (see Table 40.1).

Risk factors for ectopic pregnancy

	Relative risk
Previous history of PID	4
Previous tubal surgery	4.5
Failed sterilisation	9
Intrauterine contraceptive device in situ	10
Previous ectopic pregnancy	10–15

PID=pelvic inflammatory disease.

TABLE 40.2

Causes of infertility

Cause	Primary infertility (%)	Secondary infertility (%)
Anovulation	32	23
Tubal disease	12	14
Endometriosis	11	10
Sperm quality problems	29	24
Other	14	21
Unknown	29	30

(Adapted from Bhattacharya S, Porter M, Amalraj E et al. The epidemiology of infertility in the North East of Scotland. *Hum Reprod* 2009; 24(12): 3096–3107.)

TABLE 40.3

Infertility

Approximately 80% of normally fertile couples will conceive within a year of unprotected intercourse; when conception does not occur within 12 months the couple can be considered at risk of infertility. The median prevalence of infertility in the developed world at 12 months of unprotected intercourse is 9%, although this varies significantly in relation to age in women. Infertility is called *primary* if the woman has not previously been pregnant and *secondary* if she has had one or more previous pregnancies. Table 40.3 summarises the common causes of infertility (note that it is not uncommon for more than one factor to affect fertility in a given couple). The initial consultation should include both partners. Key questions to ask are given in Questions box 40.1.

INITIAL ASSESSMENT OF THE INFERTILE COUPLE

1. How long have you been trying to fall pregnant?
2. What methods of contraception have you or your partner used previously?
3. Have either you or your partner had a previous pregnancy together or with other partners?
4. If so, did you have any complications associated with the pregnancy?
5. Can you tell me about your periods and whether you have had any bleeding between your periods?
6. How often do you and your partner have sex? Are there any problems with pain during sex or ejaculatory / erection problems for your partner?
7. Have you ever had any sexually transmitted infections or has your partner ever had mumps orchitis (inflammation of the testes)?
8. Do you have any serious chronic illness or have you ever had surgery such as an appendectomy? Has your partner been treated for varicocele or undescended testes?

QUESTIONS BOX 40.1

Diagnosis

Clinical examination findings of significance for women include those features potentially associated with causes of amenorrhoea (see above) and endometriosis. Male examination findings include testicular size, the presence of varicocele and thickening of the epididymis (see Ch 18). Initial investigations are determined by the history; for example, if this is suggestive of previous pelvic infection, an assessment of tubal patency would be a priority. Typically, initial baseline tests include semen fluid analysis, assessment of ovulation (such as a day 21 serum progesterone level) and assessment of tubal patency (such as hysterosalpingogram or laparoscopy).

Sexual history

The amount of detail required will depend on the presenting symptom. In women complaining of disorders of sexual function and suspected sexually transmitted infection (such as vaginal discharge, PID), a full sexual history should be obtained, as described in Questions box 40.2.

Always explain the reason you need to ask questions of such a personal nature. For example, 'From what you have told me I think some of these problems may have a sexual cause. Will it be all right if I ask you some personal questions?'

Previous gynaecological history

A detailed history of any previous gynaecological problems and treatments must be recorded. The amount of detail needed about previous pregnancies will depend on the presenting symptom. In most cases the number of previous pregnancies and their outcome (miscarriage, ectopic or delivery after 20 weeks) is all that is required.

For all women of reproductive age who are sexually active it is essential to ask about contraception. This is important not only to determine the possibility of pregnancy but also because the method of contraception used may itself be relevant to the presenting symptom. For women over the age of 25, ask about the date and result of the last cervical screening test.

Previous medical history

Take particular account of any history of medical disorders of the endocrine, urinary or cardiovascular systems. Make a record of all current medications and any known drug allergies.

Family and social history

A social history is important for all problems but is particularly relevant where the presenting difficulties relate to abortion or sterilisation. Ask about smoking, alcohol and other recreational drug use. A family history of breast or ovarian cancer or both, delayed puberty or premature menopause may be relevant where the patient has the same condition.

QUESTIONS TO ASK A PATIENT COMPLAINING OF SEXUAL DYSFUNCTION OR SUSPECTED SEXUALLY TRANSMITTED INFECTION[2]

1. What is the reason for your attendance today?
2. How long have you had these symptoms?
3. Do you suffer from any of the following?
   - Urethral and vaginal discharge
   - Abnormal vaginal or rectal bleeding
   - Genital and extragenital rashes, lumps or sores
   - Itching and/or discomfort in the perineum, perianal and pubic regions
   - Lower abdominal pain or dyspareunia
   - Difficulties/pain with micturition or defecation or during intercourse
4. When was the last time you had sexual intercourse?
5. Have you had unprotected intercourse?
6. How many sexual contacts have you had in the last 3–5 months? What were the gender(s) of your sexual partners?
7. What type of sexual activity did you practise? (Oral, anal, vaginal, use of toys)
8. Did you take any steps to prevent sexually transmitted infections, such as using condoms? If so, do you use this method consistently?
9. What is your relationship with your sexual contacts (regular, casual, known, unknown)?
10. Have any of your recent sexual contacts had any symptoms of sexually transmitted infection or infections?
11. Have you previously been tested for any sexually transmitted infections? If so, what was the date of the test, and the result?
12. Do you have a current or past history of injecting drug use? Sharing of needles or syringes? Body piercing and/or tattoos? If the last-named, where and when were these done and was sterile equipment used?
13. Have you had sex overseas with anyone other than with the person you were travelling with?
14. Have you ever worked in the sex industry or had sexual contact with a sex worker?
15. Have you been vaccinated for hepatitis A and B and HPV?
16. Are you taking any current medications?
17. Do you have a history of allergies, especially adverse reaction to penicillin?
18. What contraceptives do you use?
19. When was your last menstrual period?
20. When was your last cervical screening test? What was the result? Have you ever had an abnormal result?
21. Do you have any past medical and surgical history (including any overseas medical treatment and transfusions)?
22. What is your current alcohol, tobacco and other drug use?
23. Have you ever had any concerns about your gender identity? Are you happy to tell me about these and how they have affected you?

(Adapted from NSW Sexually Transmissible Infections Programs Unit 2011. www.stipu.nsw.gov.au.)

QUESTIONS BOX 40.2

EXAMINATION

A general examination should always be performed at the first consultation, including assessment of pulse, blood pressure and temperature. Take careful note of any signs of anaemia. The distribution of facial and body hair is often important, as hirsutism may be a presenting symptom of androgen-producing tumours or PCOS. Also record the patient's body weight and height.

The intimate nature of the gynaecological examination makes it especially important to ensure that every effort is made to consider privacy and that the examination is not interrupted (see Text box 40.2). The examination should ideally take place in a separate area to the consultation. Allow the patient to undress in privacy and, if necessary, empty her bladder first. After she has undressed there should be no undue delay to the examination.

Examination of the abdomen

Inspection of the abdomen is undertaken as previously described in Chapters 14 and 18. In a patient presenting with gynaecological symptoms look for the presence of a mass as well as scars, striae and hernias. If there is a mass, try to determine whether it is fixed or mobile, smooth or regular, and whether it arises from the pelvis (you should not be able to palpate the lower edge above the pubic bone). Look for scars in the umbilicus from previous laparoscopies and in the suprapubic region where transverse incisions from caesarean sections and most gynaecological operations are found. Palpate the abdomen to assess for any guarding or rebound tenderness. Check the hernial orifices and feel for any enlarged lymph nodes in the groin. Percuss the abdomen to outline the limits of a tumour, detect the presence of a full bladder or recognise the presence of tympanic loops of bowel.

Guidelines for intimate examination[3]

When conducting intimate examinations you should:

- Explain to the patient why an intimate examination is necessary and give the patient an opportunity to ask questions.
- Explain what the examination will involve, in a way the patient can understand, so that the patient has a clear idea of what to expect, including any potential pain or discomfort.
- Obtain the patient's permission before the examination and be prepared to discontinue the examination if the patient asks you to.
- Record that permission has been obtained.
- Keep discussion relevant and avoid unnecessary personal comments.
- Offer a chaperone. If the patient does not want a chaperone, you should record that the offer was made and declined. If a chaperone is present, you should record that fact and make a note of the chaperone's identity. If for justifiable practical reasons you cannot offer a chaperone, you should explain to the patient and, if possible, offer to delay the examination to a later date.
- Give the patient privacy to undress and dress and use drapes to maintain the patient's dignity. Do not assist the patient in removing clothing unless you have clarified with them that your assistance is required.
- Obtain consent prior to anaesthetisation, usually in writing, for the intimate examination of anaesthetised patients. If you are supervising students you should ensure that valid consent has been obtained before they carry out any intimate examination.

(Adapted from General Medical Council (2013). Intimate examinations and chaperones. Available at https://www.gmc-uk.org/ethical-guidance/ethical-guidance-for-doctors/intimate-examinations-and-chaperones/intimate-examinations-and-chaperones.)

TEXT BOX 40.2

Pelvic examination

The pelvic examination should be performed *when indicated* as the final part of any complete physical examination.[4] It should not be considered an automatic and inevitable part of every gynaecological consultation. You should consider what information will be gained by the examination, whether this is a screening or diagnostic procedure and whether it is necessary at this time. In a child or in a woman with an intact hymen, speculum and pelvic examinations are not usually performed unless as part of an examination under anaesthesia. Remember that a rough or painful examination rarely produces any useful information and, in certain situations such as tubal ectopic pregnancy, may be dangerous. Throughout the examination remain alert to verbal and non-verbal indications of distress from the patient.

RULES FOR CONDUCTING A PELVIC EXAMINATION

When conducting a vaginal examination you should:

- Explain that an intimate examination is needed and why.
- Explain what the examination will involve.
- Obtain the patient's permission.
- Offer a chaperone or invite the patient to bring a relative or friend.
- Allow the patient to undress in privacy.
- Keep discussion relevant and avoid unnecessary personal comments.
- Explain findings and encourage questions and discussion.

LIST 40.4

It is essential to obtain informed consent and for male students and doctors to offer to have a female chaperone (see List 40.4). The patient's privacy must be promised and ensured.

Wear gloves on both hands during vaginal and speculum examinations. Examine the patient either in the supine position or in the left lateral position with the knees drawn up and separated (see Fig. 40.2). The left lateral position is used when the woman cannot assume the lithotomy position or when a view of the anterior vaginal wall is required—for example, when a urinary fistula is suspected (see below). The perineum should be brightly illuminated by a lamp.

Examination of the external genitalia

Parting the lips of the labia minora with the left hand, look at the external urethral meatus and inspect the vulva for any discharge, redness, ulceration or old scars or vaginal prolapse (see Table 40.4).

Bartholin's glands[a]

The Bartholin's glands lie in the posterior vaginal wall at the introitus (entrance) and secrete mucus-like fluid via a short duct into the vagina. They are normally the size of a pea but when the duct becomes blocked a cyst can form. These cysts may present acutely as an oval-shaped lump—in the posterior labia they may sometimes grow to the size of a golf ball or larger. They are usually unilateral and cause discomfort with walking, sitting and sexual intercourse. When the gland is infected, most commonly with skin or genitourinary bacteria (*Staphylococcus*, *Escherichia coli*), an abscess can develop. These abscesses arise more acutely than Bartholin's cysts and are particularly painful.

Speculum examination

Speculum examination should be performed before digital examination to avoid any contamination with lubricant. A bivalve speculum is most commonly used with the patient in the supine position as this enables a clear view of the cervix to be obtained. Where vaginal wall prolapse is suspected, a Sims' speculum should be used as an alternative with the patient in the left lateral position as this affords a better view of the anterior vaginal wall (see Fig. 40.3).

Part the labia minora with the left hand and insert the speculum into the introitus, initially with the widest dimension of the instrument in the anteroposterior orientation and turning gently to the transverse position as the tip passes the introitus, as the vagina is widest in this direction. When the speculum reaches the top of the vagina, gently open the blades to enable the cervix to be visualised. Note the presence of any discharge or bleeding from the cervix and any polyps or areas of ulceration. If the clinical history suggests possible infection (see Table 40.5), take swabs from the vaginal fornices and cervical os and place in a transport medium to look for *Candida*, *Trichomonas* and *Neisseria*; take a separate swab from the endocervix to look for *Chlamydia*.

Appearance of the vaginal wall

Ask the patient to bear down; a cystocele (descent of the bladder through the anterior vaginal wall) or rectocele (descent of the rectum through the posterior vaginal wall) or uterine prolapse may become apparent. Then ask the patient to cough; this may demonstrate stress incontinence. Note the presence of vaginal atrophy in older women.

Prolapse

Uterovaginal prolapse is the protrusion of the uterus and/or the vaginal walls beyond their normal anatomical confines. Prolapse commonly occurs in women as a result of damage to the supporting

[a] Caspar Bartholin Secundus (1655–1738), a professor of philosophy at Copenhagen at the age of 19, then professor of medicine, anatomy and physics. He described the glands in 1677.

Female reproductive anatomy.

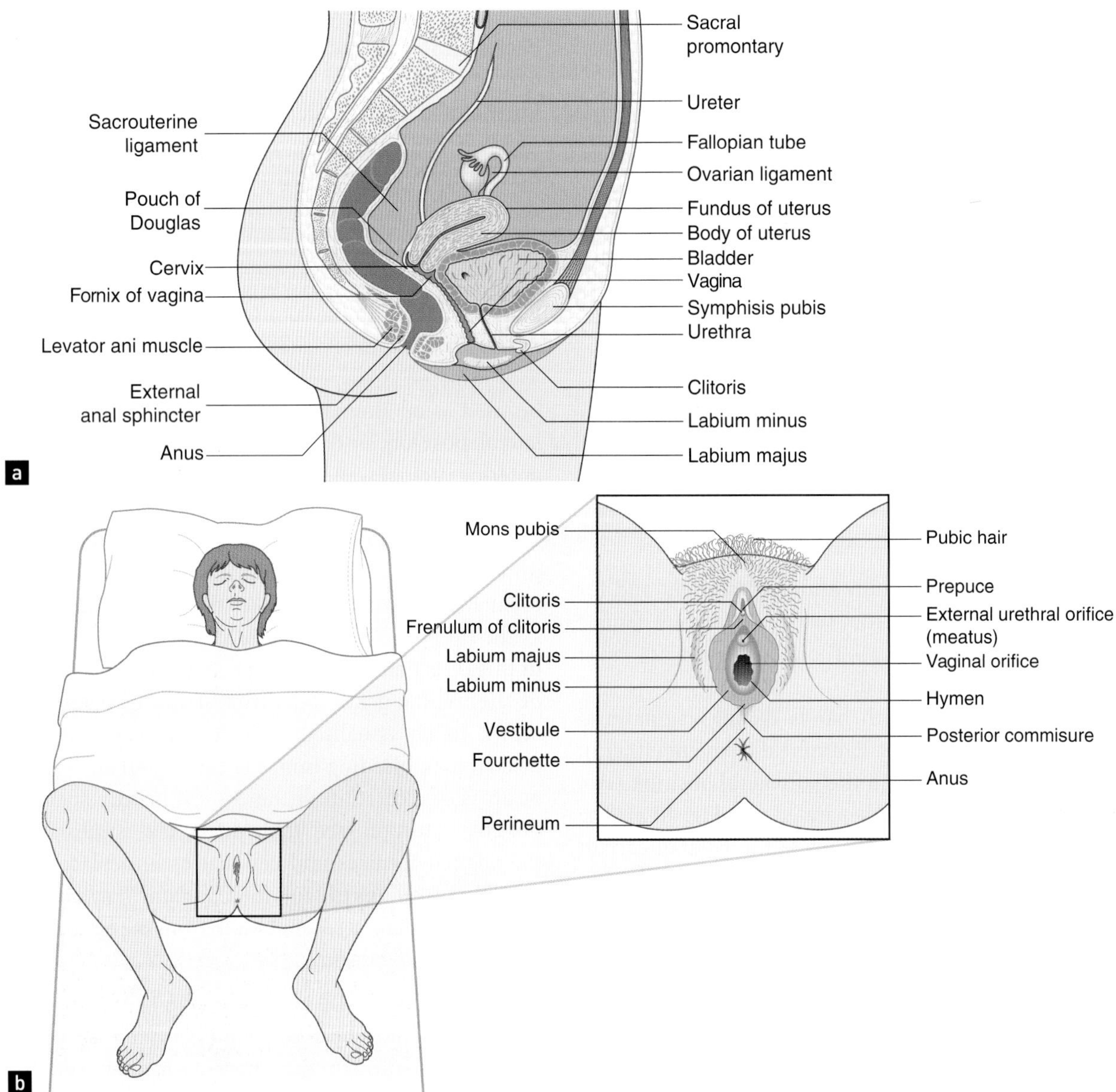

(a) Lateral view, showing the relationship of the genitals to the rectum and bladder.
(b) Position for examination

(From Douglas G, Nicol F, Robertson C. *Macleod's clinical examination*, 12th edn. Edinburgh: Churchill Livingstone, 2009.)

FIGURE 40.2

structures of the vagina and uterus following childbirth, although it may occur in women even after delivery by caesarean section. It is not unusual for minor degrees of prolapse to be asymptomatic and detected only as an incidental finding on vaginal examination. Where symptoms do occur these are commonly a feeling of fullness in the vagina or being able to feel a swelling protruding beyond the vaginal introitus.

The diagnosis of prolapse is a clinical one based on the appearances at the time of examination (see Fig. 40.6). Swelling of the anterior vaginal wall is described as a **cystocele**. Where swelling of the lower posterior

Vulval skin conditions

Presentation	Condition
Itchy, erythematous rash (endogenous) Atopic/seborrhoeic Allergic or irritant induced (exogenous)	Dermatitis
Chronic irritation, results in thickening and hypertrophy of skin, erythema, excoriations Mucosa not involved	Lichen simplex chronicus
Itch, discomfort, white discharge, dyspareunia, dysuria Hypersensitivity reaction on vulva Requires positive culture to confirm diagnosis	Candidiasis
Whitened parchment-like plaques Classic hourglass appearance involving perianal skin Loss of labial/clitoral architecture, introital narrowing May have tearing or subepithelial haemorrhage/petechiae Mucosa not involved	Lichen sclerosus (see Fig. 40.4)
Lichen simplex chronicus difficult to differentiate from lichen planus Introitus of vagina involved Adhesions and erosions may occur; not responsive to surgical division Oral/gingival involvement possible	Lichen planus
Itchy, scaly red plaques not as well demarcated as elsewhere on the skin; examine hair/scalp and nails also	Psoriasis
Itching Different patterns may be associated with red velvety area or area of lichenification	Vulvar intraepithelial neoplasia
Itch, discharge, bleeding may be painful Associated lymphadenopathy Raised ulcerated lesion	Vulvar cancer (see Fig. 40.5)

TABLE 40.4

Examination in the lateral semiprone positions with a Sims' speculum.

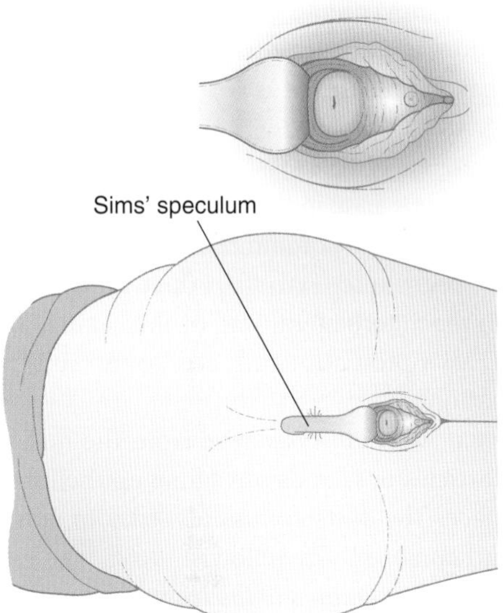

(From Symonds EM, Symonds IM. *Essential obstetrics and gynaecology*, 4th edn. Churchill Livingstone, 2004.)

FIGURE 40.3

Lichen sclerosus.

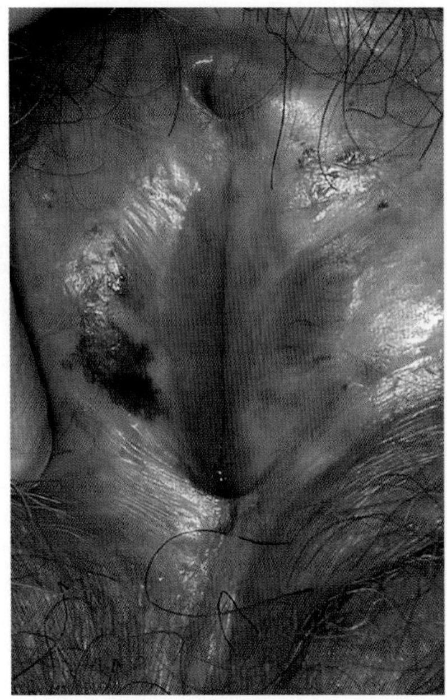

(Courtesy of Ruth Murphy, PhD, MBChB, FRCP, Nottingham, UK. In Murphy R. Lichen sclerosus. *Dermatol Clin* 2010; 28(4):707–715.)

FIGURE 40.4

Common organisms causing lower genital tract infections

Condition	Causative organism	Symptoms	Signs
Bacterial vaginosis	Anaerobic organisms including *Gardnerella* spp	Smelly vaginal discharge Vulval irritation	A typical thin homogeneous vaginal discharge
Chlamydial vulvovaginitis	*Chlamydia trachomatis*	Asymptomatic or vaginal discharge Intermenstrual bleeding	Inflamed cervix Contact bleeding Tenderness on cervical movement
Genital herpes	Herpes simplex virus (HSV) type 2	Vaginal discharge Vulval pain Dysuria Urinary retention	Skin vesicles and multiple shallow skin ulcers Inguinal lymphadenopathy
Genital warts (condyloma acuminata)	Human papillomavirus	Pruritus Vaginal discharge	Papillomatous lesions over vulva, perineum and into vagina
Gonococcal vulvovaginitis	*Neisseria gonorrhoeae*	Vaginal discharge	Mucopurulent vaginal discharge
Trichomoniasis	*Trichomonas vaginalis*	Vaginal bleeding Vaginal soreness Pruritus	Green frothy, watery discharge
Vaginal candidiasis	*Candida albicans*	Increased or changed vaginal discharge associated with soreness and itching in the vulva area	White, curd-like collections attached to the vaginal epithelium

TABLE 40.5

Carcinoma of the vulva.

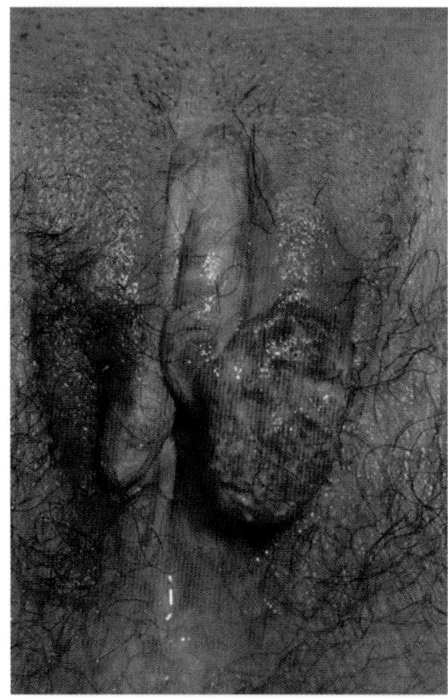

(From Arjona JE. Pregnancy following radical vulvectomy for carcinoma of the vulva: a case report and literature review. *Eur J Obstet Gynecol Reprod Biol* 2011; 158(1):113–114.)

FIGURE 40.5

wall is present this is described as a **rectocele**, and swelling of the upper posterior vaginal wall or posterior fornix is an **enterocele.** Uterine prolapse is described in terms of movement of the cervix in relation to the level of the vaginal introitus. Complete prolapse of the uterus beyond the introitus is described as **procidentia** (see Fig. 40.7).

Cystic swellings in the vagina and vulva

Congenital cysts arise in the vagina from embryological remnants. The most common varieties are those arising from Gartner's duct (Wolffian duct remnants). They occur in the anterolateral wall of the vagina. They are usually asymptomatic and are found on routine examination.

Vaginal inclusion cysts arise from the inclusion of small particles or islands of vaginal epithelium under the surface. The cysts commonly arise in episiotomy scars and contain thick yellowish fluid.

Solid benign tumours of the vagina are rare but may represent any of the tissues found in the vagina. Thus, polypoid tumours may include fibromyomas, myomas, fibromas, papillomas and adenomyomas.

Appearance of the cervix

'Normal' cervical squamous epithelium has a smooth pink appearance with a circular external os placed centrally. In practice, in women of reproductive age the external os is more irregular and slit-like and there is often a central area extending beyond the edge of the os that is a darker red and more velvety in appearance (see Fig. 40.8). This is sometimes called a cervical ectropion and represents an outgrowth of healthy columnar epithelium beyond the cervical canal. This is a normal variant, although it may be associated with an increase in clear vaginal discharge and, on occasion, contact bleeding. The columnar epithelium appears reddened because, unlike the stratified squamous epithelium of the ectocervix, there is only a single layer of columnar cells between the underlying capillaries and the surface. As the columnar epithelium is exposed to the acid pH of the vagina it tends to revert back to squamous epithelium in a process called squamous metaplasia. This sometimes traps islands of the mucus-secreting columnar epithelium below the surface of the new epithelium, leading to an accumulation of mucus in small retention cysts or Nabothian follicles.

In women with **cervicitis**, the cervix appears reddened and may be ulcerated, and there is a mucopurulent discharge as the endocervix is invariably involved. The diagnosis is established by examination and taking cervical swabs for culture.

Cervical intraepithelial neoplasia is not normally visible without the application of acetic acid or Lugol's iodine. The appearance of a raised or ulcerated lesion with irregular vessels on the surface is suggestive of cervical malignancy. Cervical polyps are common and may arise from the cervical canal or the external surface. Occasionally, an endometrial polyp may prolapse through the cervical canal and appear at the cervical os.

Cervical screening test (previously called a Pap smear)

There are two principle methods of screening for cervical neoplasia. The first is the routine cervical screening test for the detection of high-risk human papilloma virus (HPV) serotypes. The cytological examination of exfoliated cells from the squamous epithelium (previously called a Pap smear) is now performed only if the screening test is HPV positive or the patient is symptomatic. Both methods require collection of a sample from the cervix by speculum examination. The age at which routine screening starts and the frequency of testing vary from country to country. In Australia, testing commences at the age of 25, with the primary test being for the detection of HPV. A Pap smear, if indicated by an HPV-positive result, should be taken at least 6 weeks after pregnancy and not during menstruation.

The procedure is as follows. After inserting the speculum as above, wipe away any discharge from the surface of the cervix and take a 360° sweep with a suitable spatula or brush pressed firmly against the cervix at the junction of the columnar epithelium of the endocervical canal and the squamous epithelium of the ectocervix.

A liquid-based cytology test (LBC) is then performed. The sampling device is transferred into the preservative solution vial by pushing the broom into the bottom of the vial 10 times, forcing the bristles apart. In the laboratory the solution is then passed through a filter, which traps the large squamous cells but allows smaller red cells, debris and bacteria to pass through. The squamous cells are then transferred to a slide.

LBC also allows for testing for human papillomavirus and *Chlamydia* infection.

Vaginal swabs

The indications for taking vaginal swabs are symptoms of vaginal discharge (see Table 40.6), irregular bleeding and PID. Swabs may also be taken to screen for sexually transmitted infection in asymptomatic women. Cervicitis is associated with purulent vaginal discharge, sacral backache, lower abdominal pain, dyspareunia and dysuria, although in many cases the symptoms are minimal. The proximity of the cervix to the bladder often results in coexistent trigonitis and urethritis, particularly in the case of gonococcal infections.

A high vaginal swab is taken as part of the speculum examination by dipping the tip of a culture swab moistened in culture medium in the posterior vaginal fornix and then placing the swab immediately back into a suitable culture medium. This procedure is used mainly to identify organisms such as *Candida* or *Trichomonas* and in the assessment of bacterial vaginosis.

Clinical appearance of vaginal prolapse.

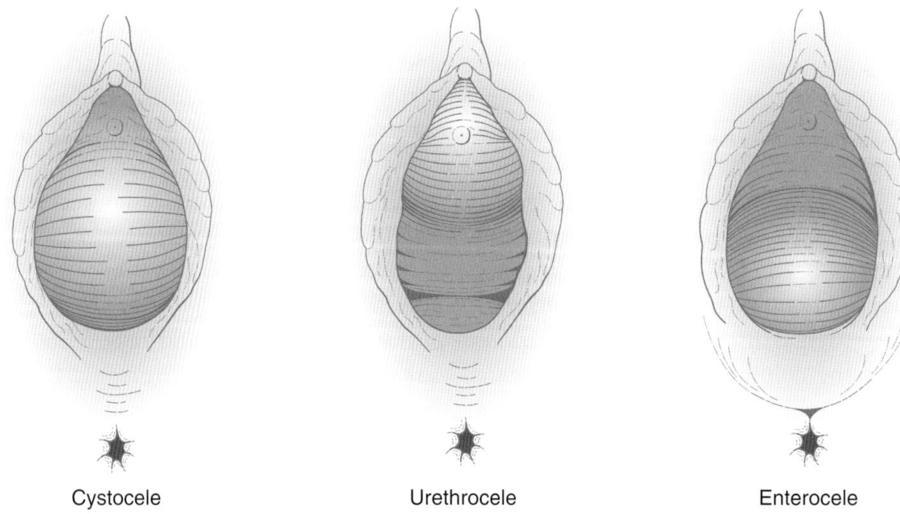

(From Symonds EM, Symonds IM. *Essential obstetrics and gynaecology*, 4th edn. Edinburgh: Churchill Livingstone, 2004.)

FIGURE 40.6

Procidentia (third-degree uterine prolapse).

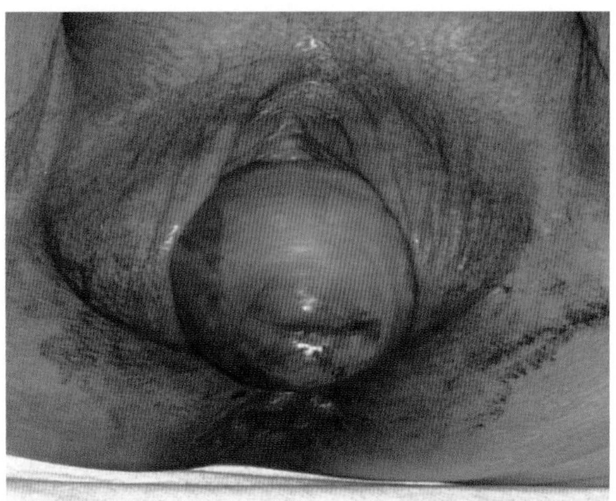

(From Lentz GM, Lobo RA, Gershenson DM. *Comprehensive gynecology*, 6th edn. Philadelphia: Elsevier Mosby, 2012, pp 453–474.)

FIGURE 40.7

Normal multiparous cervix.

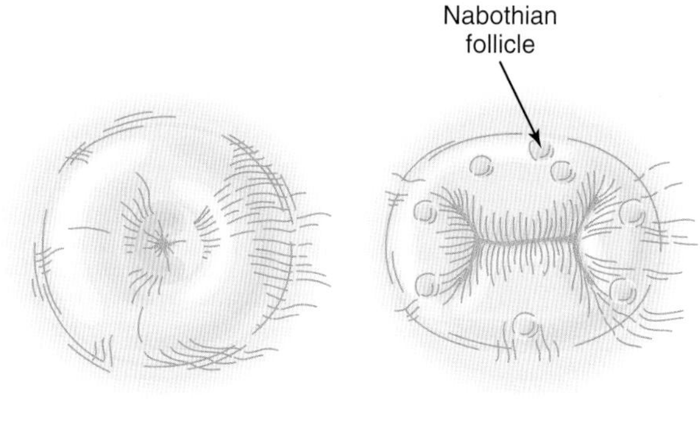

(From Hacker NF, Gambone JC, Hobel CJ. *Hacker and Moore's essentials of obstetrics and gynecology*, 5th edn. Philadelphia: Saunders, 2010.)

FIGURE 40.8

Endocervical swabs are taken by inserting the tip of the swab into the external cervical os and rotating two or three times. Using standard culture medium as for the high vaginal swab, the swab can be tested for *Neisseria gonorrhoeae*. Testing for *Chlamydia* infection can also be done by swabbing the endocervix. However, instead of culturing the organism, the presence of *Chlamydia* DNA is tested for using polymerase chain reaction by placing the swab in a specialised collection fluid in a plastic vial. The same principle can be used to test a first-pass urine sample to diagnose *Chlamydia*, so an endocervical swab is no longer necessary to test for this infection.

Bimanual examination

This is performed by introducing the middle and index fingers of your examining hand into the vaginal introitus and applying pressure towards the rectum. At the same time, place your other hand on the patient's abdomen above the symphysis pubis (see Fig. 40.9). The intravaginal portion of the cervix is tipped by your examining fingers (it can be identified by its consistency, which has a similar texture to the cartilage of the tip of the nose). Note the size, shape, consistency and position of the uterus. The uterus is commonly preaxial or anteverted, but will be postaxial or retroverted in some 10% of women. Provided that the retroverted uterus is mobile, the position is rarely significant. It is important to feel in the pouch of Douglas for the presence of thickening or nodules (a feature of endometriosis), and then to palpate laterally in both fornices for the presence of any ovarian or tubal masses (see Fig. 40.10). An attempt should be made to differentiate between adnexal and uterine masses, although often this is not possible. For example, a pedunculated fibroid may mimic an ovarian tumour, whereas a solid ovarian tumour, if adherent to the uterus, may be impossible to distinguish from a uterine fibroid. The ovaries may be palpable in the normal pelvis if the patient is thin, but the fallopian tubes are palpable only if they are significantly enlarged.

Diagnosis of vaginal discharge

Features of discharge and associated symptoms	Possible causes
Thick, white, non-itchy	Physiological
Bloody	Menstruation, a miscarriage, cancer or a cervical polyp or erosion
Thick, white, cottage cheese discharge, vulval itching, vulval soreness and irritation, pain or discomfort	*Candida albicans*
Yellow-green, itchy, frothy, foul-smelling ('fishy' smell) discharge	*Trichomonas*
Thin, grey or green, discharge with a fishy odour	Bacterial vaginosis
Thick white discharge, dysuria and pelvic pain, friable cervix	Gonorrhoea

TABLE 40.6

Pelvic mass

Table 40.7 lists the common causes of a mass arising from the pelvis in women. The uterus is palpable above the symphysis pubis on abdominal palpation in

Bimanual examination.

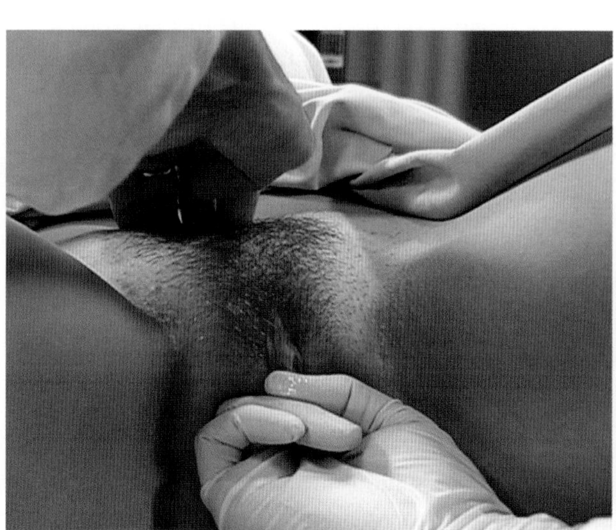

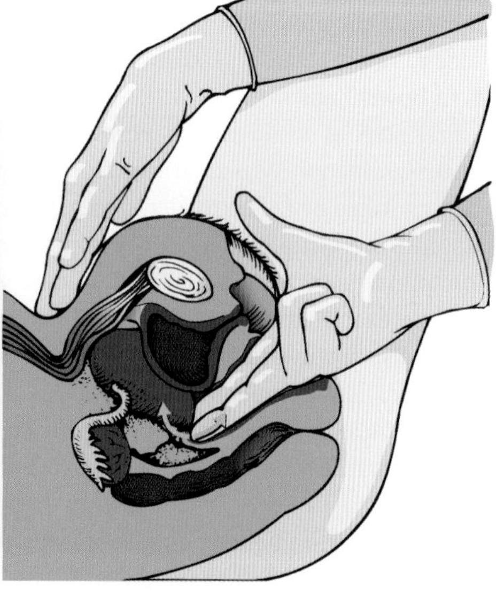

(From Seidel HM, Ball JW, Dains JE et al. *Mosby's guide to physical examination*, 7th edn. St Louis, MO: Mosby, 2011.)

FIGURE 40.9

Bimanual examination of (a) the pelvis and (b) the lateral fornix.

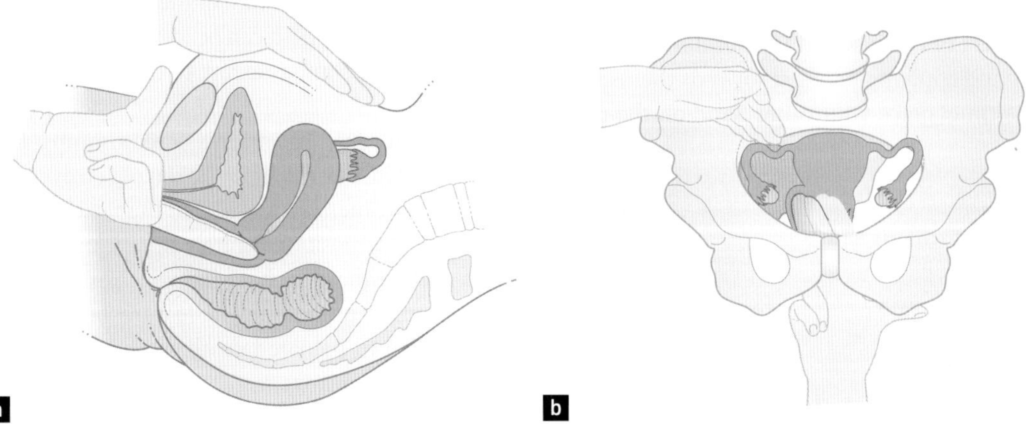

(From Symonds EM, Symonds IM. *Essential obstetrics and gynaecology*, 4th edn. Edinburgh: Churchill Livingstone, 2004.)

FIGURE 40.10

pregnancy after 12 weeks' gestation and typically uterine masses are described in terms of the equivalent uterine enlargement in pregnancy. For example, a uterine mass extending up to the umbilicus would be described as '20 weeks' in size.

Many pelvic masses cause no symptoms, even when large in size. The presence of pain most commonly occurs only when there is bleeding within or from the lesion (for example, in the case of ovarian cysts) or when the lesion becomes infarcted (for example, as a result of torsion; see Fig. 40.11). If large enough, a mass may be associated with pressure symptoms on the adjacent organs, such as urinary frequency or changes in bowel habits.

The first step in evaluating a pelvic mass is an abdominal examination. Masses arising from the pelvis can be distinguished by failure to identify a gap between the mass and the symphysis pubis. The presence of scars from previous surgery or ascites should be noted.

On pelvic examination a pelvic space-occupying lesion may cause downward pressure leading to vaginal prolapse. A speculum examination is essential to exclude a primary cervical lesion such as advanced cervical cancer, although this will normally present earlier with bleeding. The mass can then be assessed by bimanual palpation. This allows a better estimate of the size and other clinical features—in particular, whether the mass is smooth or irregular, fixed or mobile, and whether it feels cystic or solid. Further assessment is normally undertaken using pelvic ultrasound.

Special circumstances

Keep in mind the following:

- Except in an emergency situation, a pelvic examination should not be carried out on a non-English-speaking patient without an interpreter. Be aware that examination may be more difficult for women with particular cultural or religious expectations.
- Women who experience difficulty with vaginal examination should be allowed to disclose any underlying sexual difficulties or traumas. However, do not assume that all women who experience difficulty with pelvic examinations have a history of sexual abuse.
- Exceptional gentleness should be displayed in the examination of victims of alleged sexual assault. The woman should be given a choice about the gender of the doctor and be allowed to control the pace of, and her position for, the examination.
- The basic principles of respect, privacy, explanation and consent that apply to the conduct of gynaecological examinations in general apply equally to the conduct of such examinations in women who have temporary or permanent learning disabilities or mental illness.
- When examining an anaesthetised patient, treat the woman with the same degree of sensitivity and respect as if she were awake.

Differential diagnosis of pelvic mass

Origin of mass	Clinical features
Uterine	Central Uterus cannot be felt separately If uterus mobile, moves with uterus
Leiomyomata	Smooth, solid, may be single or multiple giving an irregular outline to the uterus Normally non-tender
Pregnancy	Uniform enlargement, soft and fluid-filled (the presence of fetal heart sounds is pathognomonic!)
Adenomyosis	Smoothly enlarged (rarely more than 12 weeks' size), globular shape and tender to palpation
Cancer of the corpus	Uniform enlargement, usually solid If tender, sarcoma more likely
Cervical cancer	Associated with an irregular mass arising from the cervix and extending into the vagina Often necrotic, with contact bleeding
Ovary / fallopian tubes	More likely to be adnexal than central
Inflammatory (tubo-ovarian abscess)	Tender, cervical excitation, ill-defined Solid or cystic, associated with systemic illness / fever
Ovarian cysts	May be solid (dermoid or fibroma) or cystic (epithelial tumours) Normally unilateral, smooth regular outline, mobile Tenderness suggests bleeding or torsion
Ovarian malignancy	More likely to be cystic fixed and associated with ascites
Endometriosis	May be associated with adnexal mass (usually ovarian endometrioma) More often diffuse change in the pelvis with fixed non-mobile uterus, nodules and thickening in the posterior fornix and tenderness

TABLE 40.7

Common complications of ovarian tumours causing symptoms.

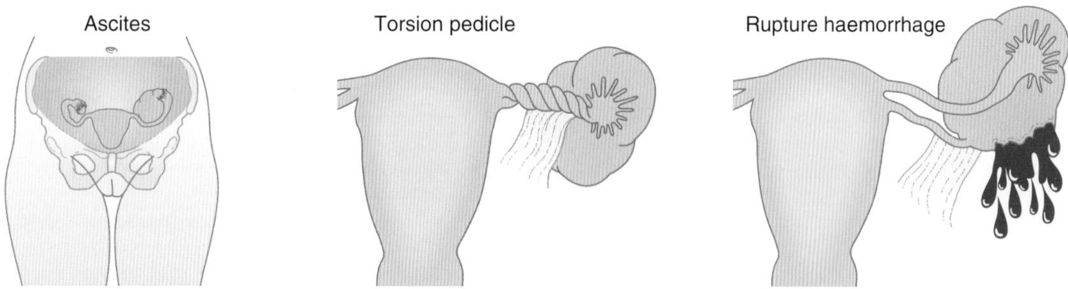

(From Symonds EM, Symonds IM. *Essential obstetrics and gynaecology*, 4th edn. Edinburgh: Churchill Livingstone, 2004.)

FIGURE 40.11

Rectal examination

Rectal examination may be indicated if there are symptoms such as a change in bowel habits or rectal bleeding, which may suggest bowel disease. It is occasionally used as a means of assessing a pelvic mass and in conjunction with a vaginal examination can provide additional information about disease in the rectovaginal septum.

OSCE REVISION TOPICS – THE GYNAECOLOGICAL HISTORY AND EXAMINATION

Use these topics, which commonly occur in the OSCE, to help with revision.

1. This woman has a history of heavy periods. Please take a full history from her and explain what further investigations you would like to perform. (pp 779–80)
2. This couple have been unable to conceive for 2 years. Please take a history and describe what features you would look for on examination that would be relevant to establishing a diagnosis. (pp 783–4, 785, 792–3)
3. This young woman presents with vaginal discharge 3 weeks after having unprotected intercourse with a new partner. Please take a full sexual history from her. (p 818)
4. Demonstrate how you would perform a pelvic examination and take a cervical screening test using this manikin. (pp 821, 825, 827)
5. Explain how you would perform a pelvic examination for a woman with vaginal discharge. (pp 791–2)
6. This woman has a pelvic mass. Please examine her. (pp 793–4)

T&O'C ESSENTIALS

1. *All women complaining of heavy periods should have a pelvic examination, full blood count and Pap smear.*
2. *Worrying features of uterine bleeding requiring further investigation include bleeding after the menopause, bleeding between periods and any abnormality of pelvic examination.*
3. *Pregnancy should be excluded in any women of reproductive age presenting with acute abdominal pain, abnormal bleeding or secondary amenorrhoea.*
4. *Atypical presentations are common in ectopic pregnancy.*
5. *The presence of a darker red area around the external cervical os on speculum examination is usually associated with an extension of the columnar epithelium onto the ectocervix and is a normal finding (ectropion).*
6. *Asymptomatic vaginal prolapse is common in multiparous women and does not require treatment.*
7. *Ovarian tumours can remain asymptomatic unless complicated by torsion, haemorrhage or rupture.*

References

1. Critchley HOD, Munro MG, Broder M, Fraser IS. A five-year international review process concerning terminologies, definitions and related issues around abnormal uterine bleeding. *Semin Reprod Med* 2011; 29:377–382.
2. NSW Sexually Transmissible Infections Programs Unit. *NSW Health Sexual Health Services standard operating procedures manual*. Sydney: NSW STI Programs Unit, 2011.
3. General Medical Council Standards Committee. Maintaining boundaries: intimate examinations and chaperones, *GMC guidelines for intimate examination ethical practice*. London: GMC, 2013. www.gmc-uk.org/Maintaining_boundaries_Intimate_examinations_and_chaperones.pdf_58835231.pdf.
4. Deneke M, Wheeler L, Wagner G et al. An approach to relearning the pelvic examination. *J Fam Pract* 1982; 14:782–783. This study provides useful hints.

CHAPTER 41

The breasts: history and examination

Blessed is the physician who takes a good history, looks keenly at his patient and thinks a bit.

WALTER C ALVAREZ (1976)

Breast examination is a vitally important part of the general physical examination. In women aged 40 and older, a screening physical examination for breast cancer may be advised (e.g. monthly self-examination by the patient and yearly examination by the doctor), but there is no convincing evidence of the value of breast self-examination.[1]

EXAMINATION ANATOMY

The attachment of the female breast extends from the clavicle superiorly to the inframammary crease (sixth rib) inferiorly and from the sternum to the midaxillary line (see Fig. 41.1). The area covered is more rectangular than circular. The axillary tail is an extension of the superolateral part of the breast up towards the axilla. This tail extends along the lower border of the pectoralis major muscle and may abut the clavipectoral fascia, which separates this from the axillary lymph nodes.

Breast tissue has fatty, glandular and fibrous components, and the distribution is variable and depends on age, weight and hormone status (e.g. use of hormone replacement therapy). Women in their twenties who are thin have very little fat. Most 80 year olds have very little fibroglandular tissue.

There is a surrounding superficial fascia attached to the skin and pectoral fascia by ligaments. The normal breast does not have a homogeneous feel but is somewhat lumpy.

There are a number of benign abnormalities of the breast that change the texture or appearance of the breast, including:

- fibroadenomas with overgrowth of connective tissue surrounding the ducts
- cysts with obstruction of collecting ducts (however, it is not simply due to obstruction; it is hormonally mediated as they are much less common in postmenopausal women not on hormone replacement therapy [HRT])
- intraductal papilloma, causing a nipple discharge on the affected side (clear or bloodstained)
- mammary duct ectasia, which causes nipple discharge.

HISTORY

The history is imperative. Essential questions to ask include the length of time any mass has been noticed, the presence of pain, any change in size or texture over time, relationship to the menstrual cycle, and any nipple discharge. Ask whether the patient has conducted regular self-examinations and has discovered a change in her breast. Ask about previous breast surgery, biopsies or cyst aspirations, or recurrent abscesses (e.g. granulomatous mastitis). Has the woman breastfed her babies and for how long? Was breastfeeding difficult or associated with breast infection (mastitis)? Has she had breast implants and have these caused any problems?

> HINT BOX
>
> Remember, pathological discharge is generally clear or bloodstained; spontaneous (i.e. not expressed), and uniduct. All other discharge—yellow/green/white, multiduct, bilateral or not spontaneous—is physiological.

Find out about risk factors for breast cancer, including any family history of breast or ovarian cancer (and age when affected), previous personal history of breast cancer, obesity, early menarche and late menopause, late first pregnancy, mantle radiation, heavy

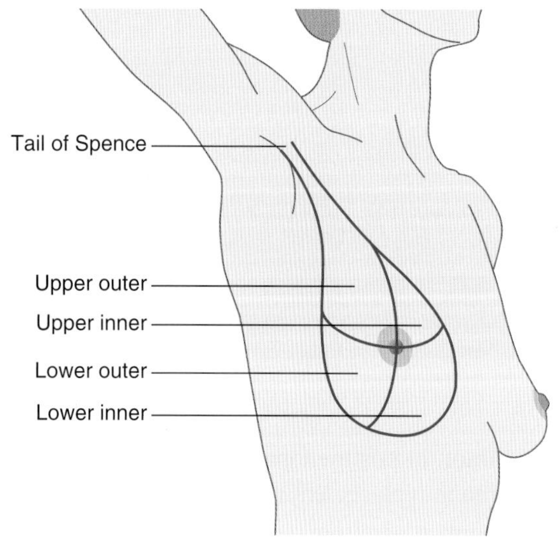

Breast anatomy

(From Douglas G, Nicol F, Robertson C. *Macleod's clinical examination*, 12th edn. Edinburgh: Churchill Livingstone, 2009.)

FIGURE 41.1

alcohol use and use of oestrogens postmenopausally. A personal history of atypical hyperplasia (ductal or lobular) increases the risk of breast cancer. However, three-quarters of patients presenting with a breast cancer have *no* known risk factors.

Ask about genetic testing and mammography if relevant. The breast cancer genes *BRCA1* and *BRCA2* are associated with a strong risk of breast (and ovarian) cancer, as well as breast cancer in men. Patients with a strong family history of breast or ovarian cancer should be asked whether genetic testing has been carried out. Screening mammography is generally recommended for all women from the age of 50 years.[2]

Enlargement of the male breasts (gynaecomastia; p 476) is often a result of hormone or drug treatment (e.g. for carcinoma of the prostate or with spironolactone or digoxin). It is often tender. Bilateral enlargement is usually benign, but unilateral enlargement may be due to malignancy. As malignancy is more common in men with gynaecomastia, asymmetrical enlargement should arouse concern. Carcinoma of the male breast is over 100 times less frequent than female breast carcinoma. As there is less breast tissue present in men and the condition is often not thought of, disease tends to be locally advanced at the time of diagnosis.

EXAMINATION

When it is done properly, the examination takes some time to perform (about 3 minutes per breast).[3] The need for examination must obviously be explained to the patient at the start. The patient should be offered a chaperone.

The examination is only just over 50% sensitive for carcinoma, but specificity is as high as 90%. The likelihood ratio (LR) of a positive examination is 14.1 and the LR of a negative examination is 0.47.[4]

Inspection

Ask the patient to sit up with the chest fully exposed. There is controversy about the value of inspection of the breasts as part of the examination, but advanced cancers may be obvious at this stage. Look at the *nipples* for retraction (due to cancer or fibrosis; in some patients retraction may be normal, so it is important to ask whether it is long-standing) and Paget's disease of the breast (where underlying breast cancer causes a unilateral rash or ulceration of the nipple). Asymmetry of breast size is common, and it is important to ask whether any asymmetry is new.

Next inspect the rest of the *skin*. Look for visible veins (which, if unilateral, suggest a cancer), skin dimpling and *peau d'orange* skin (where advanced, breast cancer causes oedematous skin pitted by the sweat glands). Look for erythema from mastitis (the area will be hot and tender). Inflammatory breast cancer is a rare cause of a similar appearance.

A persistent erythematous plaque in the nipple area may be contact dermatitis or skin irritation, but if asymmetrical or it has not responded to treatment this may be malignant *Paget's disease of the breast*.

Ask the patient to *raise the arms above the head* and then lower them slowly. Look for tethering of the nipples or skin, a shift in the relative position of the nipples or a fixed mass distorting the breast (see Fig. 41.2).

Note whether there are any obvious visible masses in the axillae.

Next ask the patient to rest the hands on the hips and then press the hands against the hips (the pectoral contraction manoeuvre). This accentuates areas of dimpling or fixation.

Conditions unrelated to the breast may be found incidentally, such as pectus excavatum or carinatum, distended veins related to inferior vena caval (IVC)

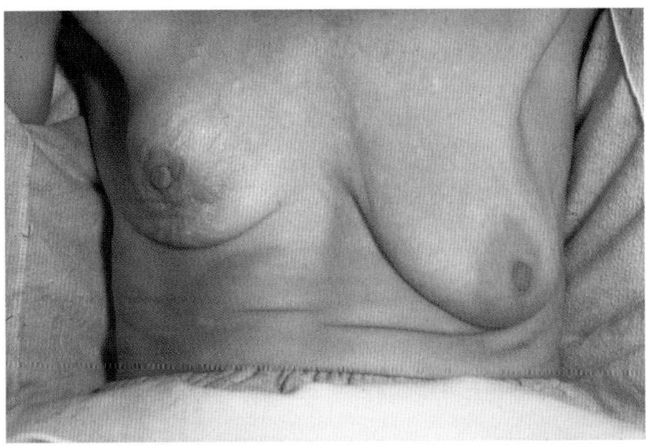

Carcinoma of the right breast, showing elevation of the breast, dimpling of the skin and retraction of the nipple

FIGURE 41.2

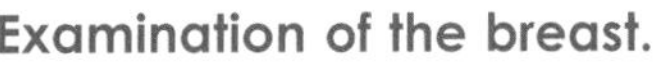

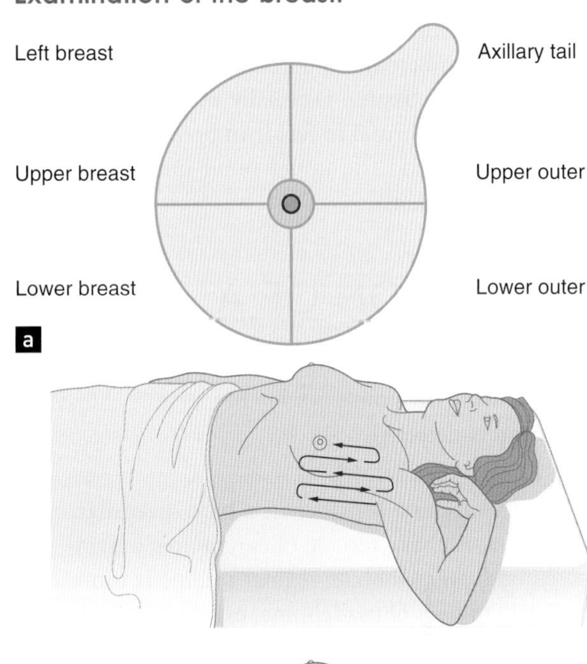

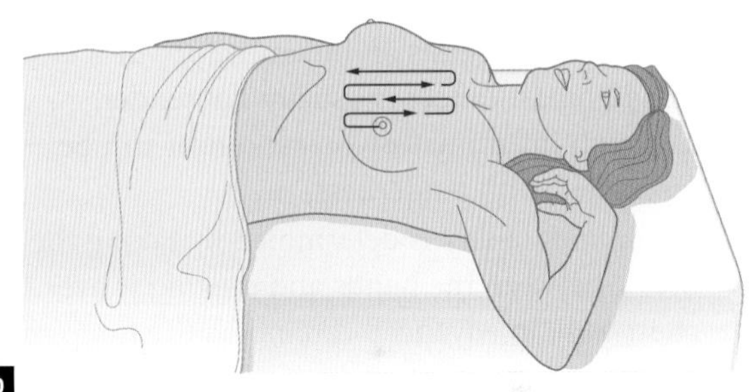

(a) Quadrants; (b) systematic examination

FIGURE 41.3

obstruction and signs of virilisation such as acne and hirsutism.

Palpation

Examine both the supraclavicular and the axillary regions for lymphadenopathy. It may be difficult, however, to distinguish an axillary fat pad from an enlarged lymph node.

Then ask the patient to lie down. The examination can be performed only if the breast tissue is flattened against the chest wall. It is helpful to have the patient place the hand behind the head for palpation of the lateral aspect of the breast and bring the elbow up level with the shoulder for palpation of the medial side of the breast.

There is no single correct way to palpate the breast, as long as all sections are palpated. We recommend palpation is performed gently with the pulps of the middle three fingers parallel to the contour of the breast supporting the breast with the other hand. The total examination should involve a rectangular area bordered by the clavicle, the sternum, the midaxillary line and the 'bra line'. Start in the axilla and palpate in a line down to the bra line inferiorly. Do not pinch the breast as you may mistakenly think you feel a mass. The pattern of palpation is like that of mowing a lawn, a series of vertical strips that cover the whole of the rectangle (see Fig. 41.3). Palpation may also be performed by quadrant, in a spiral fashion from the nipple outwards or in a 'flower petal' pattern radiating around the breast from the nipple outwards.

Palpation is more difficult when a breast implant is present. It is probably best to examine such a patient in a supine position and to keep the patient's ipsilateral arm down at the side.

Next feel behind the nipple for lumps.

Finish the examination of the breast with the patient sitting up as some lumps are easier to feel in this position. It is important to do this with two hands—that is, one (the left if right-handed) underneath and the right on top so that there is some flattening of the breast tissue.

Do not mistake normal breast structures for a mass.[5] You may feel a rib or costochondral junction normally on deep palpation. The inferior ridge of breast tissue (inframammary fold) may be felt and is symmetrical. You may feel normal rubbery-type plaques (fibroglandular tissue), especially in the upper outer quadrant. It is normal to feel firm breast tissue at the areola border, and the upper outer quadrant of the breast is often dense.

EVALUATION OF A BREAST LUMP

The following five points need to be carefully elucidated if a lump is detected.

1. *Position:* (see below).
2. *Size, shape and consistency:* a hard, irregular nodule is characteristic of carcinoma; a firm, smooth, very mobile, regular nodule is more likely to be a fibroadenoma, especially in a young woman.
3. *Tenderness:* suggests an inflammatory or a cystic lesion; breast cancer is usually not tender, although inflammatory breast cancer can be associated with tenderness.
4. *Fixation:* mobility is determined by taking the breast between the hands and moving it over the chest wall; in advanced carcinoma the lump may be fixed to the chest wall.
5. *Single or multiple lesions present:* multiple nodules suggest benign cystic disease or fibroadenosis.

Remember that lumps found on breast examination may not involve breast tissue; these include lipomas and sebaceous cysts.

Remember also that many normal breasts have palpable lumps and that, although benign lumps tend to be soft, moveable and regular, they can also have the characteristics of malignant lumps.[5] Causes of a lump in the breast are listed in Table 41.1.

In men with true gynaecomastia, a disc of breast tissue can be palpated under the areola. This is not present in men who are merely obese.

Document your findings using the 'clock system': envisage the breast like a clock with respect to the location of any lump or lesion indicated on the breast (e.g. 9 o'clock position) and the distance from the radial edge of the areola noted. The size of the mass and its other features must also be recorded (see above).

Causes of a breast lump

Non-tender	Tender
Cyst Carcinoma Fibrocystic disease* Fibroadenoma (benign highly mobile 'breast mouse')	Cyst Breast abscess Fibroadenosis Costal cartilage chondritis Inflammatory breast cancer
Uncommon causes:	
Trauma, fat necrosis Other cysts (e.g. galactocele) Other neoplasms (e.g. duct papilloma) Granulomatous mastitis (an inflammatory condition mimicking breast cancer) Chest wall (e.g. lipoma, costal cartilage chondritis [causes tenderness but not a lump])	

**Clinically lumps in the breast are often ridges of fibroglandular tissue that may become more prominent owing to changes in weight or hormonal influence. On imaging, the term 'fibrocystic change' is more commonly used to describe sonographic changes that are likely benign.*

TABLE 41.1

T&O'C ESSENTIALS

1. *A palpable breast mass is likely to be significant (called a dominant mass) if it is:*
   - *clearly three-dimensional*
   - *distinct from the surrounding tissue*
   - *asymmetrical compared with the other breast*
   - *persistent throughout a menstrual cycle*
   - *not smooth, well-demarcated or mobile.*
2. *A palpable breast mass is more likely to be malignant if it has the following characteristics:*
   - *Very firm.*
   - *Margins seem poorly defined or have an irregular edge.*
   - *Immobile or fixed.*
   - *Associated skin dimpling.*
   - *Associated retraction of the nipple, or nipple scaling.*
   - *Bloody nipple discharge history.*
   - *Draining lymph nodes are palpable.*

OSCE REVISION TOPICS – **THE BREASTS**

Take a history from this woman who has found a lump in her breast. Explain what features you would look for on examination that would suggest malignancy. (p 800)

References

1. Riley M, Dobson M, Jones E, Kirst N. Health maintenance in women. *Am Fam Physician* 2013; 87(1):30–37. Describes current guidelines for screening for breast cancer and other cancers in women.
2. Kerlikowske K, Smith-Bindman R, Ljung BM et al. Evaluation of abnormal mammography results and palpable breast abnormalities. *Ann Intern Med* 2003; 139:274–284. Discusses how to approach interpreting mammogram reports and the next steps.
3. Fenton JJ, Rolnick SJ, Harris EL et al. Specificity of clinical breast examination in community practice. *J Gen Intern Med* 2007; 22(3):332–357. Screening breast examinations in clinical practice are highly specific but insensitive. A normal exam is reassuring.
4. Barton MB, Harris R, Fletcher SW. Does this patient have breast cancer? *JAMA* 1999; 282:1270–1280. The clinical breast examination has an overall specificity that is high (94%) but the sensitivity is poor (54%). Unfortunately, inter-observer variation seems to be high.
5. Pruthi S. Detection and evaluation of a palpable breast mass. *Mayo Clin Proc* 2001; 76:641–647. Most breast masses are benign but malignancy must be excluded. If cancer is suspected but mammography is negative, further testing is indicated.

SECTION 12
Specialty system history and examination

CHAPTER 42
The eyes, ears, nose and throat

CHAPTER 43
The skin and lumps

CHAPTER 44
The older person assessment

CHAPTER 45
Approaching infectious diseases

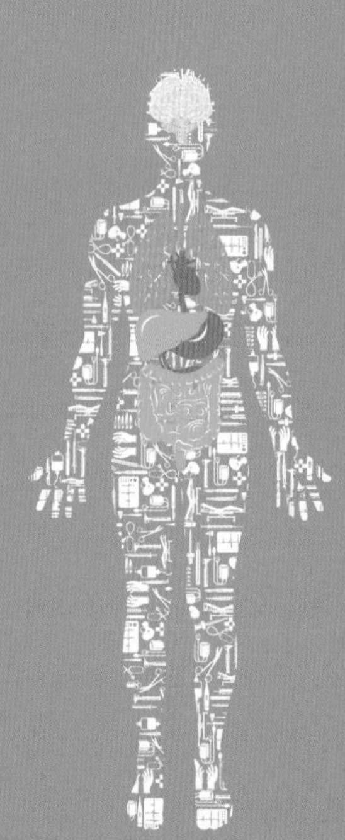

CHAPTER 42

The eyes, ears, nose and throat

Diagnosis is not the end, but the beginning of practice. MARTIN H FISCHER (1879–1962)

The examination of the eyes and ears, nose and throat is important for any medical patient because these small parts of the body may be involved in local or systemic disease.

EYES

Examination anatomy

The structure of the eye is shown in Fig. 42.1.[1] There are three layers that make up the eye ball:

- The **inner or neural layer** forms the retina itself and has inner and outer layers. The *outer layer* contains pigmented cells and the *inner layer*, which is continuous with the optic nerve, contains the photoreceptor *rod* (night and peripheral vision) and *cone* (central and colour vision) cells.
- The **central layer** is called the *uveal* tract. It forms the *iris* and *ciliary body* anteriorly and the *choroid* posteriorly. The choroid is a vascular structure. It supplies the optic nerve, the *fovea* (area of most acute vision) and the posterior two-thirds of the retina. The ciliary body produces the *aqueous humour*. This transparent fluid lies behind the cornea and fills the *anterior chamber* of the eye. The aqueous humour moves through the pupil and drains through a trabecular meshwork at the acute angle of the anterior chamber. The *lens* sits behind the cornea and is suspended from ligaments of the ciliary body.
- The **outer layer** is fibrous. The anterior part, the *cornea*, is transparent and the rest makes up the *sclera*. The main volume of the eyeball is filled with *vitreous humour*, which is a transparent gel.

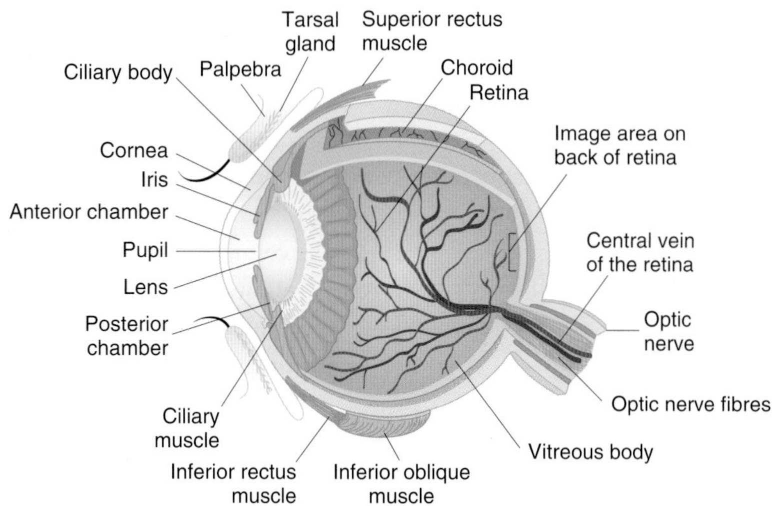

The structure of the eye

FIGURE 42.1

The anatomy of the optic nerve is described in Chapter 32.

The eyelids provide and distribute moisture to the corneas from three types of glands (two small and one large). The two types of small *lacrimal*[a] glands within the eyelids secrete tears and produce mucin and oil. These are sufficient to lubricate the eyelids and the cornea in normal circumstances. Emotion or a foreign body, however, will stimulate the large lacrimal glands that lie between the bony orbital wall laterally and the eyeball and the lateral rectus muscle medially. From each gland duct, big volumes of tears drain into the upper part of the lid. Tears either evaporate or are drained via the medial edge of the eye into the lacrimal canaliculi and on into the lacrimal sac, the lacrimal duct, the inferior nasal meatus and thence to the nose—and, if necessary, into a handkerchief. The conjunctiva is a mucous membrane that lines the eyelids and keeps them slippery on the inside.

QUESTIONS TO ASK THE PATIENT WITH A PAINFUL RED EYE

! denotes symptoms for the possible diagnosis of an urgent or dangerous problem.

1. Do you wear contact lenses? (Corneal ulceration)
2. Is it painful when you move your eyes? (Iritis or scleritis)
3. Are the lids stuck together in the morning? (Conjunctivitis)
4. ! Have you had an injury or worked with dust, metal grinders or welding equipment? (Injury, foreign body or flash burn)
5. Have you had arthritis or rashes? (Vasculitis)

QUESTIONS BOX 42.1

History

Presenting symptoms include pain or discomfort and redness (see Table 42.2 and Questions box 42.1), loss or distortion of vision and watery eyes, and infection of the eyelids and associated structures. Loss of vision and other visual symptoms (see Table 42.1 and Questions box 42.2) are also discussed in Chapter 32.

Ask about symptoms of keratoconjunctivitis sicca (dry eyes). These include dryness, burning and irritation and usually become worse as the day goes on. They are made worse by smoke, allergens and low humidity (e.g. from air conditioning). The cause may be reduced tear production or increased tear evaporation (List 42.1).

More general questions include asking about other conditions which can affect the eyes including:

- inflammatory arthritis
- thyroid disease
- atrial fibrillation
- vascular disease
- use of contact lenses
- occupation (arc welding or metal grinding)
- smoking
- measles (associated with conjunctivitis) (see Fig. 42.2)
- multiple sclerosis.

Ask about previous eye problems or surgery including laser correction surgery. Have the intraocular pressures been measured recently?

Take a drug history. Ask about eye drops and drugs such as corticosteroids (cataracts), anticholinergics (glaucoma from acute angle closure), amiodarone (corneal deposits), chloroquine and chlorpromazine (retinal toxicity) and ethambutol and isoniazid (optic neuropathy).

Examination method

Sit the patient at the edge of the bed. Stand well back at first, and note the following:

1. **Ptosis** (drooping of one or both upper eyelids).
2. The **colour of the sclerae**:
   - **yellow**, caused by deposits of bilirubin in jaundice
   - **blue**, which may be due to osteogenesis imperfecta, because the thin sclerae allow the choroidal pigment to show through; blue sclerae can also occur in families without osteogenesis imperfecta; blue-grey scleral discoloration occurs in patients with ochronosis (see Fig. 42.3(a)), resulting from the accumulation of homogentisic acid in

[a] From the Latin word for tear, *lacrima*. Hence the famous phrase in *The aeneid* when Aeneas sees the depictions of the fall of Troy on the new walls of Carthage and becomes very emotional, saying '*Refrum lacrimae sunt*'—there *are* tears for things.

Common causes of visual disturbance

Symptom	Common causes when answer is 'yes'
Sudden partial or complete loss in one eye (important to distinguish from hemianopia)	**Transient:** retinal ischaemia (amaurosis fugax), retinal migraine, optic neuritis **Prolonged:** retinal detachment, retinal embolus, diabetic retinopathy (sudden or gradual), temporal arteritis, trauma
Hemianopia	Visual cortical infarct, parieto-occipital infarct
Gradual loss of vision unilateral or bilateral	Cataract, macular degeneration, glaucoma (painless if chronic), tumour of base of skull (e.g. meningioma, pituitary adenoma)
Blurred vision	Refractive error, cataract, macular degeneration (usually a central scotoma)
Diplopia	**Monocular:** lens dislocation, cataract, astigmatism, hysteria **Binocular:** abnormal eye movements (e.g. ocular motor palsy)
Halos (distortion around the edges of bright lights)	Corneal oedema, acute glaucoma
Dry eyes (patient may feel something is in the eye)	Sjögren syndrome, blepharitis (inflammation of eyelids [e.g. from eczema]), infection of eyelids
Eye pain and headache	Cluster headache or migraine
Pain on eye movement	Optic neuritis
Eye painful and red	**Diffuse with central sparing:** conjunctivitis (lids stuck together) **No central sparing:** iritis, acute glaucoma (cornea cloudy) **Pain on moving eye:** scleritis (e.g. systemic vasculitis) Foreign body, entropion (lower lid inverted) Corneal ulceration (herpes simplex, contact lens)
Floaters in visual fields	Vitreous degeneration (associated with age and myopia)

TABLE 42.1

CAUSES OF DRY EYES

1. Reduced production: inflammation of the lachrymal glands from systemic illnesses such as rheumatoid arthritis and Sjögren syndrome
2. Increased evaporation: enlarged palpebral fissure (Grave's disease), Bell palsy

LIST 42.1

connective tissue in this inherited condition; the concha of the ear is often affected (see Fig. 42.3(b)), as are the joints and heart valves

- **red**, from *iritis* or scleritis, which causes central inflammation; or *conjunctivitis*, which causes more peripheral inflammation often with pus; or *subconjunctival haemorrhage*, which causes confluent blood as a result of trauma (see Table 42.2 and List 42.2)
- **scleral pallor**, which occurs in anaemia—pull down the lower lid and look for the normal contrast between the pearly white posterior

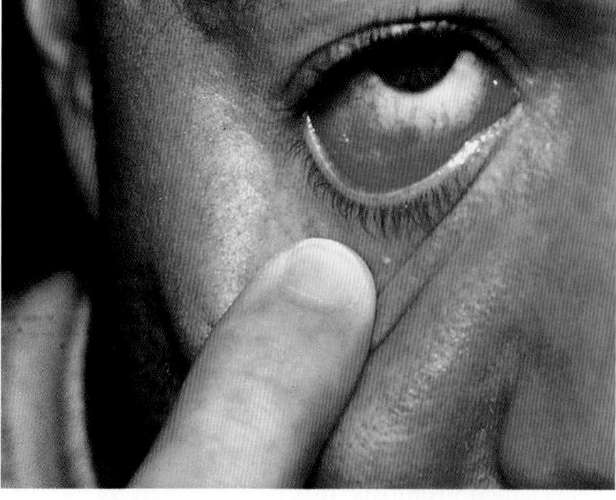

Conjunctivitis in a patient with measles

FIGURE 42.2

QUESTIONS TO ASK THE PATIENT WITH SUDDEN VISUAL LOSS

! denotes symptoms for the possible diagnosis of an urgent or dangerous problem.

1. Does the abnormality persist when you close each eye in turn? (Visual field loss)
2. Was the sensation as if a curtain was drawn across your vision? Has your vision come back? (Amaurosis fugax)
3. Have you had previous strokes or fibrillation of your heart? (Retinal embolus, cortical infarct)
4. ! Has your eye been painful? (Acute glaucoma, iritis)
5. Have you injured your eye or head? (Trauma to eye or optic nerve)
6. Have you had preceding visual disturbance, e.g. flashing lights? (Migraine)
7. Have you had severe headache on the same side? (Temporal arteritis)
8. Have you had weakness or tingling in your arms or legs, or bowel or bladder disturbance? (Multiple sclerosis and optic neuritis)
9. Are you a diabetic? (Diabetic retinopathy with haemorrhage)

QUESTIONS BOX 42.2

conjunctiva and the red anterior part; loss of this contrast is a reliable sign of anaemia (see Fig. 42.4(b)).

Look from behind and above the patient for **exophthalmos**, which is prominence of the eyes. If there is actual protrusion of the eyes from the orbits, this is called **proptosis**. It is best detected by looking at the eyes from above the forehead; protrusion beyond the supraorbital ridge is abnormal. If exophthalmos is present, examine specifically for thyroid eye disease: lid lag (the patient follows your finger as it descends—the upper lid lags behind the pupil), chemosis (oedema of the bulbar conjunctiva), corneal ulceration and ophthalmoplegia (weakness of upward gaze). Look then for any corneal abnormalities, such as band keratopathy or arcus senilis.

Ochronosis.

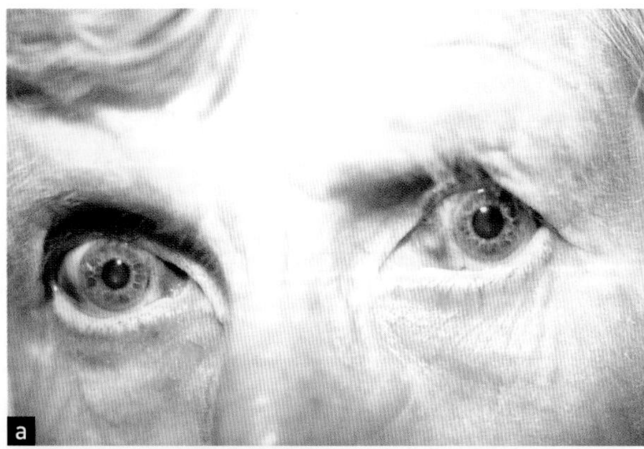

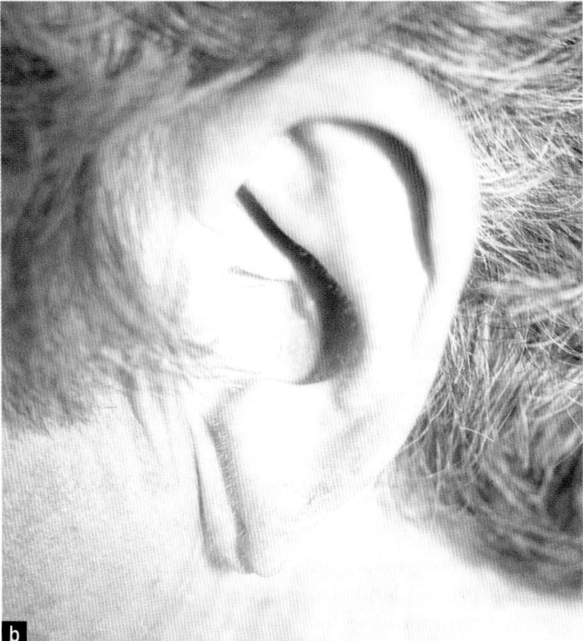

(a) Sclerae; (b) ears

FIGURE 42.3

Look for **corneal ulceration**, which may be obvious if severe. A strip coated with sterile fluorescein will stain corneal ulcers and make them easily visible. A branching (dendritic) ulcer is seen in herpes complex keratitis.

Proceed as for the **cranial nerve examination**—that is, testing *visual acuity*, *visual fields* and *pupillary responses* to light and accommodation. Interruption of the sympathetic innervation of the eye at any point results in *Horner syndrome* (*partial ptosis* and a

Distinguishing among common causes of a red and painful eye

Disease	Distribution of redness	Corneal surface	Pupil
Bacterial conjunctivitis	Peripheral conjunctiva Bilateral (central sparing)	Normal	Normal
Episcleritis	Segmental, often around cornea Unilateral	Normal	Normal
Acute iritis	Ciliary flush Unilateral	Dull (vision blurred)	Small, irregular shape, may be no light response
Glaucoma	Around cornea Unilateral	Dull	Mid-oval shape, no light response
Corneal ulcer	Around cornea Unilateral	Dull Fluorescein dye stains ulcer	Normal
Subconjunctival haemorrhage	Localised haemorrhage No posterior limit	Normal	Normal
Conjunctival haemorrhage	Localised haemorrhage Posterior limit present	Normal	Normal

TABLE 42.2

CAUSES OF UVEITIS

Iritis (anterior uveitis)

Viral

Idiopathic

Generalised disease

- Seronegative spondyloarthropathies
- Inflammatory bowel disease
- Diabetes mellitus
- Granulomatous disease (e.g. sarcoidosis)
- Infections (e.g. gonococcal, syphilis, toxoplasmosis, brucellosis, tuberculosis)

Choroiditis (posterior uveitis)

Idiopathic

Generalised disease

- Diabetes mellitus
- Granulomatous disease (e.g. sarcoidosis)
- Infections (e.g. toxoplasmosis, syphilis, tuberculosis, toxocaral infection)

The uveal tract consists of the anterior uvea (iris) and the posterior uvea (ciliary body and choroid).

LIST 42.2

T&O'C ESSENTIALS

Conjunctivitis

1. *Viral conjunctivitis (adenovirus) often begins after an upper respiratory infection. It can be unilateral and is of sudden onset. There has often been contact with other infected people.*
2. *Bacterial conjunctivitis (e.g.* Staph. aureus *in adults) usually causes thick, discoloured (green or yellow) discharge. The eyelids may be stuck together.*
3. *Allergic conjunctivitis occurs in association with sneezing, itching and excessive tear production. Bilateral redness and chemosis (conjunctival oedema) are common.*

constricted but reactive pupil). Perceptible *anisocoria* (inequality of the diameters of the pupils) has been found in 20% of healthy people. Remember also that elderly people quite often have imperceptible pupillary light reactions.

Test the **eye movements** (see Fig. 32.16, p 533). Look also for fatigability of eye muscles by asking the patient to look up at a hat-pin or finger for about half a minute. In myasthenia gravis the muscles tire and the eyelids begin to droop.

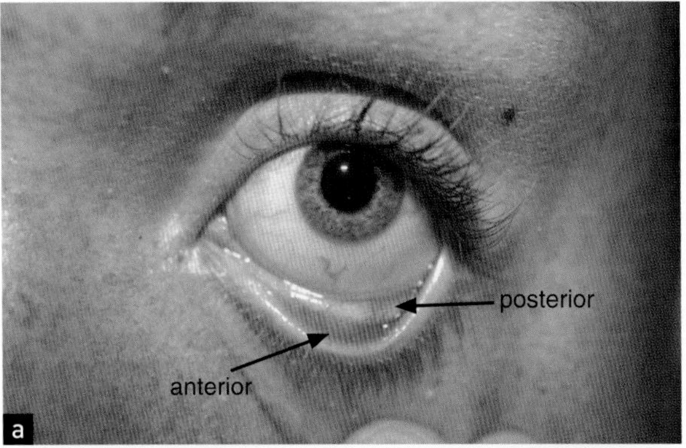

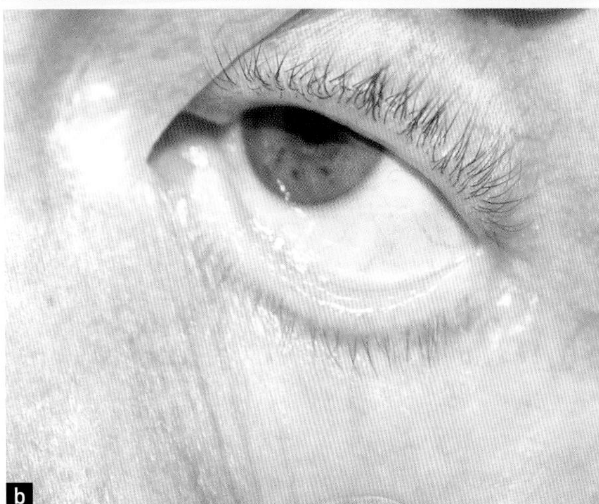

(a) Normal sclera; (b) conjunctival pallor in an anaemic patient.

Note the contrast between the anterior and posterior parts in the normal eye

FIGURE 42.4

Test **colour vision** if acuity is not poor. Ishihara test plates (where coloured spots form numbers) can be used. Red desaturation (impaired ability to see red objects) can occur with optic nerve disease. Red–green colour blindness affects 7% of males (X-linked recessive).

Test the **corneal reflex** (see also p 543).

Perform **fundoscopy**. Successful ophthalmoscopy requires considerable practice. It is important that it be performed in reduced ambient lighting so that the patient's pupils are at least partly dilated and you are not distracted. It can be easier to perform the examination, especially of the fundi, through the patient's spectacles. Otherwise, the patient's refractive error should be corrected by use of the appropriate ophthalmoscope lens. The patient should be asked to stare at a point on the opposite wall or on the ceiling and to ignore the light of the ophthalmoscope. Patients will often attempt to focus on the ophthalmoscope light and should be asked not to do this. Cataracts cause opacification of the lens and may make fundoscopy impossible. They are also associated with a reduced or absent light reflex.

T&O'C ESSENTIALS

Cataracts

1. *Cataracts are very common in old age.*
2. *They have many causes and associations (List 42.3).*
3. *They cause reduced visual acuity, poor night vision, diplopia and glare.*
4. *Surgery is indicated when loss of vision interferes with life, e.g. driving, reading.*

Begin by examining the **cornea**. Use your right eye to examine the patient's right eye, and vice versa. Turn the ophthalmoscope lens to +20 and examine the cornea from about 20 centimetres away from the patient. Look particularly for corneal ulceration. Turn the lens gradually down to 0 while moving closer to the patient. Structures, including the *lens*, the *humour* and the *retina*, at increasing distance into the eye will swim into focus.

Examine the **retina** (see Fig. 42.5, also Fig. 32.12 on p 530 and pp 128–9). Focus on one of the retinal arteries and follow it into the optic disc. The normal disc is round and paler than the surrounding retina. The margin of the disc is usually sharply outlined but will appear blurred if there is papilloedema or papillitis, or pale if there is optic atrophy. Pulsation of the retinal veins is usually most obvious at the proximal end of the central retinal veins (i.e. near the optic disc). The presence of pulsation means the intracranial pressure is not likely to be elevated. Raised intracranial pressure would make a lumbar puncture unsafe.[b,2] Look at the rest of the retina, especially for haemorrhages and the retinal changes of diabetes mellitus or hypertension.

There are four types of **haemorrhages**: *streaky haemorrhages* near the vessels (linear or flame-shaped), large *ecchymoses* that obliterate the vessels, *petechiae*, which may be confused with microaneurysms, and

[b] The positive predictive value for retinal venous pulsations and a normal ICP is 0.88 (0.87–0.9) and the negative predictive value is 0.17 (0.05–0.4).

Retinal photographs.

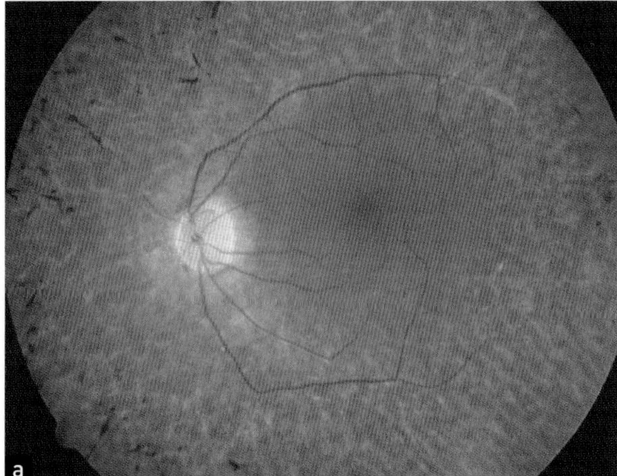

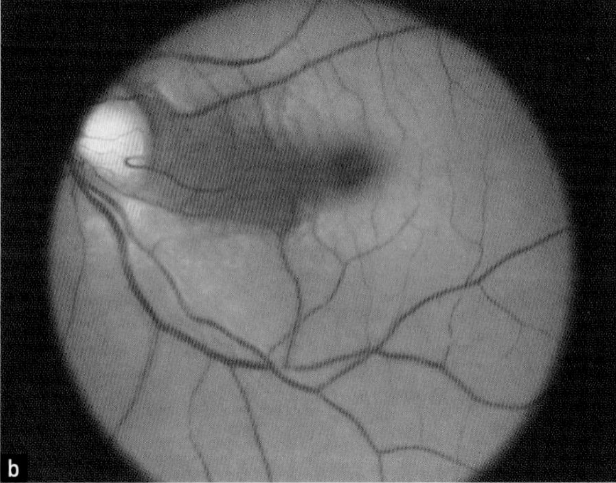

(a) Retinitis pigmentosa; (b) central retinal artery occlusion

(Courtesy of Lions Eye Institute.)

FIGURE 42.5

subhyaloid haemorrhages (large effusions of blood that have a crescentic shape and well-marked borders; a fluid level may be seen). The first two types of haemorrhage occur in hypertensive and diabetic retinopathy. They may also result from any cause of raised intracranial pressure or venous engorgement, or from a bleeding disorder. The third type occurs in diabetes mellitus, and the fourth is characteristic of subarachnoid haemorrhage.

There are two main types of retinal change in diabetes mellitus: non-proliferative and proliferative. Non-proliferative changes include: (1) two types of haemorrhages occur specifically in diabetics—*dot haemorrhages*, which occur in the inner retinal layers, and *blot haemorrhages*, which are larger and occur more superficially in the nerve fibre layer; (2) *microaneurysms* (tiny bulges in the vessel wall), which are due to vessel wall damage; and (3) two types of exudates—*hard exudates*, which have straight edges and are due to leakage of protein from damaged arteriolar walls, and *soft exudates* (cottonwool spots), which have a fluffy appearance and are due to microinfarcts. Proliferative changes include *new vessel formation*, which can lead to retinal detachment or vitreous haemorrhage.

Hypertensive changes can be classified from grades 1 to 4:

- *Grade 1* 'Silver wiring' of the arteries only (sclerosis of the vessel wall reduces its transparency so that the central light streak becomes broader and shinier)
- *Grade 2* Silver wiring of arteries plus arteriovenous nipping or nicking (indentation or deflection of the veins where they are crossed by the arteries)
- *Grade 3* Grade 2 plus haemorrhages (flame-shaped) and exudates (soft—cottonwool spots due to ischaemia, or hard—lipid residues from leaking vessels)
- *Grade 4* Grade 3 changes plus papilloedema.

It is important to describe the changes present rather than just give a grade.

Retinitis pigmentosa: causes a scattering of black pigment in a criss-cross pattern (Fig. 42.5(a)). This will be missed if the periphery of the retina is not examined.

Inspect carefully for **central retinal artery occlusion** (Fig. 42.5(b)), where the whole fundus appears milky-white because of retinal oedema and the arteries become greatly reduced in diameter. This presents with sudden, painless unilateral blindness and is a medical emergency.

Central retinal vein thrombosis: causes tortuous retinal veins and haemorrhages scattered over the whole retina, particularly occurring alongside the veins ('blood and thunder retina'). This presents with sudden painless loss of vision, which is not total.

Retinal detachment: the retina may appear elevated or folded. The patient describes a 'shade coming down', flashes of light or showers of black dots. A diagnosis requires immediate referral to try to prevent total detachment and irrevocable blindness.

White spots occur in **choroiditis** and when active have a fluffy edge (e.g. in toxoplasmosis, sarcoidosis).

Finally, ask the patient to look directly at the light. This allows you to locate and inspect the **macula**. Macular degeneration is the leading cause of blindness; central vision is lost. Drusen formation occurs in macular degeneration—small deposits are seen under the epithelium in the central retina. Macular degeneration may occur secondary to an atrophic or a neovascularisation process.

Palpate the orbits for tenderness. Auscultate the eyes with the bell of the stethoscope—the eye being tested is shut while the other is open and the patient is asked to stop breathing. Listen for a bruit that may be a sign of an arteriovenous malformation or a vascular tumour.

Feel for the preauricular node (adenoviral conjunctivitis).

Consider the possibility that the patient may have a glass eye. This should be suspected if visual acuity is zero in one eye and no pupillary reaction is apparent. Attempts to examine and interpret the fundus of a glass eye will amuse the patient but are always unsuccessful.

The causes of common eye abnormalities are summarised in List 42.3.

Diplopia

Most cases of diplopia (about 60%) are not due to a cranial nerve abnormality. It is important to have an approach to the problem that will help work out the cause.

First find out whether the diplopia is monocular (25%) or binocular. Monocular diplopia persists when one eye is covered. It is usually due to an eye problem such as astigmatism, dislocated lens, uneven contact lens surface or thick spectacles and some types of cataract. It disappears if the patient looks through a pin-hole. Although it is said to be due to hysteria, this is a very rare cause.

If the diplopia is binocular, consider the common causes:

1. Cranial nerve palsy (III, IV or VI)—look for ptosis, pupil changes (III), abnormal eye movements.
2. Eye muscle disease (myasthenia gravis)—worse later in the day, worse after prolonged upward gaze and associated with bilateral ptosis.
3. Thyroid ophthalmopathy—proptosis, lid lag, chemosis.
4. Trauma to the orbit—history or signs of trauma.
5. Internuclear ophthalmoplegia—associated neurological signs.

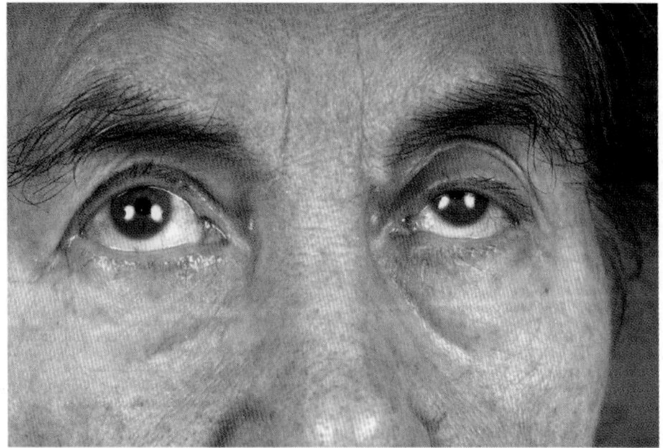

Left Horner syndrome, with partial ptosis and miosis

FIGURE 42.6

Horner syndrome

Examination anatomy

Interruption of the sympathetic innervation of the eye at any point (see Fig. 42.6) results in Horner[c] syndrome (see List 42.4).

Clinical approach

The syndrome includes partial *ptosis* (as sympathetic fibres supply the smooth muscle of both eyelids) and a *constricted* pupil (unbalanced parasympathetic action) that reacts normally to light (see Fig. 42.6). Remember the other causes of ptosis (see Table 42.3).

Test for a difference (decrease) in the *sweating* over each eyebrow with the back of the finger (absence of this sign does not exclude the diagnosis).[d]

Horner syndrome may be part of the *lateral medullary syndrome*.[e]

Next ask the patient to speak and note any hoarseness of the voice, which may be due to recurrent laryngeal nerve palsy from lung carcinoma or from a lower cranial nerve lesion.

[c] Johann Friedrich Horner (1831–86), a professor of ophthalmology at Zürich, described this in 1869.

[d] Enophthalmos, or retraction of the eye, which is often mentioned as a feature of Horner syndrome, probably does not occur in humans. It may occur in cats. Horner original paper was very specific about miosis and ptosis, but only casually mentioned that 'the position of the eye seemed very slightly inward'. Apparent enophthalmos results from a combination of ptosis and an elevated lower lid (upside-down ptosis).

[e] Occlusion of any of the following vessels may result in this syndrome: vertebral; posterior inferior cerebellar; superior, middle or inferior lateral medullary arteries.

CAUSES OF EYE ABNORMALITIES

Cataracts

1. Old age (senile cataract)
2. Endocrine (e.g. diabetes mellitus, steroids)
3. Hereditary or congenital (e.g. dystrophia myotonica)
4. Ocular disease (e.g. glaucoma)
5. Radiation
6. Trauma
7. Smoking

Papilloedema vs papillitis

PAPILLOEDEMA	PAPILLITIS
Optic disc swollen withoutvenous pulsation	Optic disc swollen
Acuity normal (early)	Acuity poor
Large blind spot	Large central scotoma
Peripheral constriction of visual field	Pain on eye movement
Colour vision normal	Onset usually sudden and unilateral
Usually bilateral	Colour vision affected (particularly red desaturation)

Causes of papilloedema

1. Space-occupying lesion (causing raised intracranial pressure) or a retro-orbital mass
2. Hydrocephalus (large cerebral ventricles)
   - Obstructive (a block in the ventricle, aqueduct or outlet to the fourth ventricle—e.g. tumour)
   - Communicating
   - Increased formation of CSF (e.g. choroid plexus papilloma—rare)
   - Decreased absorption of CSF (e.g. tumour causing venous compression, subarachnoid space obstruction from meningitis)
3. Benign intracranial hypertension (pseudotumour cerebri) (small or normal-sized ventricles)
   - Idiopathic
   - The contraceptive pill
   - Addison disease
   - Drugs (e.g. nitrofurantoin, tetracycline, vitamin A, steroids)
   - Head trauma
4. Hypertension
5. Central retinal vein thrombosis

Causes of optic atrophy

1. Chronic papilloedema or optic neuritis
2. Optic nerve pressure or division
3. Glaucoma
4. Ischaemia
5. Familial (e.g. retinitis pigmentosa, Leber* disease, Friedreich ataxia)

Causes of optic neuritis

1. Multiple sclerosis
2. Toxic (e.g. ethambutol, chloroquine, nicotine, alcohol)
3. Metabolic (e.g. vitamin B_{12} deficiency)
4. Ischaemia (e.g. diabetes mellitus, temporal arteritis, atheroma)
5. Familial (e.g. Leber's disease)
6. Infective (e.g. infectious mononucleosis)

Causes of retinitis pigmentosa

1. Congenital (associated with cataract and deaf-mutism)
2. Laurence–Moon–Biedl syndrome†
3. Hereditary trauma
4. Familial neuropathy (i.e. Refsum's disease‡)

CSF = cerebrospinal fluid.

*Theodor von Leber (1840–1917), a Göttingen and Heidelberg ophthalmologist.

†John Laurence (1830–74), a London ophthalmologist; Robert Charles Moon (1844–1914), an American ophthalmologist; Arthur Biedl (1869–1933), a professor of physiology, Prague.

‡Sigvald Refsum (1907–91), a Norwegian physician.

LIST 42.3

CAUSES OF HORNER SYNDROME

1. Carcinoma of the apex of the lung (usually squamous cell carcinoma)
2. Neck
   - Malignancy (e.g. thyroid)
   - Trauma or surgery
3. Lower trunk brachial plexus lesions
   - Trauma
   - Tumour
4. Carotid arterial lesion
   - Carotid aneurysm or dissection
   - Pericarotid tumours*
   - Cluster headache
5. Brainstem lesions
   - Vascular disease (especially the lateral medullary syndrome)
   - Tumour
   - Syringobulbia
6. Syringomyelia (rare)

*Sweating unaffected, as tumour is localised to internal carotid artery.

LIST 42.4

Important causes of ptosis

Cause	Associated features
Age-related stretching of the levator muscle or aponeurosis	Common, often asymmetrical
Orbital tumour or inflammation	Orbital abnormality
Constricted pupil, reduced sweating	Horner syndrome
Eye 'down and out', dilated pupil	Third nerve palsy
Myasthenia gravis or dystrophia myotonica	Extraocular muscle palsies, muscle weakness
Congenital or idiopathic	

TABLE 42.3

Now look at the hands for clubbing and test for weakness of finger abduction. If any of these signs is present, perform a respiratory examination, concentrating on the apices of the lungs for signs of lung carcinoma.

Examine the neck for lymphadenopathy, thyroid carcinoma and a carotid aneurysm or bruit. Syringomyelia may rarely be a cause of this syndrome, so the examination should be completed by testing for dissociated sensory loss. Remember, syringomyelia may cause a bilateral Horner syndrome.

Red eye: iritis, keratitis and scleritis

Iritis (anterior uveitis) presents with pain, photophobia and unilateral eye redness (see Table 42.2 and List 42.2). On examination of the eye, there is classically a ciliary flush with dilated vessels around the iris.

Iritis is associated with inflammatory arthropathies that are linked to HLA-B27 positivity, including ankylosing spondylitis, inflammatory bowel disease, reactive arthritis and Behçet's disease with an acute presentation. Chronic iritis can be linked to juvenile rheumatoid arthritis, as well as sarcoidosis and syphilis.

Keratitis is inflammation of the cornea and may be due to ulceration (often a result of herpes simplex infection) or injury (e.g. from metal fragments in grinders or flash burns in arc welders). Contact lens wearers who do not clean their lenses properly are also at risk. Severe proptosis or a facial nerve palsy that prevents lid closure can be a mechanical cause.

Scleritis presents similarly but with bilateral painful red eyes; it is also associated with the same HLA-B27 arthropathies. Eye movements are painful in scleritis.

Hyphaemia means blood within the eye and is usually caused by trauma. Hypopyon refers to pus in the anterior chamber; a fluid level may be seen. The pupil is usually irregular. There may also be new vessel formation over the iris.

Glaucoma

Primary open-angle glaucoma causes prolonged elevation of intraocular pressure and induces progressive visual loss. This begins in the peripheral visual fields and is painless.

Closed-angle (narrow-angle) glaucoma is due to a rapid pressure increase. Symptoms include severe eye pain, halos around lights and nausea; it is an ocular emergency. You may see a fixed mid-dilated pupil, conjunctival hyperaemia and corneal redness; intraocular pressure on measurement is increased. The condition occurs secondary to iris neovascularisation (e.g. new vessel formation in diabetes mellitus) or

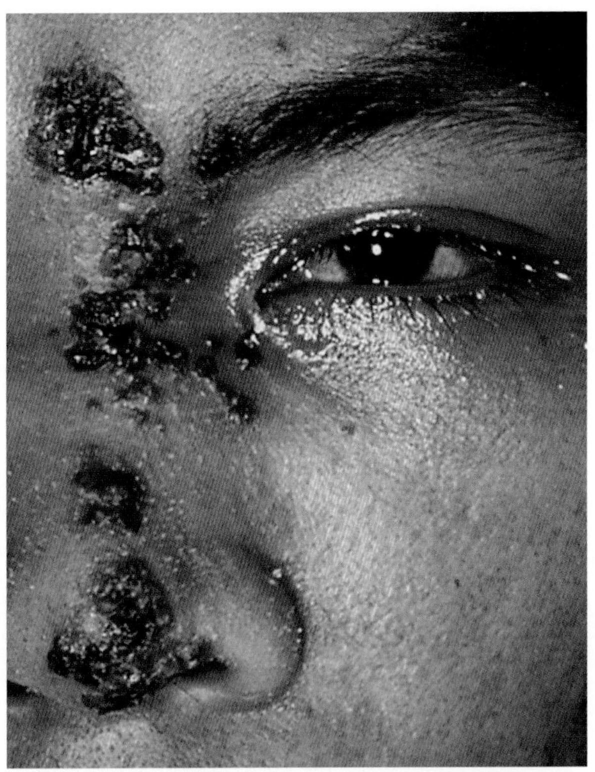

Nasociliary herpes zoster showing the distribution of the nerve

FIGURE 42.7

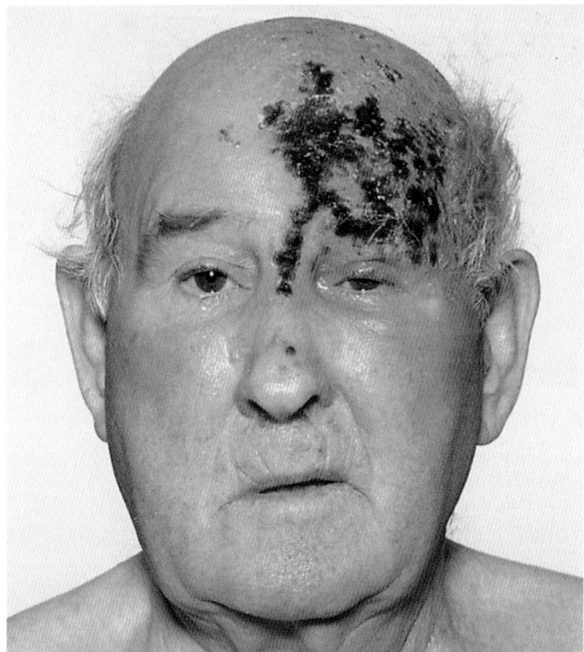

Herpes zoster, involving the eye, along the distribution of the ophthalmic branch of the fifth cranial nerve

(From Mir MA. *Atlas of clinical diagnosis*, 2nd edn. Edinburgh: Saunders, 2003.)

FIGURE 42.8

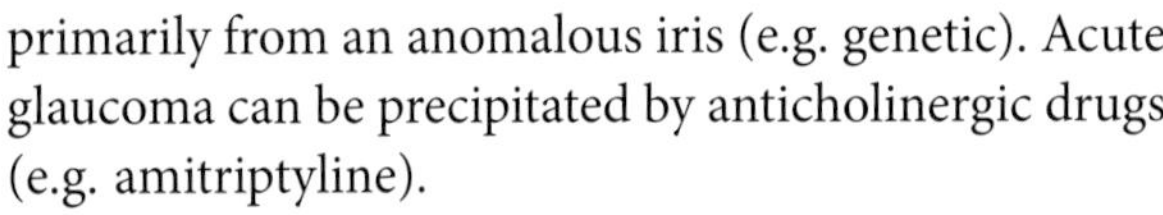

primarily from an anomalous iris (e.g. genetic). Acute glaucoma can be precipitated by anticholinergic drugs (e.g. amitriptyline).

Shingles

Herpes zoster involving the first (ophthalmic) division of the trigeminal nerve may result in uveitis and keratitis and threaten vision. The tip of the nose, cornea and iris are all innervated by the nasociliary nerve (a branch of the trigeminal nerve; see Figs 42.7 and 42.8). The appearance of vesicles on the tip of the nose (Hutchinson's[f] vesicles) in a patient with herpes zoster indicates an increased risk of ophthalmic complication (LR+ 3.5).[3]

[f] Sir Jonathon Hutchinson (1828–1913). Among other appointments he was surgeon to Moorfields Eye Hospital. He was president of the Royal College of Surgeons in 1889, elected to the Royal Society in 1882 and knighted in 1908.

Eyelid

A number of conditions of the eyelid are worth remembering:

1. Stye of the eyelid (*hordeolum*) is an infection typically caused by *Staphylococcus aureus*; it is tender.
2. *Chalazion* is a slowly enlarging non-tender nodule of the eyelid (see Fig. 42.9), resulting from sterile inflammation of the meibomian glands if deep, or of the sebaceous glands if superficial.
3. *Dacrocystitis* is infection of a lacrimal gland or of the lacrimal duct (see Fig. 42.10).
4. *Orbital cellulitis* may spread to involve the eyelid (see Fig. 42.11).
5. *Ectropion* is a drooping of the lower lid when it loses its elasticity in old age and falls away from the sclera. This interrupts tear drainage, the eye

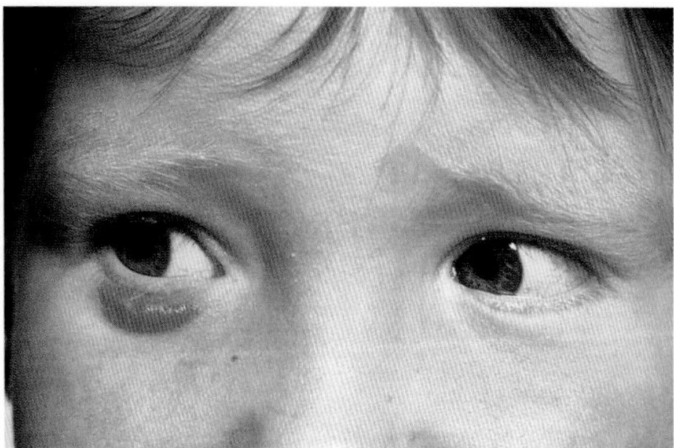

A chalazion; unlike styes, chalazions are not usually tender or painful

FIGURE 42.9

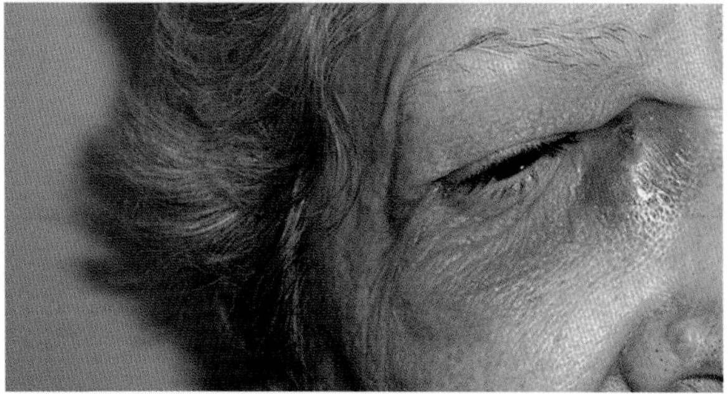

Dacrocystitis

(Courtesy of Dr A Watson, Infectious Diseases Department, The Canberra Hospital.)

FIGURE 42.10

becomes dry and tears spill over the patient's cheek.

6. *Entropion* is the opposite. Scarring or thickening of the lower lid leads to corneal abrasion from inverted lashes.

EARS

Examination anatomy

The ear is divided into three parts: the outer, middle and inner ear:

- The **outer ear** comprises the pinna, the external auditory canal and the eardrum (tympanic membrane), which are easily assessed with simple equipment (see Fig. 42.12). Glands in the skin of the auditory canal secrete cerumen.[g] As cells desquamate from the outer surface of the eardrum they combine with cerumen and migrate outwards to produce normal ear wax.
- The **middle ear** includes the inner layer of the tympanic membrane, the tympanic cavity (epimesohypotympanum), the ossicles (*malleus*, *incus* and *stapes*[h]), the *Eustachian* tube and the mastoid air cells. The Eustachian tube connects the middle ear with the nasopharynx. A branch of the facial nerve, the *chorda tympani*,[i] enters the tympanic cavity through its posterior wall and traverses the pars flaccida of the tympanic membrane, over the neck of the malleus adjacent to the mucosa, on its way back from receiving taste sensation from the front of the tongue.
- The **inner ear** (labyrinth) has vestibular (concerned with balance) and cochlear (concerned with hearing) parts. The vestibular part includes the semicircular canals that lie at right angles to each other. Movements of the head disturb the *endolymph*, a fluid that fills the canals. This stimulates hairs, which cause nerve

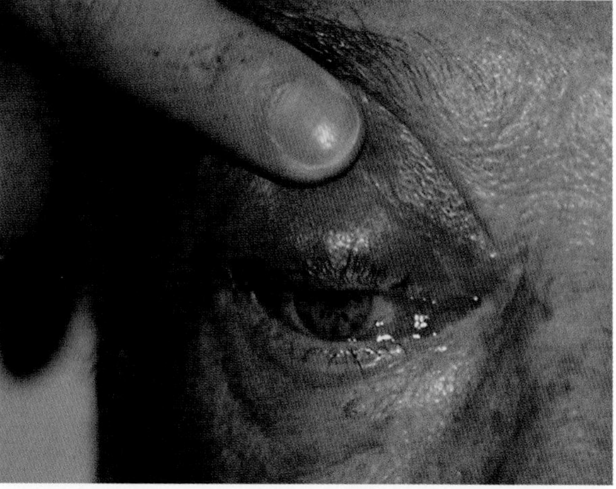

Orbital cellulitis

(Courtesy of Dr A Watson, Infectious Diseases Department, The Canberra Hospital.)

FIGURE 42.11

[g] From the Latin word for wax. *Cerula*, the diminutive, means a little piece of wax.

[h] From the Latin for hammer, anvil and stirrup.

[i] From the Latin for the string of a musical instrument and a drum.

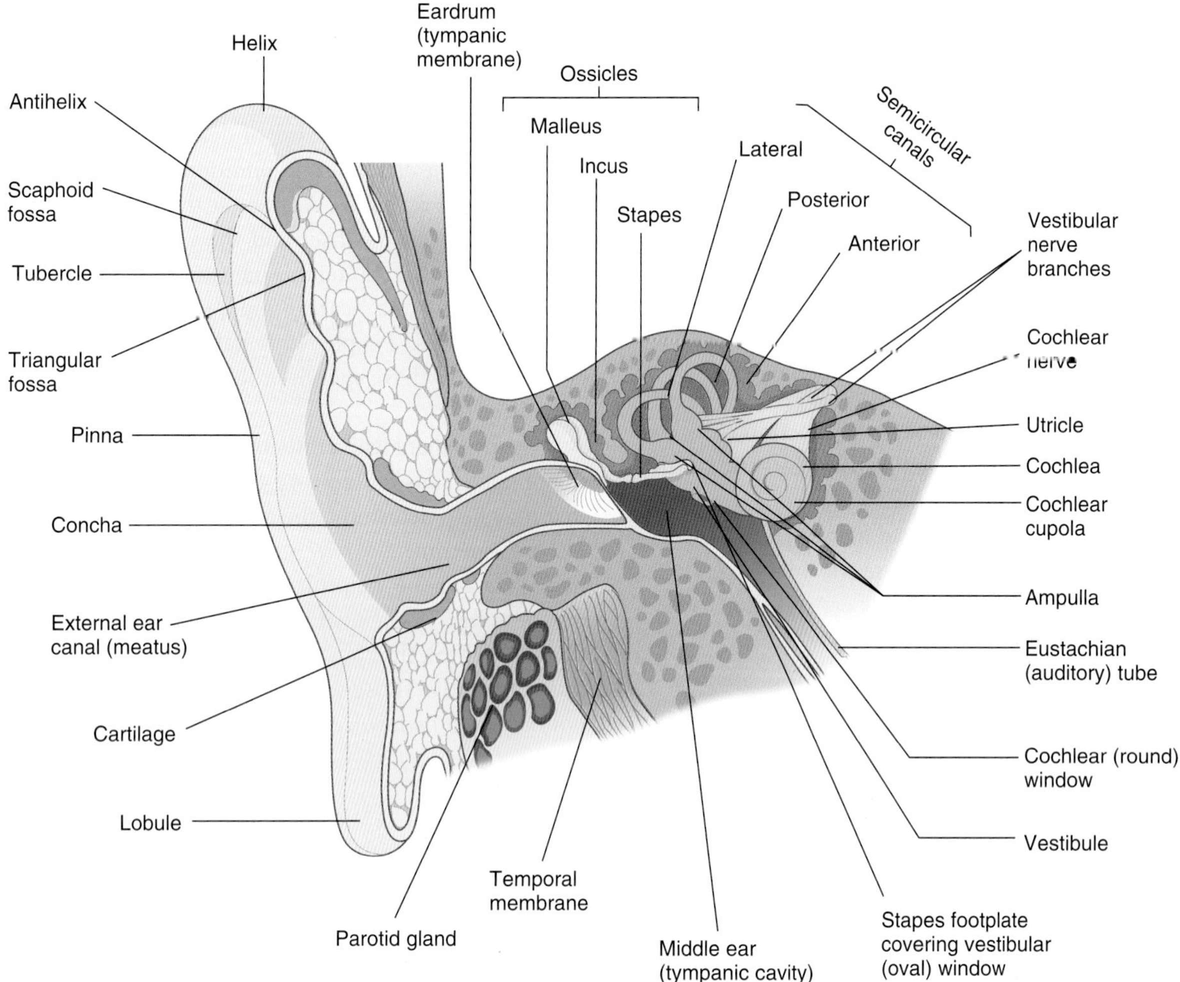

Cross-sectional anatomy of the ear showing the pinna, external auditory canal, middle and inner ear

FIGURE 42.12

impulses to travel in the vestibular part of the eighth nerve. Movement of the stapes on the *oval window* of the cochlear stimulates hair cells in the cochlear, which convert this movement into nerve impulses that travel in the cochlear part of the eighth nerve.

COMMON SYMPTOMS OF EAR DISEASE

Deafness
Vertigo
Tinnitus
Pain (otalgia)
Discharge (otorrhoea)
Itch

LIST 42.5

History

Patients may have symptoms from any of the three parts of the ear:

1. *Outer ear:* symptoms include itch, erythema and discharge (perforated drum and infection or otitis externa; see List 42.5). The pinna can be

damaged by trauma or affected by acquired or inherited diseases of cartilage. Otorrhoea is a more chronic scanty but offensive discharge. It may be due to a cholesteatoma. This is a growth of stratified squamous epithelium that begins in the middle ear or mastoid. It is a benign, slowly growing lesion that destroys bone and ear tissue as it grows. When perforation of the tympanic membrane occurs, cheesy white discharge can occur. It results in loss of hearing if the ossicles are involved. Accumulations of ear wax are a cause of deafness.

2. *Middle ear:* symptoms include infection, which is common in children, and causes pain and, if the eardrum ruptures, a purulent discharge. Otosclerosis is an inherited abnormality that affects the ossicles and causes deafness. Middle ear tumours and chronic middle ear infection are a cause of deafness.
3. *Inner ear:* deafness and balance problems including vertigo are the usual symptoms of inner ear disease. Tinnitus, which is usually described as a 'ringing in the ears', occurs with most types of inner ear disease. Drugs are a common cause (List 42.6).

Deafness may be due to a **conductive** problem because of abnormalities of the:

- outer ear
- eardrum
- ossicles, or

sensorineural, a result of abnormalities affecting the:

- inner ear
- acoustic nerve.

A patient who complains of deafness needs to be asked about the effect of the condition on work, family life and social activities. Ask about the severity of the deafness, the age of onset and the rapidity of onset. Also enquire what coping mechanisms have been tried. These may include hearing aids, sign language and support groups. People who have been deaf from childhood may have speech problems and educational difficulties.

For any patient who presents with deafness, consider the possible causes (Table 42.4) and ask the questions that may help determine the cause (see Questions box 42.3). Sometimes the way a patient speaks during the interview can be helpful. Patients with conductive deafness hear their own voices by bone conduction and often think they are speaking loudly but they tend to speak softly. Those with sensorineural deafness do not hear their own voices well and tend to speak loudly.

DRUG CAUSES OF TINNITUS

1. Antibiotics, especially aminoglycosides but also vancomycin, erythromycin and neomycin
2. Antimalarials: quinine, chloroquine
3. Benzodiazapines
4. Carbamazepine
5. Chemotherapeutic drugs: vincristine, carboplatin, cisplatin
6. Loop diuretics
7. Aspirin and non-steroidal anti-inflammatory drugs
8. Tricyclic antidepressants

LIST 42.6

QUESTIONS TO ASK THE PATIENT WITH DEAFNESS

1. How long has your hearing been a problem? (e.g. congenital)
2. Does your job or any of your hobbies expose you to noise?
3. Have you been treated with drugs that could damage your hearing? (Ask about salicylates, cisplatin and gentamicin)
4. Is there a history of deafness in your family? (e.g. otosclerosis)
5. Have you had recurrent ear infections? (Especially common in Aboriginal children)
6. Have you had problems with wax in your ears in the past?
7. Have you had any injury to your ears or head or a serious infection such as meningitis?
8. Have you also got ringing in your ears? (e.g. Ménière's disease)

QUESTIONS BOX 42.3

Causes of deafness

Conductive	Notes
Ear wax (cerumen)	Cerumen may completely block the external ear canal and reduce sound conduction
Perforation of eardrum (tympanic membrane)	A result of infection or trauma, reduces sound conduction to the ossicles
Otosclerosis	Bony overgrowth of the footplate of the stapes and reduces movement. There is often a family history of the condition
Cholesteatoma	This is a mass of keratinising epithelial cells which expands and invades locally and can affect the cochlear, ossicles and tympanic membrane
Sensorineural	
Meniere's disease	Patient may have tinnitus, sensorineural hearing loss and vertigo
Presbycusis	Loss especially of high-frequency hearing in old age very common
Sudden sensorineural hearing loss	The cause is not known but it may respond to treatment with corticosteroids
Industrial (boilermaker's) deafness*	Chronic noise exposure or exposure to sudden extreme noise
Drug-induced	Ototoxic drugs include aminoglycoside antibiotics and some chemotherapeutic agents, aspirin and loop diuretics
Acoustic neuroma	Can also cause tinnitus and vertigo
Both	
Infection	Middle ear infection can interfere with tympanic membrane or ossicle function; viral cochleitis can cause sensorineural deafness
Head injury	Can damage the eardrum ossicles, cochlear or acoustic nerve

**Perhaps more common now in ageing popular musicians*

TABLE 42.4

Tests of hearing can also provide information about the severity and anatomical site of hearing loss.

Sudden hearing loss (30 dB over 3 days) is an emergency. Causes include:

- viral infection
- bacterial meningitis
- migraine
- acoustic neuroma
- head injury
- drug reactions
- sarcoidosis, but
- 90% are idiopathic.

Examination method

Ear examination consists of inspection and palpation, otoscopy, tuning fork assessment, testing hearing and peripheral vestibular examination. In some cases lower cranial nerve assessment is indicated.

Inspect the position of the **pinna** and note its size and shape. Note any scars or swelling around the ears. Look for an obvious accessory auricle (separate piece of cartilage away from the pinna), cauliflower ears (haematomas from recurrent trauma, which obscure the normal anatomical features of the pinna) and bat ears (protrusion of the ears from the side of the head).

Look for **inflammation externally** and any obvious ear *discharge*. Inspect the auditory meatus and outer ear. There are four types of *otitis externa*, a condition associated with inflammation of the skin of the external canal:

1. *Acute localised otitis externa* involves the outer third of the auditory canal where the skin overlies cartilage and hair follicles are present. It is a form of furunculosis and is usually a result of *S. aureus* infection.
2. *Acute diffuse otitis externa* is often called swimmer's ear although it occurs in people who have not been swimming. Excessive moisture, heat and humidity, loss of protective cerumen and an increase in pH are responsible for skin

maceration and irritation. Infection may occur with *Pseudomonas aeruginosa*. The initial symptom is itching, which can progress to pain and is made worse by movement of the pinna. The appearance on examination ranges from mild erythema to severe erythema and swelling. There may be a small amount of white, clumpy discharge.

3. *Chronic otitis externa* is usually the result of repeated local irritation. This may be due to persistent drainage of a chronic middle ear infection but can also be caused by the insertion of foreign bodies into the ear (e.g. cotton swabs, ear picks). Itch is a more prominent symptom than pain. The appearance is of scaly erythematous dermatitis. Other forms of dermatitis such as psoriasis, atopic dermatitis and seborrhoeic dermatitis can also cause chronic otitis externa.
4. *Malignant (invasive) otitis externa* is an aggressive and sometimes life-threatening condition. It affects elderly diabetics and immunocompromised patients. It begins in the external auditory canal and spreads slowly inwards. Untreated it can cause osteomyelitis of the base of the skull and reach the meninges and the brain. *Pseudomonas* infection is the most common cause but other organisms can be responsible. Deep otalgia is the most predominant symptom. The appearance at first is like that of severe chronic otitis externa. On examination there is discharge and the canal appears swollen and erythematous.

Then look for signs of **gouty tophi** (nodular, firm, pale and non-tender chalky depositions of urate in the cartilage of the ear, specific but not sensitive for gout).

Palpate the pinna for swelling or nodules. Pull it down gently; the manoeuvre is often painful when there is infection of the external canal.

Otoscope examination of the ears requires use of an earpiece that fits comfortably in the ear canal to allow inspection of the ear canal and tympanic membrane (see Fig. 42.13). This examination is essential for any patient presenting with an upper respiratory tract infection, any symptom related to the ears, dizziness, facial weakness or head injury. Always examine both ears!

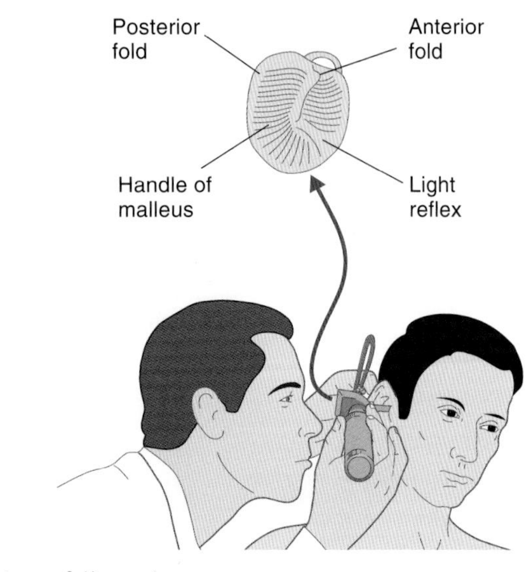

Use of the otoscope

FIGURE 42.13

The correct technique is as follows. Ask the patient to turn his or her head slightly to the side, then pull the pinna up, out and back to straighten the ear canal and provide optimal vision. Stretch out the fingers of your hand holding the otoscope to touch the patient's cheek, to steady the instrument and to prevent sudden movements of the patient's head. When examining the patient's right ear, the otoscope is preferably held in a *downward position* with the right hand, while using the left hand to pull the pinna. An alternative position involves holding the otoscope upwards, but there is a risk that if the patient moves suddenly injury is more likely to occur.

Look at the **external canal** for any evidence of inflammation (e.g. redness or swelling) or discharge. There should be no tenderness unless there is inflammation. *Ear wax* is usually white or yellowish, and translucent and shiny; it can be moist or hard and impacted. It may obscure the view of the tympanic membrane. *Blood* or *cerebrospinal fluid* (watery, clear fluid) may be seen in the canal if there is a fracture at the base of the skull. In patients with herpes zoster, there may be *vesicles* (fluid-filled blisters) on the posterior wall around the external auditory meatus.

Inspect the **tympanic membrane** (eardrum) by introducing the speculum further into the canal in a forward but downward direction. The normal tympanic

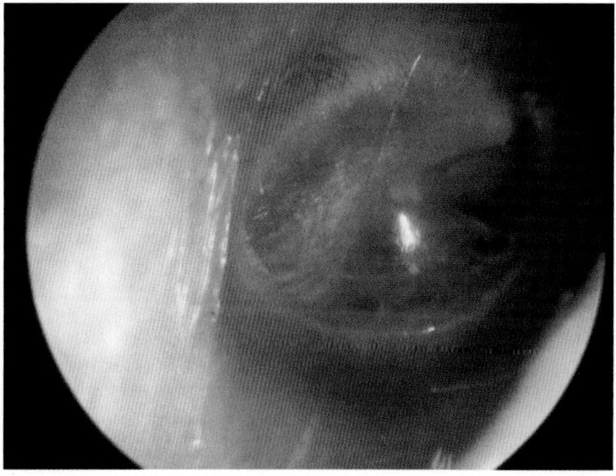

The tympanic membrane as viewed through an otoscope

(From Mir MA. *Atlas of clinical diagnosis*, 2nd edn. Edinburgh: Saunders, 2003.)

FIGURE 42.14

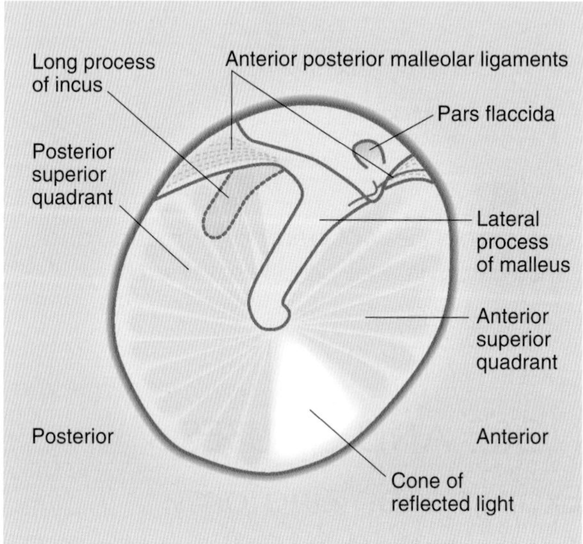

The detail of the tympanic membrane

(From Mir MA. *Atlas of clinical diagnosis*, 2nd edn. Edinburgh: Saunders, 2003.)

FIGURE 42.15

membrane is a pearly grey colour. It is ovoid in shape and semitransparent (see Fig. 42.14). The upper fifth is called the *pars flaccida* and the lower four-fifths are called the *pars tensa* (see Fig. 42.15). The handle of the malleus is often visible near the centre of the latter.

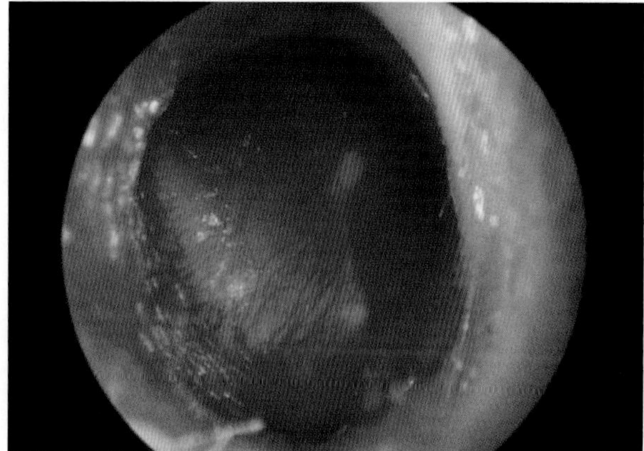

Otitis media with hyperaemia of the tympanic membrane

(From Mir MA. *Atlas of clinical diagnosis*, 2nd edn. Edinburgh: Saunders, 2003.)

FIGURE 42.16

From the lower end of the handle a bright cone of light should be visible: the light reflex. The presence or absence of the light reflex is not a sensitive or a specific sign of disease. Note the colour, transparency and any evidence of *dilated blood vessels* (hyperaemia—a sign of otitis media; see Fig. 42.16). Look for *bulging* or *retraction* of the tympanic membrane. Bulging can suggest underlying fluid or pus in the middle ear. Retraction means a reduction in pressure in the middle ear and is a sign of a blocked Eustachian tube. Perforation of the tympanic membrane should be noted (see Fig. 42.17).

If a middle ear infection is suspected, **pneumatic auriscopy** can be useful. Use a speculum large enough to occlude the external canal snugly. Attach a rubber squeeze bulb to the otoscope. When the bulb is squeezed gently, air pressure in the canal is increased and the tympanic membrane should move promptly inwards. Absence of, or a decrease in, movement is a sign of fluid in the middle ear.

To test hearing, whisper numbers or words such as 'mark' or 'park' into one of the patient's ears while the other ear is distracted by movement of your finger in the auditory canal or the canal is occluded by pressure on the tragus. It is important to stand behind the patient to prevent lip reading. Then repeat the process with the other ear. With practice, the normal range of hearing is appreciated. If a patient says he or she is deaf, or the

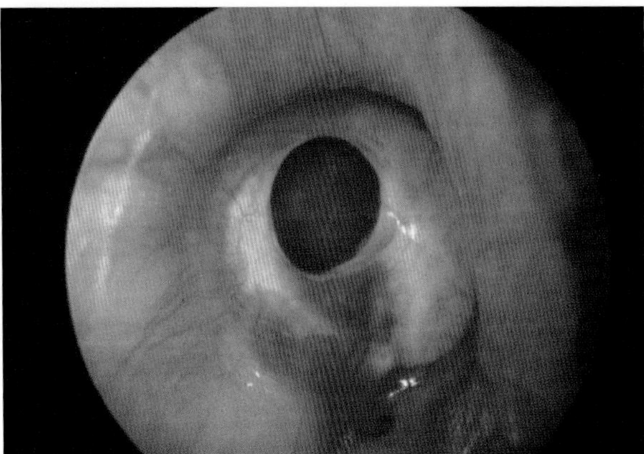

Perforated tympanic membrane

(From Mir MA. *Atlas of clinical diagnosis*, 2nd edn. Edinburgh: Saunders, 2003.)

FIGURE 42.17

whisper test is positive, formal hearing testing (audiometry) is indicated.[4]

Traditionally, Rinné's and Weber's tests are performed if deafness is suspected, but these are not very useful screening tests:[4]

1. *Rinné's test:* place a vibrating 512 Hz tuning fork on the mastoid process. When the sound is no longer heard, move the fork close to the auditory meatus where, if air conduction is (as is normal) better than bone conduction, it will again be audible.
2. *Weber's test:* place a vibrating 512 Hz fork at the centre of the patient's forehead. Nerve deafness causes the sound to be heard better in the normal ear, but with conduction deafness the sound is heard better in the abnormal ear.

T&O'C ESSENTIALS

If the patient or a relative says he or she is deaf then he or she is deaf. This can be confirmed by testing in 90% of cases.

Sudden hearing loss requires urgent assessment and investigation.

Anatomy of the nose.

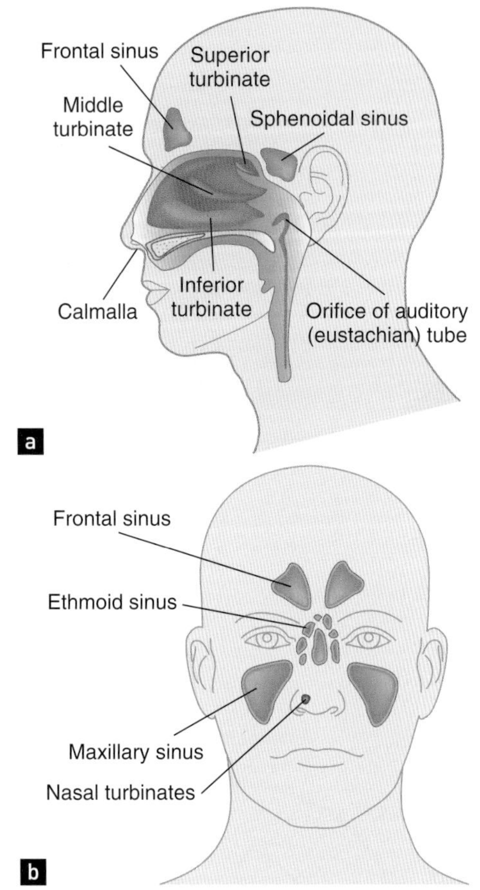

(a) Coronal view of paranasal sinuses; and (b) sagittal view of paranasal sinuses

FIGURE 42.18

NOSE AND SINUSES

Examination anatomy

The upper one-third of the nose is formed by the two nasal bones and the lower two-thirds are formed from cartilage (see Fig. 42.18). Cartilage divides the nose into its two cavities. The nasal bones articulate with the frontal bones and the maxilla. On the lateral walls of the nose the three pairs of nasal turbinates (superior, middle and inferior) cause turbulence as air enters the nose. This makes small particles drop onto the nasal mucosa, where cilia sweep them into the nasopharynx. The air is also warmed and humidified in the nose. Below each turbinate is a meatus named for the turbinate above it.

The frontal, maxillary and anterior ethmoid sinuses drain via the middle meatus. The posterior ethmoid sinus drains via the superior meatus. Drainage is assisted as a result of action of the ciliated epithelium. The maxillary sinus drains upwards against gravity through its ostium into the nasal cavity. This explains the importance of postural drainage for the treatment of bacterial sinusitis and why water drips from swimmers' noses when they bend over to dry their hair. The nasolacrimal duct drains into the inferior meatus. Drainage can be interrupted as a result of oedema (e.g. allergic rhinitis), mechanical obstruction (e.g. nasal polyps) or impaired ciliary function (Kartagener syndrome).

The turbinates are vascular structures and their blood supply is under autonomic control. Sympathetic stimulation causes vasoconstriction and shrinkage of the turbinates. Parasympathetic stimulation causes vasodilation, swelling and sometimes obstruction of airflow and a watery discharge. The blood supply to the nose is from the internal and external carotid arteries. The blood vessels of the anterior nasal septum meet at *Little's*[j] *area*. This is about 2 centimetres from the nares (nostrils). Nose bleeds often come from this vascular area.

The nerve supply of the nose includes the olfactory nerve, which supplies the olfactory epithelium in the upper part of the nose. Fibres of the olfactory nerve pass through the cribriform plate of the ethmoid bone to reach the olfactory bulb in the brain. The rest of the inside of the nose is supplied by branches of the trigeminal nerve.

The vascular nasal mucosa produces mucus, which contains immunoglobulins. Mucus and the nasal hairs (*vibrissae*) trap particles and prevent them entering the lungs. The mucus is swept backwards by cilia and swallowed.

History

Common presenting problems include the following:

- *Nasal discharge (a runny nose):* consider allergy (watery discharge), a cold (coryza: more viscous discharge with or without fever and systemic symptoms) or sinusitis or a foreign body (purulent discharge)—see Questions box 42.4.
- *Blocked nose:* cold, foreign body, deviated nasal septum.
- *Epistaxis:* trauma (or nose picking), allergy, neoplasm or a cold. Ask about assault. Ask about anticoagulation and use of antiplatelet drugs. Haematological malignancies and haemophilia are sometimes causes. Ask about the amount of blood loss, which can occasionally be severe. Have blood transfusions been required?
- *Anosmia or reduced sense of smell (often with apparent loss of taste):* consider mechanical obstruction due to polyps, infection (including SARS-CoV-2 infection) or trauma if there is complete anosmia.
- *Symptoms of sinusitis:* 'sinus trouble again', cough, nasal congestion, sneezing, facial pain or headache worse with bending forwards, purulent discharge—see Table 42.5.
- *Big nose:* rhinophyma.

QUESTIONS TO ASK THE PATIENT WITH A BLOCKED NOSE

1. How long has your nose been blocked? (Acute problem suggests infection)
2. Are both sides of your nose affected or only one? (Deviation of nasal septum)
3. Have you had a problem with allergies?
4. Have you had polyps in your nose in the past?
5. Is the problem worse at different times of the year? (Allergic rhinitis)
6. Is it associated with sneezing? (Allergic rhinitis)
7. Have you had any injuries to your nose? Could there be anything in there? (Foreign body)
8. Are there any other symptoms? (Loss of sense of smell—polyps; headache and fullness in the head—sinusitis; fever)

QUESTIONS BOX 42.4

[j] William Little (1810–94), a surgeon at St Luke's hospital in New York, described this area in 1843.

Assessment for sinusitis

Sinusitis more likely	Sinusitis less likely
Maxillary toothache Blocked nose Purulent discharge Cough and sneezing Headache Pain worse with bending Pain above the eye (frontal sinusitis) Periorbital pain (ethmoid sinusitis)	Sore throat Itchy eyes **Not helpful either way** Malaise

TABLE 42.5

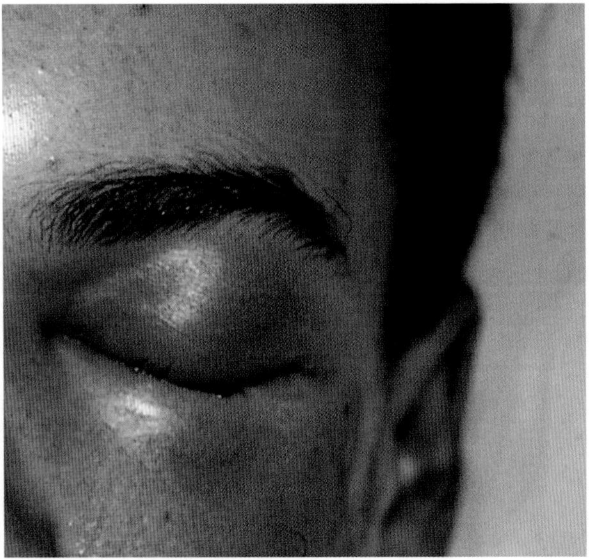

Bacterial ethmoidal sinusitis

(Courtesy of Dr A Watson, Infectious Diseases Department, The Canberra Hospital.)

FIGURE 42.19

Examination method

Nose and sinus examination consists of inspection, palpation and testing the sense of smell. Inspect the **skin**. The patient concerned about a big nose may have a rhinophyma.[k] This enlargement and distortion of the skin of the nose is due to sebaceous gland enlargement. It is often associated with rosacea. Note any nasal deviation (best seen from behind the patient and looking down). Note any periorbital swelling (e.g. from sinusitis). Inspect the nares by pressing the tip of the nose upwards with the thumb.

Palpate the **nasal bones**. Then feel for facial swelling or signs of inflammation. Block each nostril to assess any obstruction by asking the patient to inhale. If there is a history of anosmia (loss of smell), test smell as described in Chapter 32 (cranial nerve I).

A saddle-nose deformity (collapse of the nasal septum) can occur in granulomatosis with polyangiitis (GPA) and relapsing polychondritis.

Examine **inside the nose** using a nasal speculum. This simple device with two blades can be used to open the nares. Hold the device in your left hand and introduce it into the patient's nose with the blades facing up and down. The blades should not rest or be pushed against the nasal septum. Use your other hand to steady and move the patient's head so that the inside of the nose can be seen. Your left index finger should rest against the patient's nose to steady the upper blade. Note:

1. deviation or perforation of the anterior septum
2. the colour of the mucosa—usually a rich dark-red colour (darker than the oral mucosa) and smooth, moist and clean
3. the presence of bleeding, swelling or exudate
4. the presence of polyps—most often seen near the middle meatus
5. a foreign body
6. signs of bleeding at Little's area if epistaxis has occurred
7. the presence and nature of discharge (e.g. watery, purulent, bloody)
8. the size and colour of the turbinates.

Sinusitis

Sinusitis is inflammation of the paranasal sinuses. Pain and tenderness over the sinuses occurs, which in adults is classified as acute if less than 4 weeks in duration, subacute if 4–12 weeks in duration and chronic if greater than 12 weeks in duration. Most acute sinusitis is secondary to viral infection.[5]

Acute bacterial sinusitis (see Fig. 42.19) can occur after viral infection or in the setting of allergic rhinitis, in patients with anatomical abnormalities such as nasal septal deformity or polyps in the nose, or in immunocompromised patients. The most common

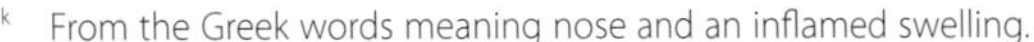

[k] From the Greek words meaning nose and an inflamed swelling.

bacterial causes of sinusitis are *Streptococcus pneumoniae* and *Haemophilus influenzae*. The four key clinical features suggesting that sinusitis may be bacterial are: (1) worsening symptoms after early improvement (a biphasic illness pattern), (2) purulent discharge from the nose, (3) tooth or facial pain over the maxillary sinus (especially if unilateral), and (4) tenderness over the maxillary sinus (unilaterally). Fever may occur.

Complications of acute bacterial sinusitis can include orbital cellulitis, meningitis, cavernous sinus thrombosis, brain abscess and osteolitis of the sinus bones. Therefore, if patients present with any of the following warning signs—periorbital oedema, visual changes or changes in mental status—you should be concerned about complicated bacterial sinusitis. Orbital cellulitis typically presents with erythema of the eyelid, oedema of the eyelid and proptosis. Periorbital cellulitis (septal cellulitis) is a more benign condition caused by primary infection of the skin around the orbit.

Potential mimickers of acute bacterial sinusitis include GPA, carcinoma or lymphoma, sarcoidosis and, in immunocompromised or diabetic patients, fungal sinusitis. Chronic sinusitis presents with chronic sinus congestion, postnasal drip, cough, headache and bad breath.

Rhinocerebral mucormycosis is a fungal infection that destroys the sinuses. A black eschar may be seen on the nasal mucosa or palate.

Examination

There are two commonly used ways of illuminating the sinuses. The simpler method is to place a bright torch or proprietary transilluminoscope in the patient's mouth. The room must be completely dark and the patient must seal the lips around the device. Normal sinuses are visible through the skin of the face and appear as a warm glow. This method has the advantage that the two sides can be compared. The second method avoids the need to clean the torch between examinations. Place the torch over the infraorbital rim and shield your eyes from the light while peering into the patient's mouth to look for illumination of the hard palate.

MOUTH AND THROAT

Examination anatomy

The main structures of the oral cavity (see Fig. 42.20) are as follows:

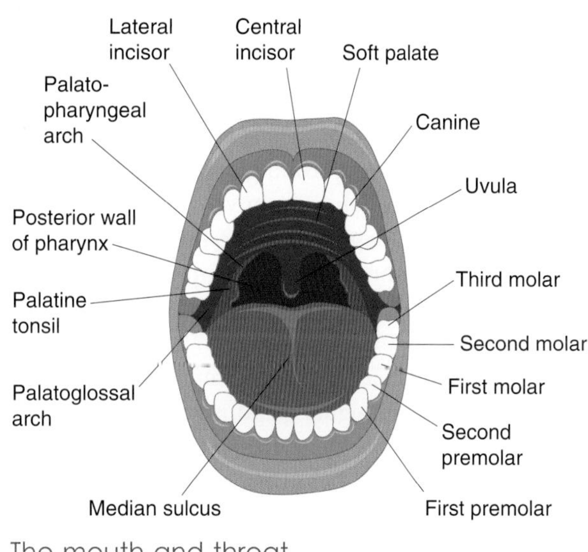

The mouth and throat

FIGURE 42.20

- The *lips* are covered in a thin epidermis and have numerous vascular papillae (the cause of their red colour).
- The *tongue* is attached to the hyoid bone. Its functions include eating and speech and it is the main area where taste is detected. It has a central sagittal median sulcus that ends posteriorly at the foramen caecum. The surface is rough because of its covering of papillae. The fungiform papillae are found on the tip and sides of the tongue. The largest papillae lie in front of the caecum and are called the circumvallate papillae. They divide the tongue into the posterior one-third and the anterior two-thirds.
- The *teeth*.
- The *hard palate* is a concave bony structure. Anteriorly its mucosa has raised folds called *rugae*. The *soft palate* is muscular and flexible. It ends at the uvula, which helps close off the nasopharynx during swallowing.
- The *taste buds* are found on the sides of the papillae. The chorda tympani, which is a division of the facial nerve, receives taste input from the anterior two-thirds of the tongue and the glossopharyngeal nerve from the posterior one-third. Salty taste is detected at the sides of the tongue, sweet taste at the tip of the tongue

and sourness and bitterness from the posterior third (glossopharyngeal nerve).

- The *salivary glands* lubricate the mouth and contain digestive enzymes including amylase. The largest are the parotid glands, which lie in front of the ears. They drain via Stensen's duct and through a papilla opposite the upper first molars. The submandibular glands are next in size. They are located below the angle of the mandible. They drain through Wharton's duct to papillae on either side of the frenulum below the tongue. The sublingual gland is found on the floor of the mouth beneath the tongue and drains through numerous small ducts.

History

The important symptoms of mouth and throat disease include the following:

- Pain in the mouth or throat (see Questions box 42.5).
- Ulceration (see Questions box 42.6).
- Bleeding: ask where the blood seems to be coming from (e.g. gums, throat or coughed up). Find out whether the patient is aware of a mass in the mouth or throat, whether there is bleeding anywhere else and whether he or she is taking antiplatelet or anticoagulant drugs.
- A mass or lump in the mouth: ask whether this is painful (infection) or not, how long it has been present and whether it has been bleeding (neoplasm).
- Dry mouth: ask about medications (e.g. antidepressants, antihistamines, steroid inhalers), previous radiotherapy (damage to salivary glands), dry eyes (sicca syndrome) and thrush (*Candida* infection is an association).
- Dysphagia: ask whether the patient has difficulty in swallowing only solids (oesophageal stricture or tumour) or liquids and solids (oesophageal motility problems). Is the problem associated with a sore throat (tonsillitis)?
- Dysphonia (difficulty with speech; see Questions box 42.7).

Examination method

Throat examination consists of inspection and palpation.

Inspect the **lips** for herpetic ulcers, Peutz–Jeghers syndrome, cyanosis and masses. The most common cause is a mucocele. These cystic painless lesions can be as large as a few centimetres in diameter. They are

QUESTIONS TO ASK THE PATIENT WITH PAIN IN THE MOUTH OR THROAT

1. Is the pain in your mouth? (Dental disease, ulcers)
2. What is the pain like? (Constant: toothache; only during exercise: angina; when eating: temporomandibular joint disease)
3. Is it painful when you swallow? (Tonsillitis, pharyngeal ulcers)
4. How long has it been there? (Acute problem suggests infection)
5. Have you had problems with your teeth?

QUESTIONS BOX 42.5

QUESTIONS TO ASK THE PATIENT WITH MOUTH ULCERS

1. Do you have more than one ulcer? (Multiple suggests systemic disease is possible, e.g. Crohn's disease, coeliac disease)
2. Are they painful? (Painless suggests malignancy)
3. Have you had ulcers or lesions anywhere else: penis, vagina, anus? (Sexually transmitted infection, Crohn's disease)
4. Have you been unwell and are your lips involved? (Herpes simplex primary infection)
5. Have you had these many times before? (Aphthous ulcers)
6. Do you smoke or drink alcohol? (Malignant ulcers)

QUESTIONS BOX 42.6

QUESTIONS TO ASK THE PATIENT WITH HOARSENESS CAUSING DIFFICULTY WITH SPEECH (DYSPHONIA)

1. How long have you been hoarse? (Short history suggests laryngitis)
2. Is it getting worse?
3. Have you had an injury to your neck?
4. Are you a smoker? (Laryngeal carcinoma, carcinoma of the lung and recurrent laryngeal nerve palsy)
5. Do you use a steroid inhaler?
6. Do you have to use your voice extensively? (Overuse, vocal cord papilloma)
7. Have you had a recent anaesthetic? (Intubation injury)
8. Have you had thyroid disease? (Hypothyroidism)

QUESTIONS BOX 42.7

caused by traumatic damage or obstruction of a small salivary gland.

Look at the **buccal mucosa, palate and teeth**. Using a light, push the buccal mucosa out of the way with a tongue depressor. Note any signs of inflammation (e.g. redness, swelling). Look at the parotid duct opening (for inflammation). White painless plaques (leucoplakia) may be present on the gingivae, tongue or buccal mucosa. This is a precancerous condition. Lichen planus also causes a white painless lesion in the mouth. It has a reticulated pattern. Look for masses and ulcerated lesions. Inspect the teeth for obvious decay and infection.

Look at the **gingivae** for hypertrophy (associated with phenytoin use, leukaemia and pregnancy), bleeding and inflammation. Erythroplakia is a mucosal abnormality characterised by red granular papules that bleed easily. It has more malignant potential than leucoplakia.

Inspect the **tongue** first in the mouth, then ask the patient to poke it out to one side and then the other. Weakness of the tongue due to neurological or muscular disease may be seen. Look for masses and mucosal changes as with the rest of the mouth. The surface of the tongue may show localised red areas denuded of papillae surrounded by white or yellow margins and looking rather like a map. This is called *geographical tongue* and is quite benign. Elongation and pigmentation (from food or tobacco staining or certain microorganisms) of the papillae makes the tongue look black and hairy. This is also benign. A tongue with exaggerated fissures is called a *scrotal tongue*; it is also benign. Look for evidence of *Candida* infection (see Fig. 42.22). These white lesions cover an inflamed mucosa and may be the result of immunodeficiency or recent antibiotic use.

Inspect the **floor of the mouth** and under the tongue. Ask the patient to lift the tongue up onto the hard palate to give you a good view. Large veins may be visible under the tongue in elderly people. These are benign and are not a cause of bleeding. Inspect the mucosal surfaces for the abnormalities described above. There may also be a *ranula*.[l] This is a large mucus retention cyst. These can be quite large and although painless eventually interfere with eating and speech.

Inspect the hard and soft **palates** for similar mucosal lesions and the hard palate for petechiae. A common benign finding is a bony swelling of the posterior part of the hard palate. This occurs in the midline and is often lobulated. It is called a *torus palatinus*.[m]

Palpate the tongue with your gloved hand. Hold it with some gauze with one hand and feel with the other. The anterior two-thirds can usually be palpated without provoking the gag reflex. Feel for induration (hardening) of any lesion (a sign of malignancy).

Now palpate the floor of the mouth. Using both gloved hands, feel with your right index finger pointing downwards under the tongue and your left index finger under the chin and pushing upwards. Use the thumb and third finger of your left hand to push the patient's cheeks in between the teeth; this is a precaution that prevents your finger being bitten. Feel between your fingers for masses and tenderness. Feel the submandibular salivary glands.

Ask the patient to say 'Ah', then inspect the **oropharynx and uvula** (there is often a need to press a tongue depressor on the tongue to see properly—and using two tongue depressors can help even further). The tongue should be pushed forwards behind the front teeth. Applying the depressor too far back will cause

[l] From the Latin word for tadpole or little frog.

[m] From the Latin for a swelling or protuberance.

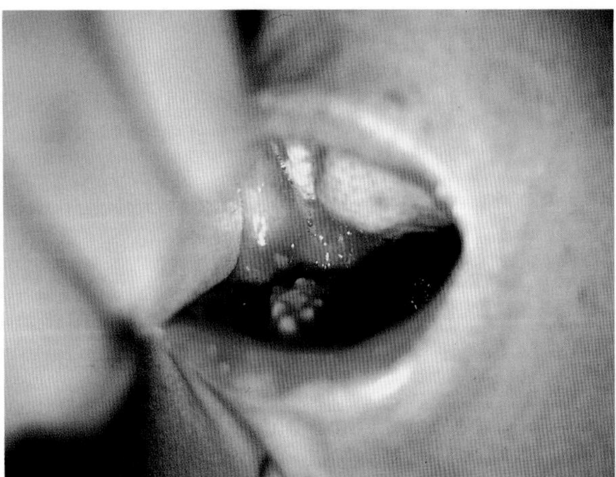

Buccal ulcer

(Courtesy of Dr A Watson, Infectious Diseases Department, The Canberra Hospital.)

FIGURE 42.21

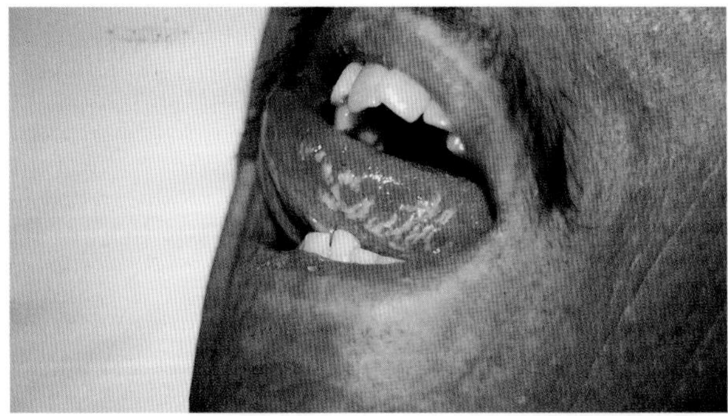

Candidiasis

(Courtesy of Dr A Watson, Infectious Diseases Department, The Canberra Hospital.)

FIGURE 42.22

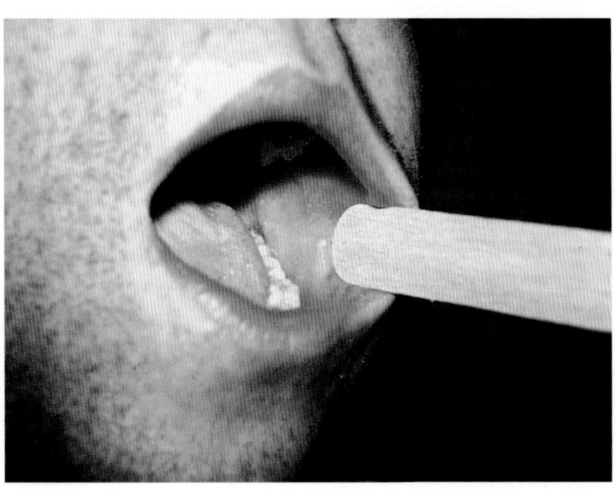

Koplik's spot (measles)

(Courtesy of Dr A Watson, Infectious Diseases Department, The Canberra Hospital.)

FIGURE 42.23

gagging; too far forward and the tongue will roll up and obscure the pharynx. Inspect the tonsils (note the size, shape and colour, and any discharge or membrane—they involute in adults and may not be seen). Enlarged tonsils with a covering of membrane or pus are typical of viral or bacterial tonsillitis. Enlargement may occur in patients with leukaemia and lymphoma.

Examine the **cervical lymph nodes**.

Abnormalities to look and feel for in the mouth and throat examination include:

1. angular stomatitis
2. the state of the teeth and gums
3. gum and tongue ulcers (herpes simplex, aphthous ulcers [see Fig. 42.21], candidiasis [see Fig. 42.22])
4. mucosal mass (consider malignancy)
5. parotid duct pus
6. Koplik's spot (measles; see Fig. 42.32)
7. tongue: smooth (iron, B_{12} deficiency), big (acromegaly, tumour), wasted and fasciculating (motor neurone disease), ulcers and white patches
8. tonsils: present or absent, inflamed or covered in pus; enlarged (lymphoma)
9. salivary glands: size and tenderness; squeeze to express pus through the salivary duct
10. the draining lymph nodes: tenderness and enlargement (see Fig. 42.24)
11. stridor and cough
12. the appropriate cranial nerves, if indicated.

Pharyngitis

A sore throat due to an exudative pharyngitis in adults is usually secondary to infection. The specific causes of pharyngitis include viruses in about 50% of cases (especially Epstein–Barr virus [EBV] in adolescents—1 in 13 cases) (see Good signs guide 42.1).[6] About 10% of cases are due to the group A beta-haemolytic streptococci (see Fig. 42.25). *Neisseria gonorrhoea* is an

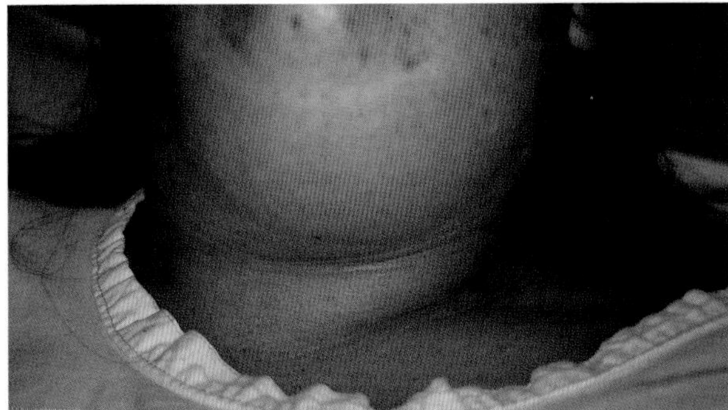

Submandibular abscess

(Courtesy of Dr A Watson, Infectious Diseases Department, The Canberra Hospital.)

FIGURE 42.24

GOOD SIGNS GUIDE 42.1
Infectious mononucleosis (glandular fever)

Symptom or sign	Sensitivity or positive likelihood range (LR)
Sore throat and tiredness	Sensitivity range 0.81–83 (not specific)
Absence of any lymphadenopathy	LR +ve range 0.23–0.44
Posterior cervical lymphadenopathy	LR +ve 3.1
Inguinal or axillary lymphadenopathy	LR +ve 3
Petechiae on the palate	LR +ve 5.3
Splenomegaly	LR +ve range 1.9–6.6

uncommon cause of pharyngitis in adults, and primary human immunodeficiency virus (HIV) infection is an occasional cause; typically, there are sexual risk factors present in the history. The other two most important viruses are herpes simplex and adenovirus. Many cases of pharyngitis are of unknown cause. Clinically, there is redness of the pharynx with or without ulceration. Swabs of an ear discharge may grow the causative organism.

Clinical criteria help to determine whether or not pharyngitis may be due to beta-haemolytic streptococcus (the four-item Centor score):[7]

- absence of cough
- fever
- pharyngeal exudate
- anterior cervical adenopathy.

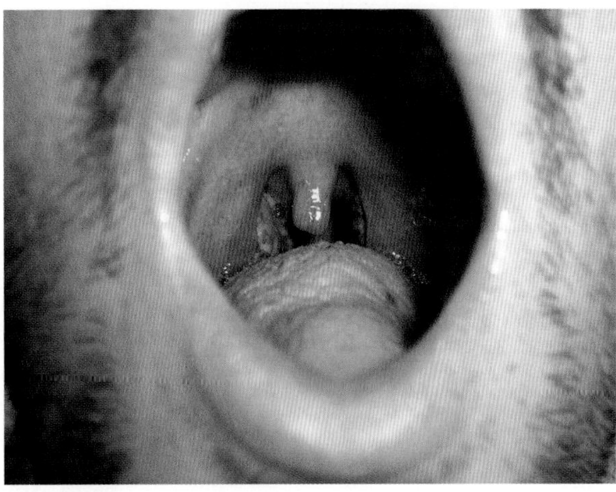

Streptococcal throat

(Courtesy of Dr A Watson, Infectious Diseases Department, The Canberra Hospital.)

FIGURE 42.25

If all four criteria are present, this helps predict the presence of this infection, while the absence of the last three strongly suggests that the infection is *not* due to beta-haemolytic streptococcus.

Despite these criteria it is difficult to distinguish viral from bacterial pharyngitis in many cases. Antibiotic therapy should be reserved for patients who are at high risk of rheumatic fever and those who are very unwell.

Supraglottitis (epiglottitis)

Supraglottitis is a rare but important cause of sore throat.[8] This disease classically presents with a triad of sore throat, painful swallowing (odynophagia) and fever. The patient may uncommonly have stridor, which may be misdiagnosed as asthma; here there is inspiratory wheeze due to the inflammation above the epiglottis. Pooling of secretions is another clue to the diagnosis. Urgent medical attention is indicated to prevent airway obstruction.

COMMON INVESTIGATIONS

CT scans can be commonly used in the diagnosis of nasopharyngeal tumours and sinusitis (see Figs 42.26 and 42.27). They can help identify the spread of infection into the brain and orbits.

The visual fields can be mapped accurately with a visual field chart. Retinal photographs are often used for the screening of diabetic patients.

Nasopharyngeal carcinoma.

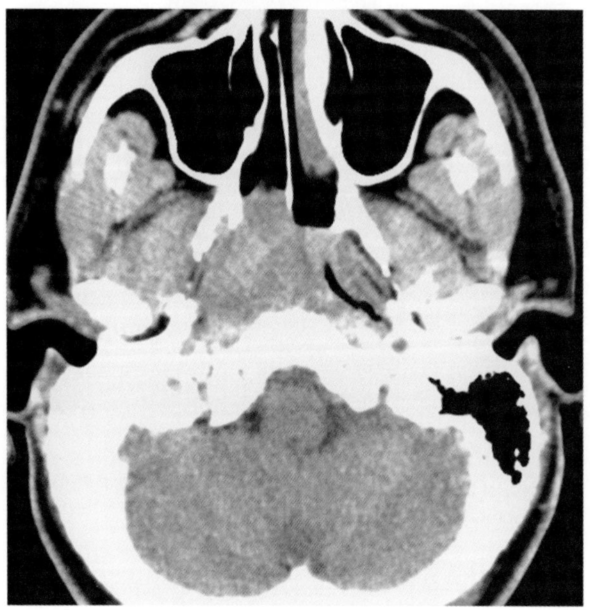

This CT scan shows a soft-tissue mass obstructing the right nasopharynx and right Eustachian tube

(From Haaga JR, Boll D, Dogra VS et al. *CCT and MRI of the whole body*, 5th edn. Maryland Heights MO: Mosby, 2008.)

FIGURE 42.26

T&O'C ESSENTIALS

1. *Important local and systemic disease will be missed unless the eyes and ears are examined as part of a general medical examination.*
2. *Accurate fundoscopy with the ophthalmoscope requires practice. Dilating the patient's pupils may be necessary to obtain an adequate view.*
3. *Subtle eye signs, such as Horner syndrome, will be missed unless time is taken to stand back and compare the two sides.*

Acute sinusitis.

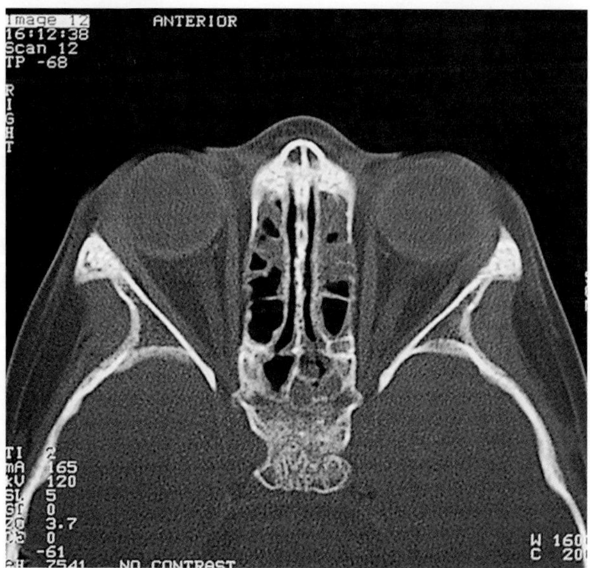

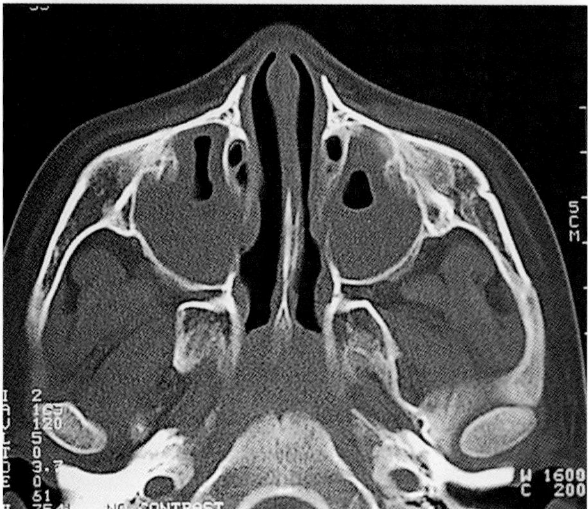

This CT scan coronal view shows opacification of the right maxillary sinus; the left is almost completely opacified, with only a small air pocket visible

(From Zitelli BJ, Davis HW. *Atlas of pediatric physical diagnosis*, 5th edn. Philadelphia: Saunders, 2007.)

FIGURE 42.27

OSCE EXAMPLES

A. EYE EXAMINATION

Mrs Baker has had painful eyes. Please examine her sclerae and conjunctivae.

1. Stand back to look. This is probably a spot diagnosis.
2. Look for scleral icterus. Proceed accordingly if present.
3. Look for conjunctival pallor or injection, or chemosis or subconjunctival haemorrhage.
4. Note the distribution of any redness (e.g. single red eye in iritis). Decide whether conjunctival injection is central (iritis) or spares the central region (conjunctivitis).
5. If there is conjunctival injection, ask for gloves before pulling down the lower lid. Note any ocular discharge (conjunctivitis).
6. If there is pallor, pull down the lower lid and compare the pearly white posterior part of the conjunctiva with the red anterior part.
7. If there is chemosis, look for proptosis and other signs of thyrotoxicosis.
8. Look at the iris (haziness indicates oedema or inflammation).
9. Look and test the pupils (e.g. small irregular pupil in iritis, dilated oval poorly reactive pupil in acute glaucoma).
10. Assess eye movements (painful in scleritis).
11. Fundoscopy (e.g. corneal ulceration looks black examining the red reflex).
12. Look for systemic evidence of vasculitis (e.g. urinalysis).

B. FUNDOSCOPY

Mr Abbott has diabetes. Please look in his fundi.

1. The pupils will probably have been dilated.
2. Use the ophthalmoscope in the approved manner.
3. Look for changes of hypertension or diabetes.

C. VISUAL LOSS

Ms Jenny Elder has experienced sudden loss of vision in one eye. Please examine her.

1. Test *each* eye for visual acuity, and fully assess the visual fields.
2. Assess each pupil's reaction to light and accommodation, and for an afferent pupillary defect (optic nerve damage).
3. Test eye movements and ask about any pain on movement (optic neuritis).
4. Examine the fundi. Note whether the disc is swollen and is abnormally pink or white (ischaemic optic neuropathy). Note any retinal fundal pallor (arterial occlusion), haemorrhages (venous occlusion) or an obvious embolus (at an arterial bifurcation).
5. Test colour vision (for optic nerve damage) if red–green test plates are available.
6. Auscultate for a carotid bruit (stenosis).
7. Take the pulse (atrial fibrillation) and blood pressure (hypertension).
8. Test the urine for blood or protein (vasculitis).

D. EAR EXAMINATION

Mr Li complains of a sore ear. Please examine his auditory canal and eardrum.

1. Note whether the patient looks unwell or feverish.
2. Look at the pinna and external auditory meatus for gouty tophi, dermatitis, cellulitis, signs of trauma (e.g. haematoma), scars (e.g. surgery) and discharge.
3. Look at both ears.
4. Ask the patient whether the ear is painful before using the otoscope to examine the canal and drum.
5. Look for erythema or blisters in the canal and for wax, pus or discharge from the drum.
6. Inspect the tympanic membrane (eardrum) for perforation, grommets or loss of the normal shiny appearance.

Continued

OSCE EXAMPLES *continued*

7. Test hearing, and perform Weber's and Rinné's tests.
8. Palpate the temporomandibular joint for tenderness and crepitus (referred pain).
9. Examine the throat for inflammation (referred pain).

E. THROAT EXAMINATION

Ms Peta Smith complains of recurrent sore throat. Please examine her.

1. Put on gloves and remove any dentures. Note any drooling or flushing or whether the patient appears ill.
2. Take a torch and ask the patient to open wide.
3. Inspect the mouth and pharynx using a tongue depressor. Note tonsillar enlargement and any erythema or other signs of inflammation.
4. Note whether the patient cannot open the mouth fully (trismus).
5. Feel the oral cavity and tongue gently with a gloved finger.

OSCE REVISION TOPICS – **EYES, EARS, NOSE AND THROAT**

Use these topics, which commonly occur in the OSCE, to help with revision.

1. This woman has experienced some loss of vision. Please take a history and then examine her. (pp 806, 831)
2. This woman complains of painful red eyes. Please examine her. (pp 806, 831)
3. This man has double vision. Please examine him. (pp 525–6)
4. This man with diabetes mellitus has problems with his vision. Please examine his fundi. His pupils have been dilated. (pp 810, 831)
5. This woman has a sore throat. Please examine her. (pp 826, 832)
6. This woman reports that she has sinusitis again. Please examine her. (p 824)
7. This man has mouth ulcers. Please take a history and then examine him. (p 826)
8. This man has noticed a problem with deafness. Please take a history and then examine him (speak loudly). (p 817)

References

1. Robinett DA, Kahn DH. The physical examination of the eye. *Emerg Med Clin North Am* 2008; 26:1–16. An excellent summary of eye anatomy and examination.
2. Nair BK, Chen CY, Browne W, McKay D. Central retinal venous pulsations. *Med J Aust* 2016; 205(7):299.
3. McGee S. *Evidence-based clinical diagnosis*, 3rd edn. St Louis: Saunders, 2012.
4. Bagai A, Thavendiranathan P, Detsky AS. Does this patient have hearing impairment? *JAMA* 2006; 295(4):416–428.
5. Gwaltney JM, Sydnor A, Sande MA. Etiology and antimicrobial treatment of acute sinusitis. *Ann Otol Rhinol Larygol Suppl* 1981; 90(3 pt 3):68–71.
6. Ebell MH, Call M, Shinholser J, Gardner J. The Rational Clinical Examination Systematic Review. Does this patient have infectious mononucleosis? *JAMA* 2016; 315(14):1502–1509.
7. McIsaac WJ, Kellner JD, Aufricht P et al. Empirical validation of guidelines for the management of pharyngitis in children and adults. *JAMA* 2004; 291(13):1587–1595.
8. Cirilli AR. Emergency evaluation and management of the sore throat. *Emerg Med Clin North Am* 2013; 31(2):501–515.

CHAPTER 43

The skin and lumps

For one mistake made for not knowing, ten mistakes are made for not looking. J A LINDSAY (1856–1931)

EXAMINATION ANATOMY

Fig. 43.1 shows the three main layers of the skin: the epidermis, dermis and subcutaneous fat. These layers can all be involved in skin diseases in varying combinations. For example, most skin tumours arise in the epidermis (see Fig. 43.2), some bullous eruptions occur at the dermoepidermal junction (DEJ), and lipomas are tumours of subcutaneous fat. The skin appendages, which include the sweat (eccrine and apocrine) glands, hair follicles (see Fig. 43.3) and the nails, are common sites of infection.

The eccrine glands are present everywhere except in the nail beds and on some mucosal surfaces. They are able to secrete over 5 litres of sweat per day. The apocrine glands are found in association with hair follicles but are confined to certain areas of the body, including the axillae, the pubis, the perineum and the nipples. They secrete a viscous fluid whose function is unclear in humans.

The nails are formed from heavily keratinised cells that grow from the nail matrix. The matrix grows in a semilunar shape and appears as the lunules in normal finger- and toenails. Hair is also the product of

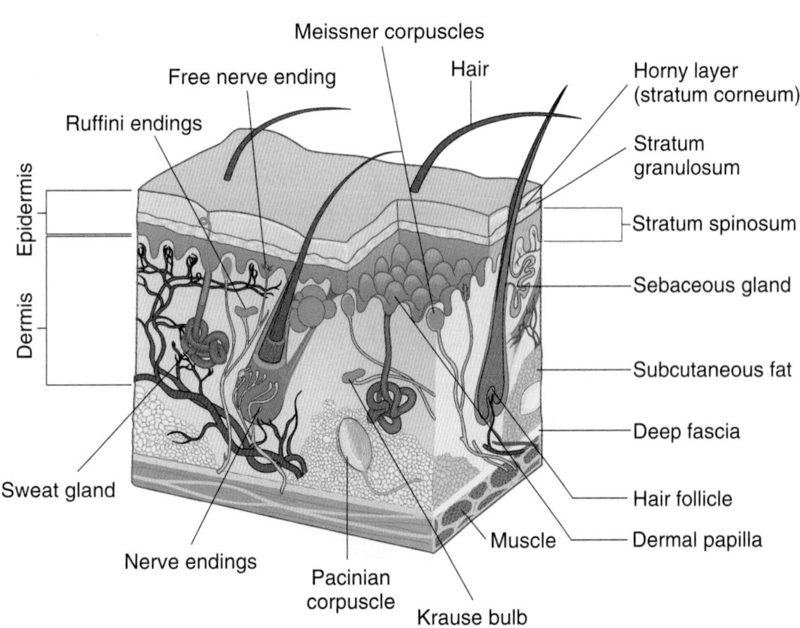

The layers of the skin

FIGURE 43.1

specialised epithelial cells and grows from the hair matrix within the hair follicle.

DERMATOLOGICAL HISTORY

For any patient with a rash or skin condition, it is important to determine when and where it began, its distribution, whether it has changed over time, its relationship to sun exposure or other environmental conditions and any treatments tried[1] (see Questions box 43.1). Ask whether pruritus is associated; localised pruritus is usually due to dermatological disease, but generalised pruritus can be present without a primary rash—such as in liver or renal disease and haematological malignancies. If an infestation is the suspected cause of pruritus it is useful to ascertain whether other household members are affected. Determine also whether pain or disturbed sensation has occurred; for example, inflammation and oedema can produce pain in the skin, whereas disease involving neurovascular bundles or nerves can produce burning or anaesthesia (e.g. leprosy, syphilis, cutaneous neural tumours). Constitutional symptoms such as fever, headache, fatigue, anorexia, weight loss and depression also need to be documented.

Ask about a past personal or family history of rashes, allergic reactions or medical conditions. Asthma, eczema or hay fever suggests atopy. Similarly, evidence of systemic disease in the past may be important in a patient with a rash (e.g. diabetes mellitus, connective tissue disease, inflammatory bowel disease).

A detailed social history needs to be obtained regarding occupation and hobbies, as chemical exposure and contact with animals or plants can all induce dermatitis. All medications that have been taken must be documented. Orally ingested or parenteral

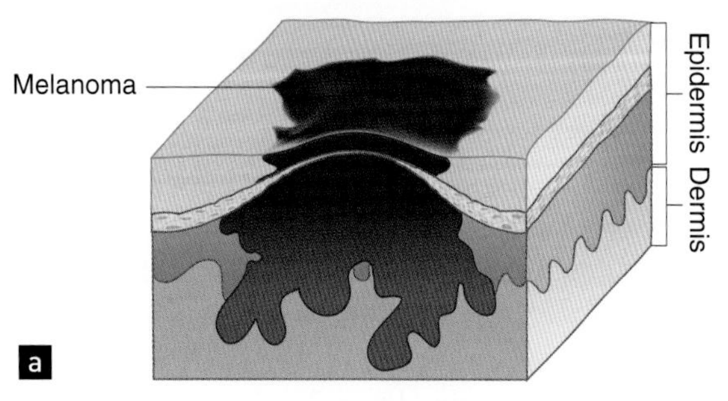

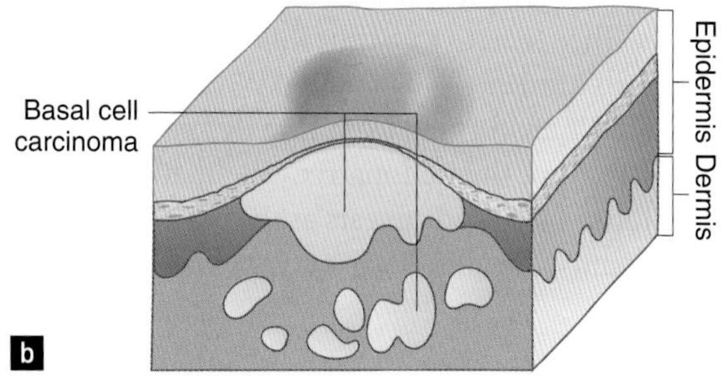

(a) Melanoma; (b) basal cell carcinoma

FIGURE 43.2

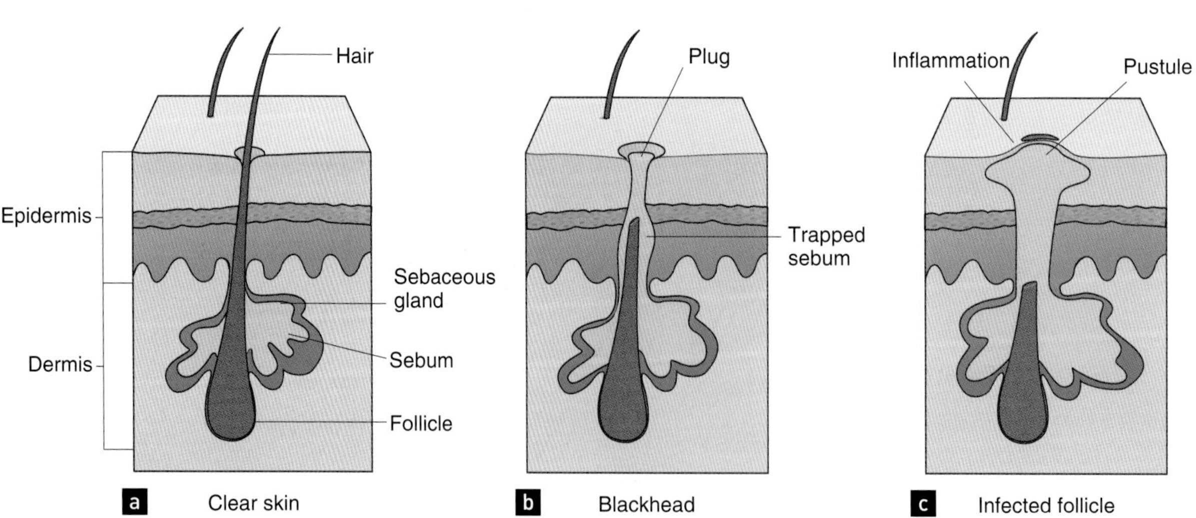

Common sites of infection in the skin

FIGURE 43.3

QUESTIONS TO ASK THE PATIENT WITH A RASH

1. How long have you had the rash?
2. Have you ever had it before?*
3. Is it getting worse?
4. What parts of your skin are affected (e.g. sun-exposed areas, areas in contact with clothing or chemicals)?
5. Was the rash flat or raised to begin with, or was it blistered?
6. Is the area itchy?
7. Does anything seem to make it better, or worse?
8. Has your diet changed recently?
9. What treatment have you tried for it?
10. Have you had a fever or any joint pains?
11. Have you had problems with allergies?
12. Are you taking any tablets or medicines? Are any of these new (in the last 6 weeks)?
13. Have you changed your soap, shampoo, deodorant or washing powder recently?
14. What sort of work do you do? Do you come into contact with chemicals at work or with your hobbies?
15. Have you travelled recently? Where to?
16. Has anyone you know got a similar rash?
17. Have you any other problems with your health?

*When a dermatologist cannot decide the cause of a rash this question can help. If the patient says that he or she has had the rash before, the clinician can then say with confidence 'Well, you've got it again'.

QUESTIONS BOX 43.1

medications can cause a host of cutaneous lesions and can mimic many skin diseases (see Table 43.1).

GENERAL PRINCIPLES OF PHYSICAL EXAMINATION OF THE SKIN

The aim of this chapter is to provide an approach to the diagnosis of skin diseases.[2,3] Particular emphasis

Types of cutaneous drug reactions

1. Acne (e.g. steroids)
2. Hair loss (alopecia; e.g. cancer chemotherapy)
3. Pigment alterations: hypomelanosis (e.g. hydroxyquinone, chloroquine, topical steroids), hypermelanosis
4. Exfoliative dermatitis or erythroderma (p 847)
5. Urticaria (hives; e.g. non-steroidal anti-inflammatory drugs, radiographic dyes, penicillin)
6. Maculopapular (morbilliform) eruptions (see Fig. 43.4; e.g. ampicillin, allopurinol)
7. Photosensitive eruptions (e.g. sulfonamides, sulfonylureas, chlorothiazides, phenothiazines, tetracycline, nalidixic acid, anticonvulsants)
8. Drug-induced lupus erythematosus (e.g. procainamide, hydralazine, minocycline)
9. Vasculitis (e.g. propylthiouracil, allopurinol, thiazides, penicillin, phenytoin)
10. Skin necrosis (e.g. warfarin)
11. Drug-precipitated porphyria (e.g. alcohol, barbiturates, sulfonamides, contraceptive pill)
12. Lichenoid eruptions (e.g. antimalarials, beta-blockers)
13. Fixed drug eruption (e.g. sulfonamides, tetracycline, phenylbutazone)
14. Bullous eruptions (e.g. frusemide, nalidixic acid, penicillamine, clonidine)
15. Erythema nodosum (p 850) or erythema multiforme (p 851)
16. Toxic epidermal necrolysis (e.g. allopurinol, phenytoin, sulfonamides, non-steroidal anti-inflammatory drugs)
17. Pruritus (e.g. opiates, antibiotics, ACE inhibitors, monoclonal antibodies)
18. Psoriasiform (e.g. lithium, beta-blockers)

TABLE 43.1

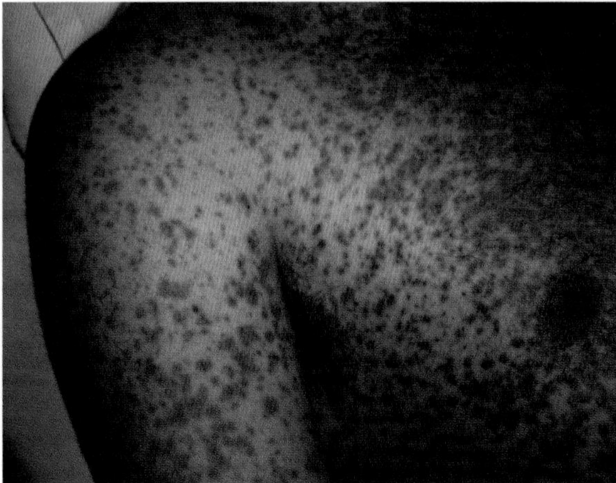

Maculopapular eruption

FIGURE 43.4

will be placed on cutaneous signs as indications of systemic disease. Other chapters have included the usual clues that can be used to arrive at a particular diagnosis. This chapter tries to unify the concept of 'inspection' as a valuable starting point in the examination of the patient. Text box 43.1 gives a suggested method for the dermatological examination.

Ask the patient to undress down to their undergarments and provide a gown for modesty. The whole surface of the skin and its appendages should be carefully inspected (see List 43.1). The genitals are not routinely inspected unless directed by the patient or a specific pathology is being investigated.

The dermatological examination: a suggested method

Even if the patient shows the examiner only a small single area of abnormality, proceed to examine all the skin, mucous membranes and nails (Fig. 43.5).

After obtaining good lighting conditions and asking the patient to disrobe, begin by looking at the **nails and hands**. Paronychia is an infection of the skin surrounding the nails. Other changes to note include pitting (psoriasis, fungal infections) and onycholysis (e.g. thyrotoxicosis, psoriasis). Dark staining under the nail may indicate a subungual melanoma. Linear splinter haemorrhages (e.g. vasculitis) or telangiectasias (e.g. systemic lupus erythematosus) may be seen in the nail bed.

A purplish discoloration in streaks over the knuckles may indicate dermatomyositis (Gottron's papules). Also look at the backs of the hands and forearms for the characteristic blisters of porphyria, which occur on the exposed skin. Papules and scratch marks on the backs of the hands, between the fingers and around the wrists may indicate scabies. Viral warts are common on the hands.

Look at the palms for Dupuytren's contracture, pigmented flat junctional moles (which have a high risk of becoming malignant) and xanthomata in the palmar creases.

Next look at the **forearms**, where lichen planus may occur on the flexor surfaces (characterised by small shiny, violaceous flat-topped polygonal papules) and psoriasis may be present on the extensor surfaces. Palpable purpura—raised bruising that indicates bleeding into the skin—may be seen on the arms and indicates vasculitis. Acanthosis nigricans can occur in the axillae.

Inspect the patient's **hair and scalp**. Decide whether or not the hair is dry and whether the distribution is normal. Alopecia may indicate male pattern baldness, recent severe illness, hypothyroidism or thyrotoxicosis. Patches of alopecia occur in the disease alopecia areata. Short broken-off hairs occur typically in systemic lupus erythematosus. In psoriasis there are silvery scales, which may be seen on the skin of the scalp. Metastatic deposits may rarely be felt as firm nodules within the skin of the scalp. Sebaceous cysts are common. The unfortunate examiner may find nits sticking to the head hairs.

Move down now to the **eyebrows** and look for scaling and greasiness, which are found in seborrhoeic dermatitis. A purplish erythema occurs around the eyelids in dermatomyositis (heliotrope rash). Xanthelasmata are seen near the eyelid.

Look at the **face** for rosacea, which causes bright erythema of the nose, cheeks, forehead and chin, and occasionally pustules and rhinophyma (disfiguring swelling of the nose). Acne causes papules, pustules and comedones involving the face, neck and upper trunk. The butterfly rash of systemic lupus erythematosus occurs across the cheeks but is rare. Spider naevi may be present. Ulcerating lesions on the face may include basal cell carcinoma, squamous cell carcinoma or, rarely, tuberculosis (lupus vulgaris).

Other tumours of the face include keratoacanthoma (a volcano-like lesion from a sebaceous gland) and congenital haemangiomas.

Look for the blisters of herpes zoster, which may occur strictly in the distribution of one of the divisions of the trigeminal nerve.

Inspect the **neck**, which is prone to many of the lesions that occur on the face. Rarely, the redundant loose skin of pseudoxanthoma elasticum will be seen around the neck.

Go on to inspect the **trunk**, where any of the childhood exanthema produce characteristic rashes. Look for spider naevi. Campbell de Morgan spots are commonly found on the abdomen (and chest), as are flat, greasy, yellow-coloured seborrhoeic keratosis. They may also be pigmented (brown or black) or skin-coloured.

TEXT BOX 43.1

The dermatological examination: a suggested method *continued*

Sites of some important skin lesions of the limbs, face and trunk.

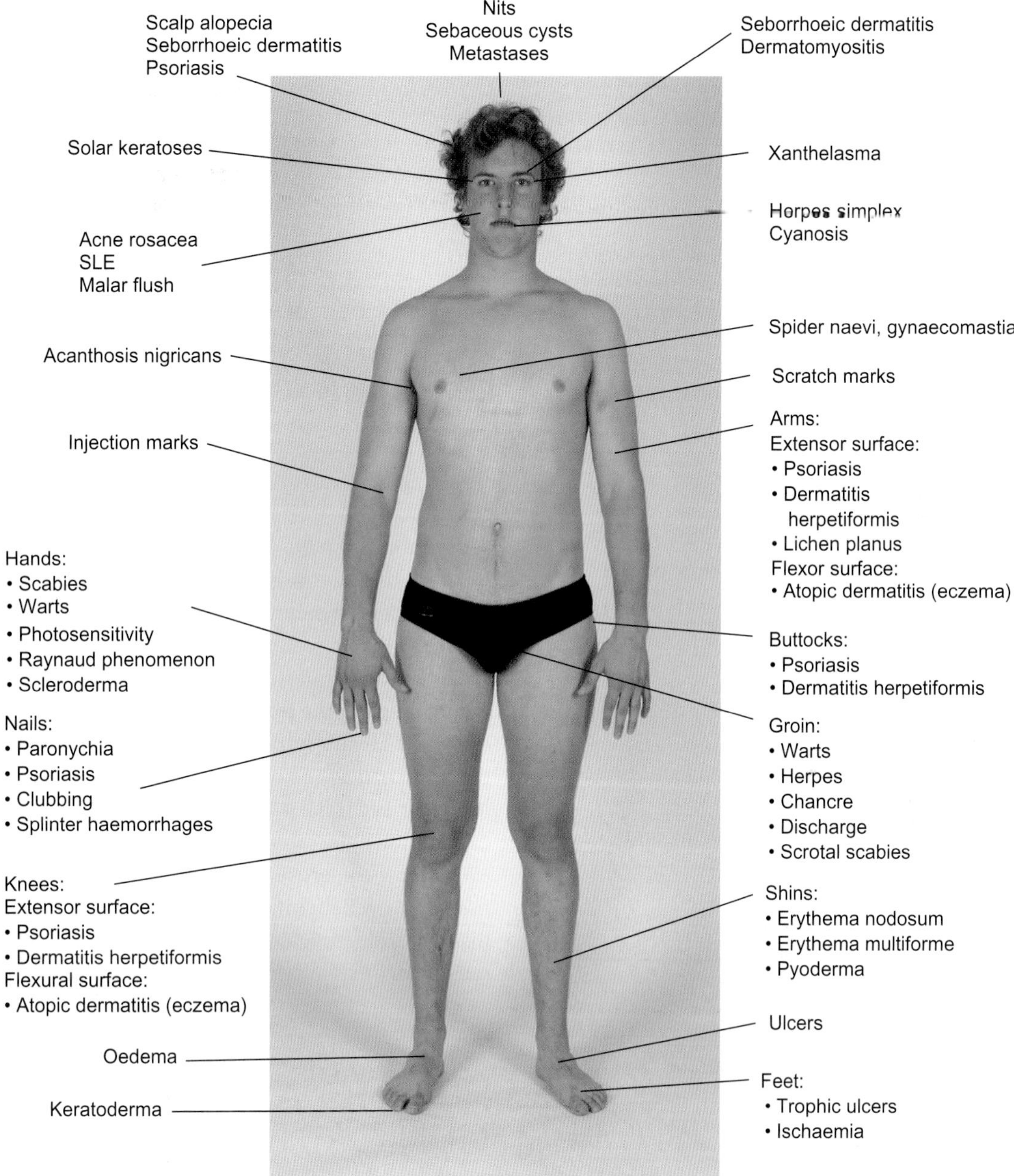

SLE=systemic lupus erythematosus

FIGURE 43.5

TEXT BOX 43.1

Continued

The dermatological examination: a suggested method *continued*

Erythema marginatum (rheumatic fever) occurs on the chest and abdomen. Herpes zoster may be seen overlying any of the dermatome distributions.

Metastases from internal malignancies may rarely occur anywhere on the skin. Neurofibromas are soft flesh-coloured tumours; when associated with more than five 'café-au-lait' spots (brownish, irregular lesions) they suggest neurofibromatosis. Pigmented moles are seen on the trunk and these should be assessed for signs of melanoma. The patient's buttocks and sacrum must be examined for bedsores, and the abdomen and thighs may have areas of fat atrophy or hypertrophy from insulin injections.

Go to the **legs**, where erythema nodosum or erythema multiforme may be seen on the shins. Necrobiosis lipoidica diabeticorum affects the skin over the tibia in diabetics. Pretibial myxoedema also occurs over the shins. Look for ulcers on either side of the lower part of the leg. Livedo reticularis is a net-like, red reticular rash that occurs in vasculitis, the antiphospholipid syndrome and with atheroembolism.

Inspect the **feet** for the characteristic lesion of reactive arthritis called keratoderma blennorrhagicum, where crusted lesions spread across the sole because of the fusion of vesicles and pustules. Look at the foot for signs of ischaemia, associated with wasting of the skin and skin appendages. Trophic ulcers may be seen in patients with peripheral neuropathy (e.g. diabetes mellitus). Always separate the toes to look for melanomas.

TEXT BOX 43.1

CONSIDERATIONS WHEN EXAMINING THE SKIN

1. Hair
2. Nails
3. Sebaceous glands—oil-producing and present on the head, neck and back
4. Eccrine glands—sweat-producing and present all over the body
5. Apocrine glands—sweat-producing and present in the axillae and groin
6. Mucosa

LIST 43.1

When examining actual skin lesions, a number of features should be documented. First, the morphology of each lesion should be *described* precisely. Use the appropriate dermatological terminology (see Table 43.2), even though this may seem to make dermatological diseases more, rather than less, mysterious. As many dermatological diagnoses are purely descriptive, a good description will often be of considerable help in making the diagnosis. Second, the *distribution* of the lesions should be noted, as certain distributions suggest specific diagnoses. Third, the *pattern* of the lesions—such as linear, annular (ring-shaped), reticulated (net-like), serpiginous (snake-like) or grouped—also helps establish the diagnosis. Then *palpate* the lesions, noting texture, consistency, tenderness, temperature, depth and mobility.

Types of skin lesions are shown in Fig. 43.8 and a clinical algorithm for diagnosis is presented in Fig. 43.9. It is always important to keep in mind whether the skin changes are primary (i.e. caused by the disease itself) or secondary (i.e. caused by the patient—like excoriations [scratch marks]—or by the lesion's evolution—e.g. erosion or ulceration, crusting, eschar, fissuring or lichenification). Remember that if the history and clinical examination do not lead to a satisfactory explanation for a rash or lesion then a skin biopsy is a simple procedure of immense diagnostic utility.

HOW TO APPROACH THE CLINICAL DIAGNOSIS OF A LUMP

First, determine the lump's site, size, shape, consistency, mobility and tenderness. Next, evaluate in what tissue layer the lump is situated. If it is in the *epidermis or dermis* (e.g. epidermoid cyst, verruca), it should move when the skin is moved, but if it is in the *subcutaneous tissue* (e.g. neurofibroma, lipoma, lymph node), the skin can

Dermatological terms

Term	Definition	Descriptive terms	
Atrophy	Thinning of the skin with loss of normal markings	Annular	Ring-shaped (clear centre; e.g. tinea infection)
Bulla	A large collection of fluid below the epidermis (>1 cm)	Arcuate	Curved (e.g. secondary syphilis)
Crust	Dried serum, exudate, blood or pus	Circinate	Circular
Ecchymoses	Bruises	Confluent	Lesions that have coalesced (e.g. measles)
Excoriations	Lesions caused by scratching that results in loss of the epidermis	Discoid	Circular without a clear centre (e.g. lupus)
Keloid (see Fig. 43.6)	Persistent thickened scar that extends beyond the original wound margins	Eczematous	Inflamed scaly poorly defined plaques (e.g. atopic dermatitis)
Macule	A flat, non-palpable circumscribed alteration of skin colour (<1 cm)	Keratotic	Thickened from increased keratin (e.g. psoriasis, keratoacanthoma)
Nodule	A circumscribed palpable mass (>1 cm)	Lichenified	Thickening and roughening of the epidermis associated with accentuated skin markings
Papule	A circumscribed palpable elevation (<1 cm)	Linear	In lines (e.g. contact dermatitis)
Petechiae	Purpuric, non-blanching spots (<5 mm)	Papulosquamous	Plaques associated with scaling
Pigment alterations	Increased (hyperpigmentation) or decreased (hypopigmentation)	Reticulated	In a network pattern (e.g. cutaneous parasite)
Plaque	An elevated circumscribed thickened epidermis (>1 cm)	Serpiginous	Sinuous
Purpura	Purple, non-blanching spots (>5 mm)	Zosteriform (see Fig. 43.7)	Following a dermatomal distribution
Pustule	A visible collection of pus		
Scale	An accumulation of excess keratin (hyperkeratosis)		
Sclerosis	Fibrosis of subcutaneous tissues, which may involve the dermis		
Ulcer	Full thickness loss of epidermis, which may also include the dermis and subcutis		
Vesicle	A small collection of fluid below the epidermis (<1 cm)		
Wheal	An area of dermal oedema		

TABLE 43.2

be moved over the lump. If it is in the *muscle* or *tendon* (e.g. tumour), then contraction of the muscle or tendon will limit the lump's mobility. If it is in a *nerve*, pressing on the lump may result in pins and needles being felt in the distribution of the nerve, and the lump cannot be moved in the longitudinal axis but can be moved in the transverse axis. If it is in *bone*, the lump will be immobile.

Determine whether the lump is *fluctuant* (i.e. contains fluid). Place one forefinger (the 'watching' finger) halfway between the centre and the periphery of the lump. Place the forefinger from your other hand (the 'displacing' finger) diagonally opposite the watching finger at an equal distance from the centre of the lump. Press with the displacing finger and keep the watching finger still. If the lump contains fluid, the watching

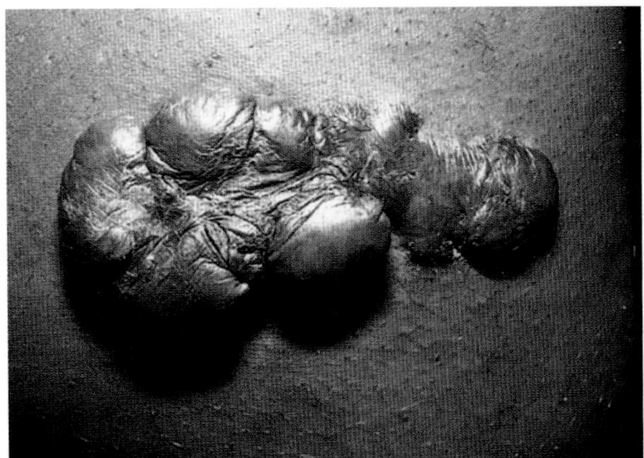

Keloid: excess collagen deposition in the skin forming a raised scar known as keloid

(From Murphy GF, Herzberg AJ. *Atlas of dermatopathology*. Philadelphia: WB Saunders, 1996, p 219.)

FIGURE 43.6

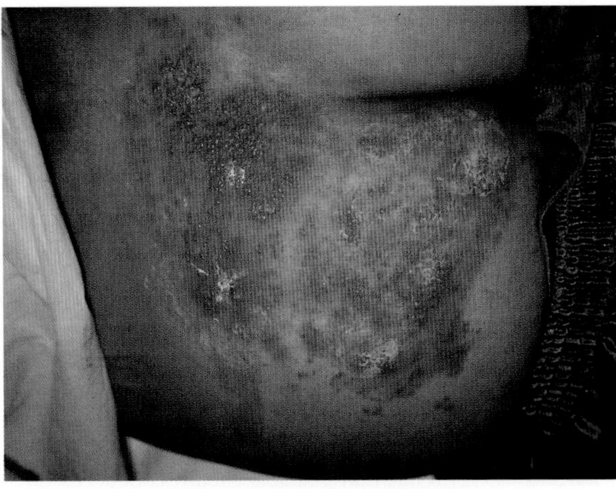

Zosteriform rash of the left buttock

(Courtesy of Dr A Watson, Infectious Diseases Department, The Canberra Hospital.)

FIGURE 43.7

finger will be displaced in *both* axes of the lump (i.e. fluctuation is present).

Place a small torch behind the lump to determine whether it can be *transilluminated*. Light will be transmitted through a cystic lump, which will appear to glow when transilluminated.

Note any associated signs of *inflammation* (i.e. heat, redness, tenderness and swelling[a]).

Look for similar lumps elsewhere, such as multiple subcutaneous swellings from neurofibromas or lipomas. Neurofibromas are smaller than lipomas. They look hard but are remarkably soft; they occur in neurofibromatosis type 1 (von Recklinghausen's[b] disease). They continue to increase in number throughout life and are associated with café-au-lait spots and occasionally spinal neurofibromas.

If an inflammatory or a neoplastic lump is suspected, remember always to examine the regional lymphatic field and the other lymph node groups.

[a] These four cardinal signs were described by Celsus in the 8th volume of his medical book, which taught those who were interested surgical techniques. After performing surgery, readers were warned to look out for the four cardinal signs of postsurgical inflammation—'calor, rubor, dolor and tumor'. Modern surgeons have added loss of function to these signs.

[b] Frederich von Recklinghausen (1833–1910) was Virchow's assistant in Berlin and then a professor of pathology in Strasbourg from 1872. He described this disease in 1882 and haemochromatosis in 1889.

CORRELATION OF PHYSICAL SIGNS AND SKIN DISEASE

There are many different skin diseases with varied physical signs (see Fig. 43.9). With each major sign the groups of common important diseases that should be considered will be listed.

Pruritus

Pruritus simply means itch, and is the most commonly reported skin symptom. It may be either generalised or localised. Scratch marks are generally present. Localised pruritus is usually caused by a dermatological condition such as dermatitis or eczema. Generalised pruritus may be caused by primary skin disease, systemic disease or psychogenic factors.

To determine the cause of the pruritus it is essential to examine the skin in detail (see List 43.2). Excoriations are caused by scratching, regardless of the underlying cause. Specific features of cutaneous diseases such as dermatitis, urticaria, scabies (see Fig. 43.10) or the blisters of dermatitis herpetiformis and bullous pemphigoid should be looked for.

When primary skin diseases have been excluded, a detailed history and examination should be undertaken

Types of skin lesion.

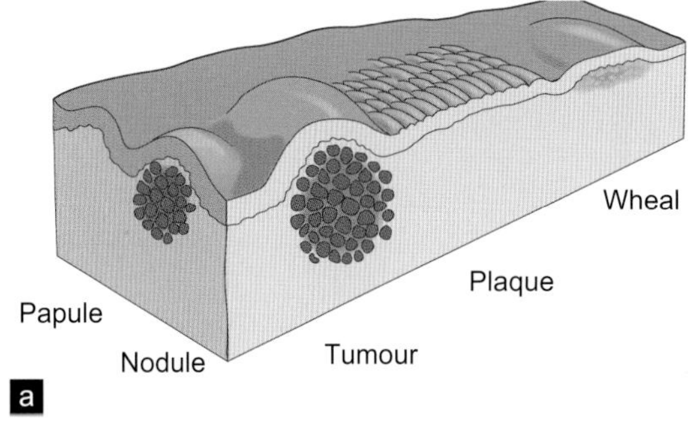

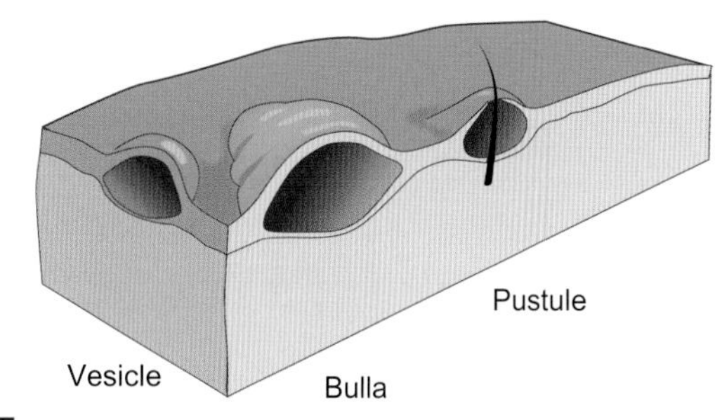

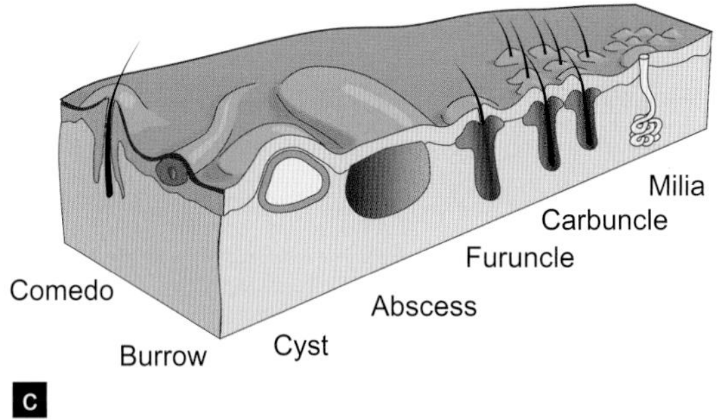

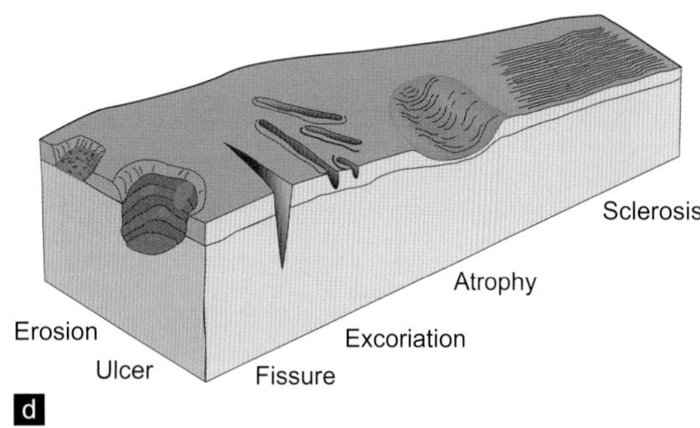

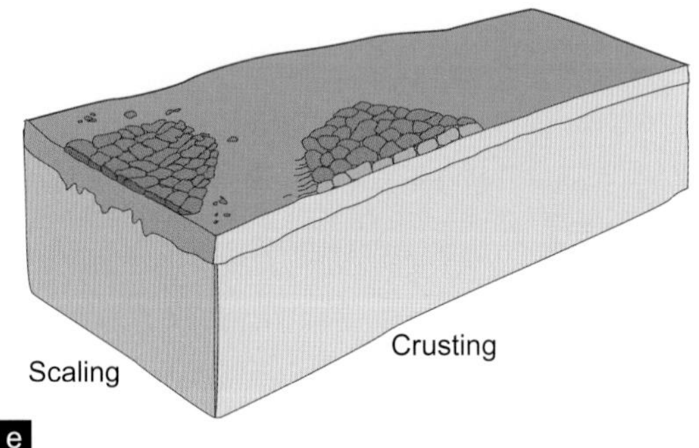

(a) Primary skin lesions, palpable with solid mass; (b) primary skin lesions, palpable and fluid-filled; (c) special primary skin lesions (milia are white papules due to keratin retention); (d) secondary skin lesions, below the skin plane; (e) secondary skin lesions, above the skin plane

(Adapted from Schwartz M. *Textbook of physical diagnosis*, 4th edn. Philadelphia: Saunders, 2002.)

FIGURE 43.8

to consider the various systemic diseases outlined in List 43.3.

Erythrosquamous eruptions

Erythrosquamous eruptions are made up of lesions that are red and scaly. They may be well demarcated or have ill-defined borders. They may be pruritic or asymptomatic.

When attempting to establish a diagnosis of an erythrosquamous eruption, the history is very important. Ask about the time course of the eruption, about a family history of similar skin diseases and whether or not there is a family history of atopy. The presence or absence of itching and the distribution of the lesions (often on the extensor surfaces of the limbs) also give clues about the diagnosis (List 43.4).

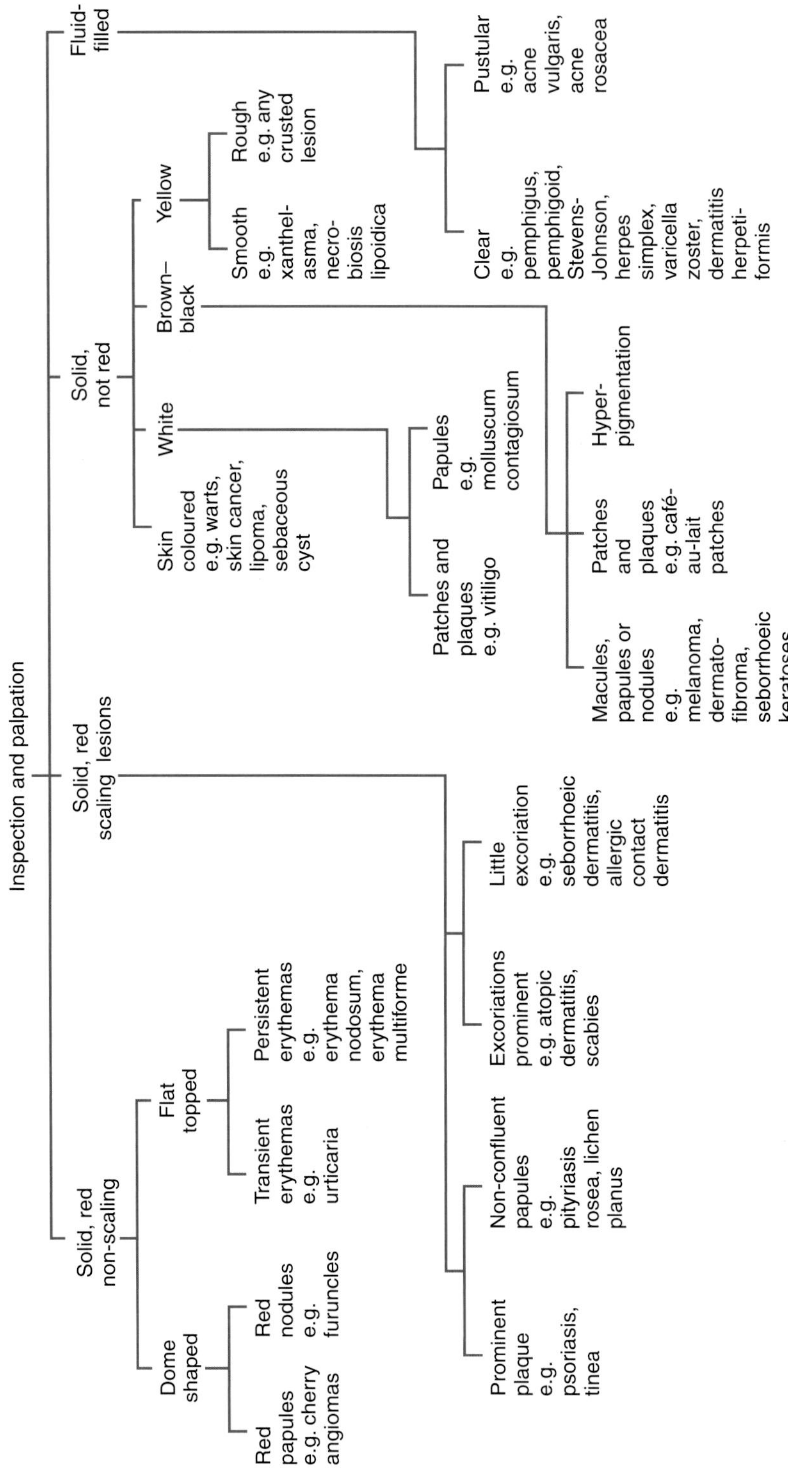

Diagnosis of skin disease: an algorithm

(Adapted from Lynch PJ. *Dermatology for the house officer*, 2nd edn. Baltimore: Williams & Wilkins, 1987.)

FIGURE 43.9

PRIMARY SKIN DISORDERS CAUSING PRURITUS

1. Asteatosis (dry skin)
2. Atopic dermatitis (erythematous, oedematous papular patches on head, neck, flexural surfaces)
3. Psoriasis
4. Lichen planus
5. Urticaria
6. Scabies
7. Dermatitis herpetiformis
8. Bullous pemphigoid

LIST 43.2

SYSTEMIC CONDITIONS CAUSING PRURITUS

1. Cholestasis (e.g. primary biliary cirrhosis)
2. Chronic kidney disease
3. Pregnancy
4. Lymphoma and other internal malignancies
5. Iron deficiency, polycythaemia rubra vera
6. Endocrine diseases (e.g. diabetes mellitus, hypothyroidism, hyperthyroidism, carcinoid syndrome)

LIST 43.3

Scabies.

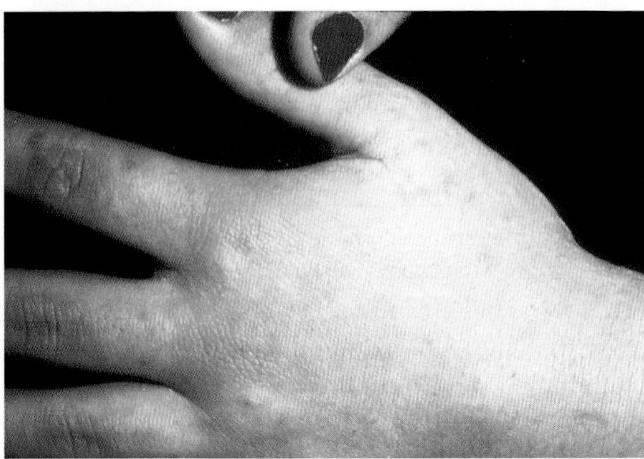

Scattered fine papules with severe itching. Finger web involvement is common

(From Reeves JT, Maibach H. *Clinical dermatology illustrated: a regional approach*, 3rd edn. Sydney: McLennan & Petty, ©2000.)

FIGURE 43.10

CAUSES OF ERYTHROSQUAMOUS ERUPTIONS

1. Psoriasis (salmon-pink plaques with silvery scale)
2. Atopic eczema (diffuse erythema with fine scaling)
3. Pityriasis rosea (pink, scaly, itchy macular lesions in a Christmas tree pattern; herald patch;* self-limited; young adults)
4. Nummular eczema (round patches of subacute dermatitis)
5. Contact dermatitis (irritant or allergic)
6. Dermatophyte infections (ringworm)
7. Lichen planus (violet-coloured, small, polygonal papules)
8. Secondary syphilis (flat, red, hyperkeratotic lesions)

*The herald patch is a single lesion that looks like tinea corporis. It appears several days before the generalised eruption of pityriasis occurs.

LIST 43.4

Asymptomatic lesions on the palms and soles are suggestive of secondary syphilis, whereas pruritic lesions on the anterior wrist would be more suggestive of lichen planus (see Figs 43.11 and 43.12) or scabies infestation. Lichen planus is occasionally associated with primary biliary cirrhosis and other liver diseases, chronic graft-versus-host disease and drugs (e.g. penicillamine, angiotensin-converting enzyme [ACE] inhibitors). Scattered lesions of recent origin on the trunk would be more suggestive of pityriasis rosea (see Fig. 43.13), whereas more widespread, diffuse and intensely pruritic lesions would be more suggestive of nummular eczema (see Fig. 43.14).

Erythematous lesions with a well-demarcated border and overlying silvery scale over the extensor surfaces are usually due to psoriasis (see Figs 43.15 and 43.16).

Blistering eruptions

There are a number of different diseases that will present with either vesicles or bullae (see List 43.5). Dermatitis can present as a blistering eruption, particularly allergic

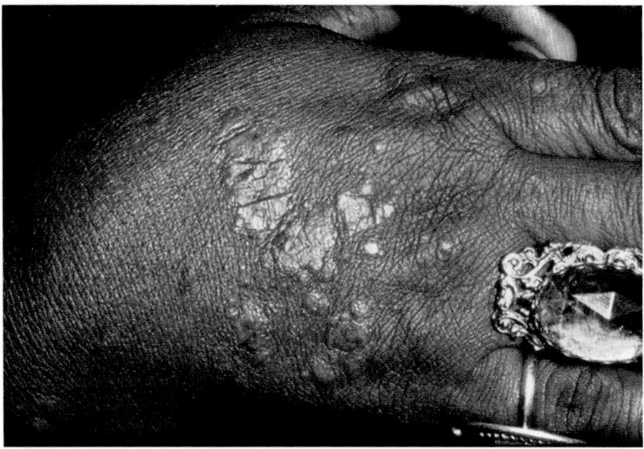

Lichen planus, with polygonal flat-topped violaceous lesions

(From Reeves JT, Maibach H. *Clinical dermatology illustrated: a regional approach*, 2nd edn. Sydney: MacLennan & Petty Pty Ltd, ©1991.)

FIGURE 43.11

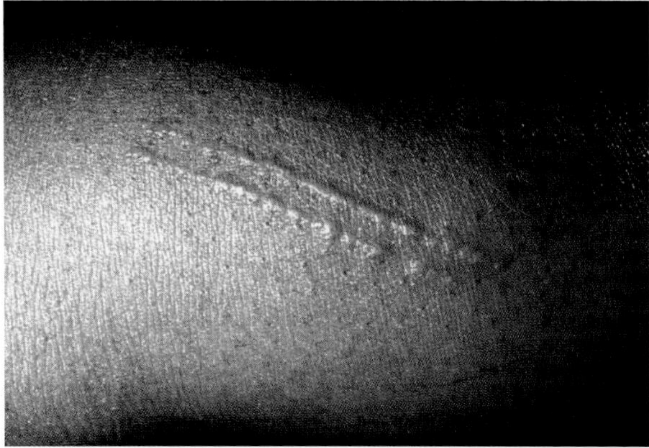

Lichen planus, with development of lesions in an area of trauma—the 'Koebner' phenomenon

(From Reeves JT, Maibach H. *Clinical dermatology illustrated: a regional approach*, 2nd edn. Sydney: MacLennan & Petty Pty Ltd, ©1991.)

Figure 43.12

Pityriasis rosea, with scattered scaly oval lesions on the trunk and a larger 'herald' patch

(From Reeves JT, Maibach H. *Clinical dermatology illustrated: a regional approach*, 2nd edn. Sydney: MacLennan & Petty Pty Ltd, ©1991.)

FIGURE 43.13

CAUSES OF BLISTERING ERUPTIONS

1. Traumatic blisters and burns
2. Bullous impetigo (due to a particular strain of *Staphylococcus aureus*)
3. Viral blisters (e.g. herpes simplex, varicella)
4. Bullous erythema multiforme
5. Bullous pemphigoid
6. Dermatitis herpetiformis
7. Pemphigus
8. Porphyria
9. Epidermolysis bullosa
10. Dermatophyte infections
11. Acute contact dermatitis
12. Necrotising fasciitis
13. Insect bites

LIST 43.5

contact dermatitis (see Fig. 43.17 and also Questions box 43.2).

Clinical features of bullous eruptions

Viral blisters such as those of herpes simplex virus infection (see Fig. 43.18) have a distinctive morphology (small grouped vesicles on an erythematous background, described as 'herpetiform').

Bullous pemphigoid is a rare autoimmune blistering disease usually affecting older patients. Blisters are widespread and tense, have a thick roof and tend not to rupture easily (see Fig. 43.19).

Pemphigus vulgaris is another autoimmune blistering disease (see Fig. 43.20). Patients are often younger than those affected by bullous pemphigoid, and the disease can be more severe. It has thin-roofed

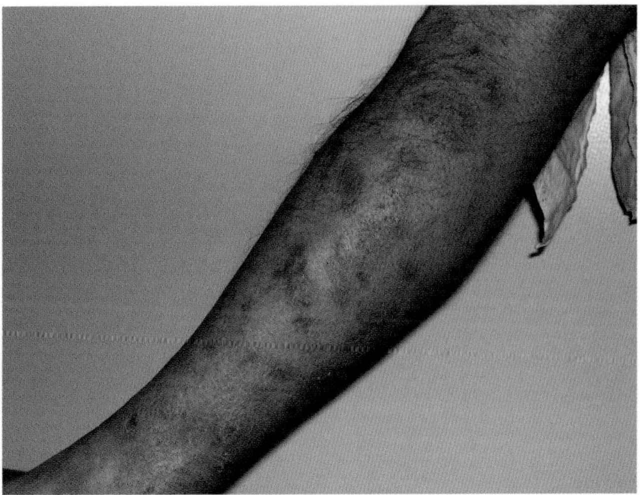

Nummular eczema—pink oval scaling, slightly crusted patches

(From Miller JJ, Marks JG. *Lookingbill and Marks' principles of dermatology*, 6th edn. Philadelphia: Elsevier, 2019.)

FIGURE 43.14

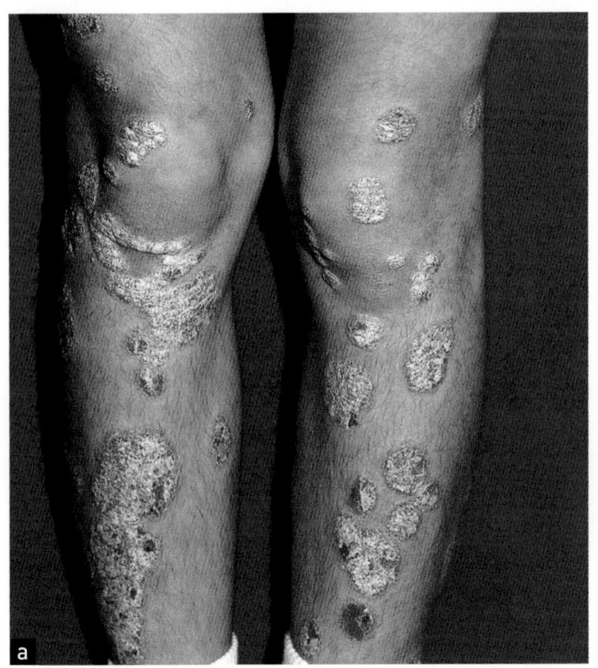

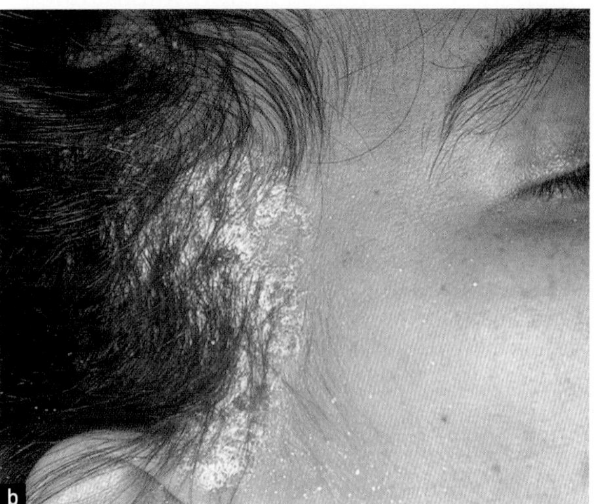

(a) Psoriasis—typical bright-red, scaly plaque with silvery scale over a joint; (b) psoriasis of the scalp in the hair line

((a) From Paller AS, Mancini AJ. *Hurwitz Clinical pediatric dermatology: a textbook of skin disorders of children and adolescence*, 5th edn. Philadelphia: Elsevier; 2016; (b) from Giddens JF, Wilson SF. *Health assessment for nursing practice*, 6th edn. Philadelphia: Elsevier, 2017.)

FIGURE 43.15

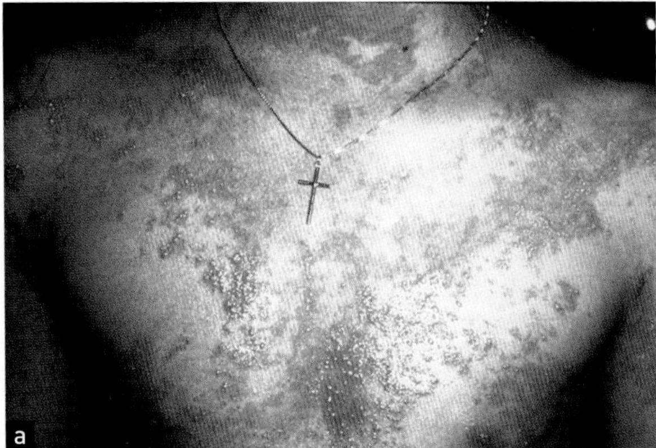

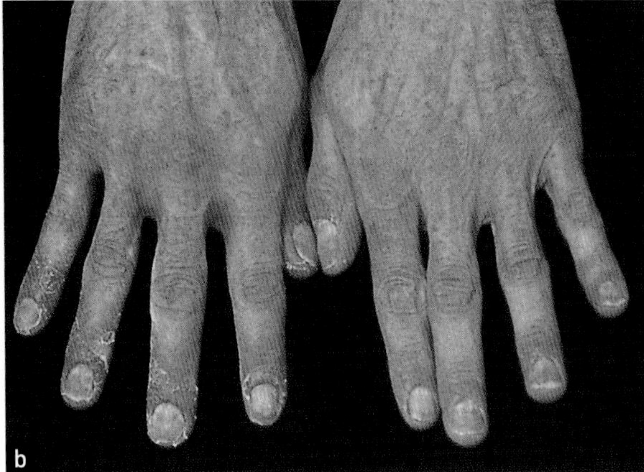

(a) Acute widespread pustular psoriasis. Often the eruption is bright red with bizarre patterns and pustules predominantly at the margins. (b) Pustular psoriasis of the hands

((a) From Reeves JT, Maibach H. *Clinical dermatology illustrated: a regional approach*, 2nd edn. Sydney: MacLennan & Petty Pty Ltd, ©1991; (b) from Hochberg M, Silman AJ, Smolen J et al. *Rheumatology*, 5th edn. Maryland Heights: Mosby, 2010.)

FIGURE 43.16

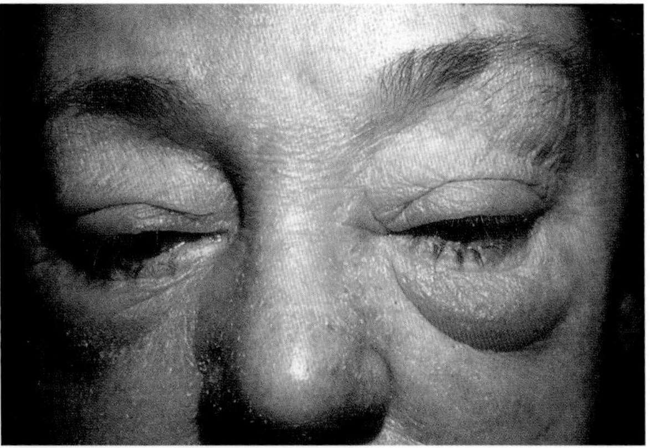

Allergic contact dermatitis from over-the-counter topical medication rubbed over congested sinuses

(Courtesy of Dr A Watson, Infectious Diseases Department, The Canberra Hospital.)

FIGURE 43.17

blisters that readily rupture and form erosions and crusts. The epidermis is fragile and can sometimes shear with lateral pressure (Nikolsky's[c] sign). Almost all patients will have oral mucosal involvement, and many will have other mucosal sites such as eyes and genitals affected.

Dermatitis herpetiformis is a cutaneous manifestation of gluten sensitivity characterised by a pruritic papules or vesicles favouring the extensor surfaces, back and buttocks (see Fig. 43.21).

[c] Pyotr Vasilyevich Nikolsky (1855–1940), a Kiev and Warsaw dermatologist. Nikolsky's sign also occurs in staphylococcal scalded-skin syndrome and toxic epidermal necrolysis.

QUESTIONS TO ASK THE PATIENT WITH A BLISTERING ERUPTION

! denotes symptoms for the possible diagnosis of an urgent or dangerous problem.

1. Have you had blisters on the backs of your hands that break easily and are worse if you have been in the sun? (Porphyria cutanea tarda)
2. Have you had sores or blisters in your mouth that came on before the skin blisters? (Pemphigus vulgaris)
3. **!** Did the inside of your mouth become ulcerated and painful suddenly? Have your eyes become painful? (Stevens–Johnson syndrome; see Fig. 43.22)
4. Was the blister on your lip or genitals, and was it preceded by itching or burning? (Herpes simplex)
5. **!** Were the blisters preceded by some days of severe pain and burning in the areas where the blisters have broken out? (Herpes zoster)
6. Did you notice pink spots on the skin that were itchy before the blisters appeared? (Bullous pemphigoid)

QUESTIONS BOX 43.2

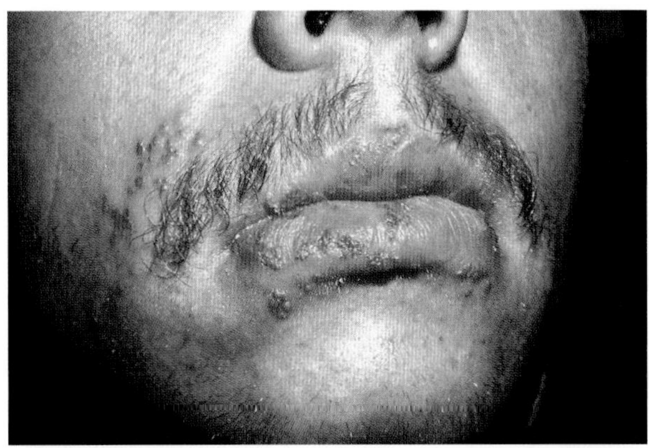

Primary herpes simplex virus infection in an adult; shows typical widespread distribution around the mouth

(From Reeves JT, Maibach H. *Clinical dermatology illustrated: a regional approach*, 2nd edn. Sydney: MacLennan & Petty Pty Ltd, ©1991.)

FIGURE 43.18

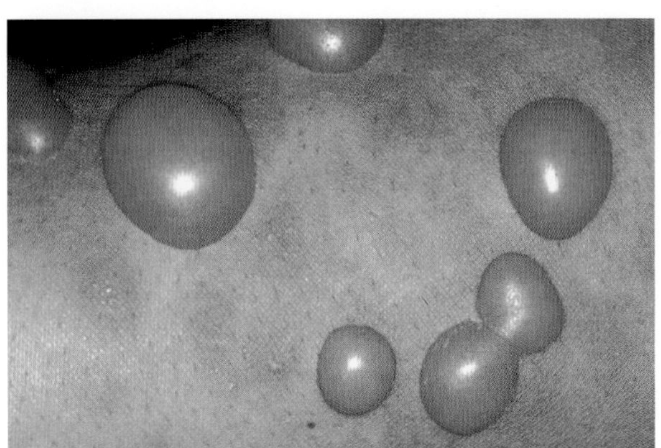

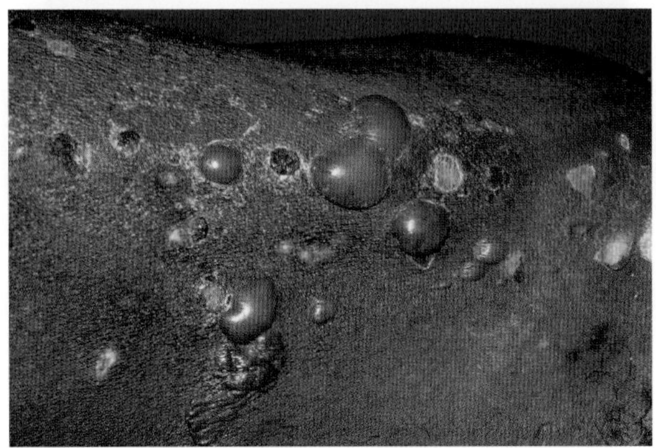

Bullous pemphigoid

(From Schwarzenberger K. *General dermatology*. Philadelphia: Saunders, 2008.)

FIGURE 43.19

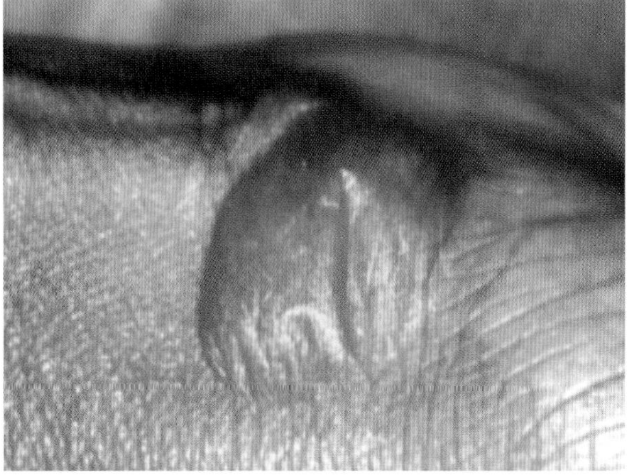

Pemphigus vulgaris

(From Reeves JT, Maibach H. *Clinical dermatology illustrated: a regional approach*, 2nd edn. Sydney: MacLennan & Petty Pty Ltd, ©1991.)

FIGURE 43.20

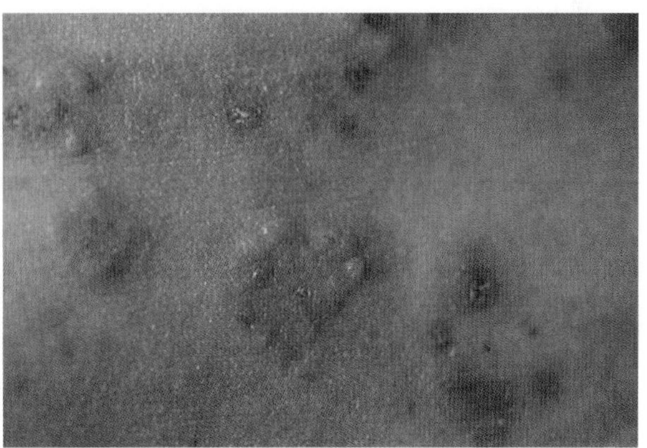

Dermatitis herpetiformis

FIGURE 43.21

Porphyria cutanea tarda is a metabolic disorder characterised by clear or haemorrhagic tense blisters on the dorsal hands and other sun-exposed areas, hyperpigmentation and increased facial hair; hepatic insult from hepatitis C, alcohol, haemochromatosis and the oral contraceptive pill can induce symptoms (due to decreased uroporphyrinogen decarboxylase).

Erythroderma

Erythroderma is best thought of as the end stage of numerous skin conditions (see List 43.6). The

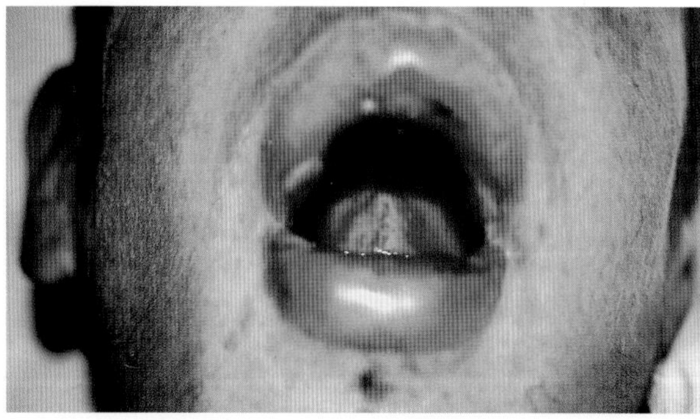

Stevens–Johnson syndrome

(Courtesy of Dr A Watson, Infectious Diseases Department, The Canberra Hospital.)

FIGURE 43.22

CAUSES OF ERYTHRODERMA

1. Eczema
2. Psoriasis
3. Drugs (e.g. phenytoin, allopurinol)
4. Pityriasis rubra pilaris
5. Mycosis fungoides, leukaemia, lymphoma
6. Lichen planus
7. Pemphigus foliaceus
8. Hereditary disorders
9. Dermatophytosis
10. Toxic shock syndrome—generalised erythroderma

LIST 43.6

erythrodermic patient has involvement of >90% of the skin with an erythematous inflammatory process, often with exfoliation. This represents that most unusual occurrence: a dermatological emergency.

An attempt should be made to determine the underlying cause of the erythroderma, and this is best done based on the history and examination. Specific treatment can then be directed at the underlying cause. Patients with erythroderma may develop systemic manifestations such as peripheral oedema, tachycardia, metabolic changes (including hypoalbuminaemia and extrarenal fluid loss) and disturbances in thermoregulation. Therefore these patients require close medical supervision and monitoring until they have recovered from the acute phase of their illness.

Livedo reticularis and medical conditions

Condition	Example
Haematological	Polycythaemia rubra vera, leukaemia, thrombocytosis
Hypercoagulable states	Antiphospholipid syndrome, factor V Leiden mutation, protein S or C deficiencies
Paraprotein	Multiple myeloma
Autoimmune diseases	Systemic lupus erythematosus, dermatomyositis, scleroderma, rheumatoid arthritis
Infections	Hepatitis C, syphilis, meningococcal disease, tuberculosis
Vasculitides	Polyarteritis nodosa, granulomatosis with polyangiitis
Endocarditis	
Cryoglobulinaemia, cryofibrinogenaemia	
Neurohumoral diseases	Carcinoid, phaeochromocytoma

TABLE 43.3

The most common cause is eczema, which is usually of the atopic variety. These patients often have an intense pruritus. Some of them will develop a chronic unremitting erythroderma.

Livedo reticularis

This is a net-like pattern of blue or reddish blood vessels visible through the skin and is common particularly

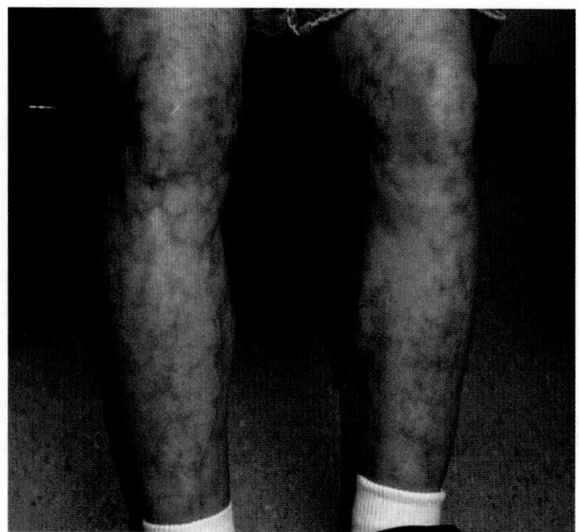

Livedo reticularis

FIGURE 43.23

on the lower extremities (see Fig. 25.10 on p 434). It is usually the result of slow flow through subcutaneous vessels due to cold temperatures (physiological). Physiological livedo can be elicited by cooling the leg and will disappear on warming (see Fig. 43.23). Less commonly it can be secondary to an underlying disease (Table 43.3). There is no extravasation of blood, which distinguishes it from ecchymoses or purpura. Therefore it blanches upon pressure, unless vessel occlusion (e.g. thrombosis) with ischaemia has occurred.

Pustular and crusted lesions

The clinical appearance of a *pustular* lesion results from accumulation of neutrophils. Such collections usually indicate an infective process; however, sterile pustules may form as part of a number of skin diseases owing to the release of chemotactic factors following an immunological reaction.

A *crust* is dried serum, blood or pus that is found on the skin's surface. It may include bacteria (usually *Staphylococcus*); an example of where this occurs is a honey-yellow crust in impetigo.

It is essential to determine whether or not a pustular lesion (or a group of pustular lesions) represents a primarily infectious process or an inflammatory dermatological condition. For example, pustular lesions on the hands and feet may be due to tinea infection, a sterile primary pustular psoriasis or palmoplantar pustulosis (see List 43.7 and Questions box 43.3). Skin scrapings of desquamating skin flakes or a swab of pustule contents sent for microscopy and culture will help to differentiate infectious from inflammatory causes of pustules. If pustules, vesicles or crusts are herpetiform or haemorrhagic in morphology, swabs for herpes simplex and herpes zoster should be taken.

CAUSES OF PUSTULAR AND CRUSTED LESIONS

1. Acne vulgaris (comedones, papules, pustules, cystic lesions, ice-pick scars—no telangiectasias)
2. Acne rosacea (acne-like lesions, erythema and telangiectasias on central face—no comedones)
3. Impetigo
4. Folliculitis
5. Viral lesions
6. Pustular psoriasis
7. Drug eruptions
8. Dermatophyte infections
9. Sweet syndrome (pustular dermatosis)

LIST 43.7

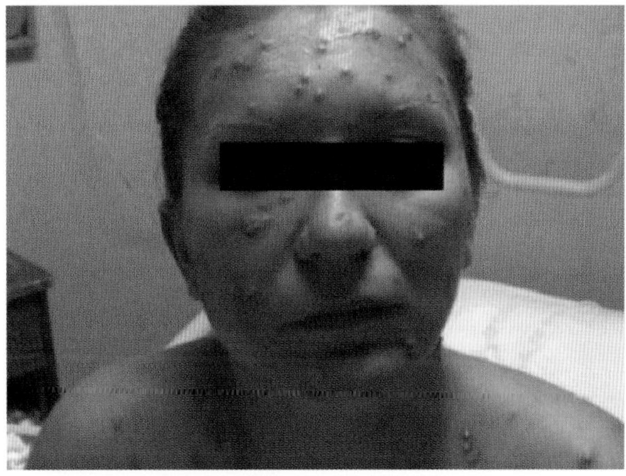

Sweet's syndrome

(From Fazili T, Duncan D, Wani L. Sweet's syndrome. *Am J Med* 2010; 123(8):694–696.)

FIGURE 43.24

QUESTIONS TO ASK THE PATIENT WITH PUSTULAR LESIONS

1. Are you taking cortisone tablets? (Steroid acne)
2. Has your skin been painful or have you had a fever? (Pustular psoriasis)
3. Have you had psoriasis in the past?
4. Do you find your face becomes flushed easily, for example if you drink hot drinks? (Acne rosacea)
5. Are you a diabetic? (Cutaneous candidiasis)
6. Do you sweat excessively? (Folliculitis)

QUESTIONS BOX 43.3

Dermal plaques

Dermal plaques are localised thickenings of the skin that are caused by changes in the dermis or subcutaneous fat. These may be due to chronic inflammatory processes or scarring sclerotic processes (see List 43.8).

CAUSES OF DERMAL PLAQUES

1. Granuloma annulare (see Fig. 43.25)
2. Necrobiosis lipoidica
3. Sarcoidosis
4. Erythema nodosum
5. Lupus erythematosus
6. Sweet syndrome
7. Morphoea and scleroderma
8. Tuberculosis
9. Leprosy

LIST 43.8

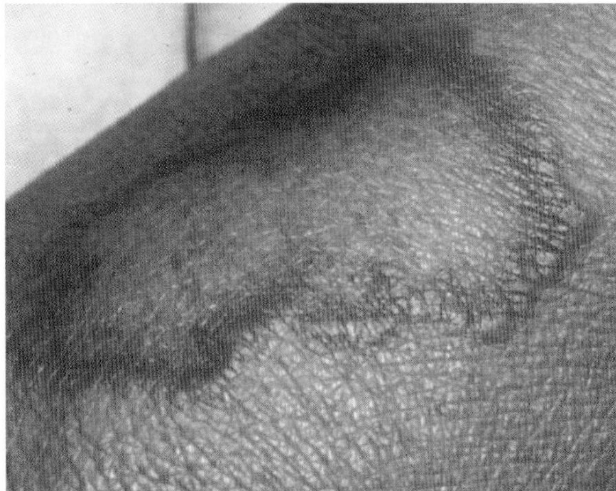

Granuloma annulare

(From James W. *Andrews' diseases of the skin: clinical dermatology*, 11th edn. Philadelphia: Saunders, 2011.)

FIGURE 43.25

The pattern of involvement of the plaques, the age of the patient and other clinical features should enable a diagnosis to be established.

Neutrophilic dermatoses are a group of conditions characterised by neutrophilic infiltrates without any identifiable infectious cause. Sweet's syndrome[d] (acute febrile neutrophilic dermatosis) is a condition involving painful red plaques and nodules that are well demarcated from surrounding skin. There is often an associated fever. Sweet's syndrome may be idiopathic or occur in association with haematological disease (myelodysplastic disorders and acute myeloid leukaemia), solid organ tumours, infections, inflammatory bowel disease, autoimmune disease, pregnancy and some drugs (e.g. granulocyte-stimulating factor).

[d] Dr Robert Sweet from Plymouth, England, first described this in 1964.

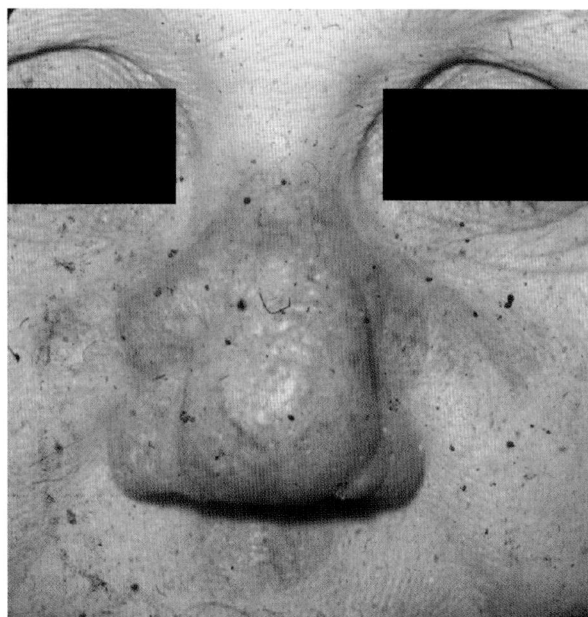

Lupus pernio

(From Holmes J, Lazarus A. Sarcoidosis: extrathoracic manifestations. *Disease-a-month* 2009; 55(11):675–692.)

FIGURE 43.26

There are a number of other neutrophilic dermatoses including pyoderma gangrenosum and Behçet's disease.

Lupus pernio (see Fig. 43.26) appears as violaceous papules and plaques on the nose, cheeks and ears. Despite its name this condition is not associated with systemic lupus erythematosus: it is a manifestation of cutaneous sarcoidosis. Lupus pernio on the nose is more commonly associated with pulmonary and upper respiratory tract sarcoidosis than with other forms of cutaneous sarcoidosis.

Erythema nodosum

This is the best known of the group of diseases classified as panniculitis (inflammation of the subcutaneous fat). Nodular vasculitis is another type of panniculitis causing painful nodules on the lower legs, usually on the calves. In contrast the lesions of erythema nodosum are usually found in the pretibial area and are erythematous, palpable and tender (p 285). Systemic symptoms may include fever, arthralgia, arthritis and malaise. A significant percentage

CAUSES OF ERYTHEMA NODOSUM

1. Sarcoidosis
2. Streptococcal infections
3. Inflammatory bowel disease
4. Drugs (e.g. sulfonamides, penicillin, sulfonylurea, oestrogen, iodides, bromides)
5. Tuberculosis
6. Other infections (e.g. lepromatous leprosy, toxoplasmosis, histoplasmosis, *Yersinia*, *Chlamydia*)
7. Systemic lupus erythematosus
8. Behçet syndrome

LIST 43.9

of cases—more than one-third—are idiopathic; other common causes include upper respiratory tract infections (both streptococcal and viral), drugs such as the oral contraceptive and sulfonamides, inflammatory bowel disease, tuberculosis and sarcoidosis (see List 43.9).

Erythema multiforme (EM)

This is a distinctive inflammatory reaction of skin and mucosa. The characteristic skin lesion is a *target lesion* that has a well-defined border and consists of three distinct zones of colour change (see Fig. 43.27). The centre develops a dusky appearance over time and has been likened to a 'bulls eye'. The central zone can form a bulla or crust. When the mucosal membranes are significantly involved the condition is referred to as EM major; in the purely cutaneous form it is called EM minor. In most cases the condition is precipitated by viral infections, especially clinical or subclinical herpes simplex virus. Other causes include *Mycoplasma pneumoniae*, histoplasmosis and drugs. Sometimes no underlying cause will be established.

It is now known that this condition is a distinct disorder from *Stevens–Johnson*[e] *syndrome* (SJS) (see Fig. 43.18) and *toxic epidermal necrolysis* (TEN). These are two rare, potentially fatal variants within a continuous spectrum of adverse drug reactions. They are characterised by differing severity of mucocutaneous involvement, erythema and exfoliation. The medications most frequently implicated are antibiotics, anticonvulsants,

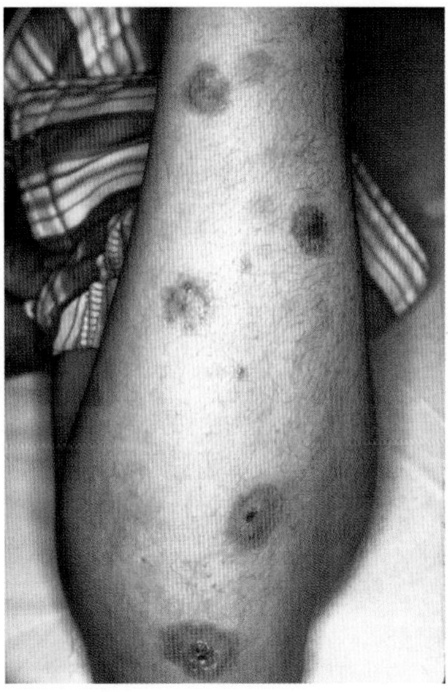

Erythema multiforme; shows classic iris or target lesions, secondary to herpes simplex virus infection of the lips

(From Reeves JT, Maibach H. *Clinical dermatology illustrated: a regional approach*, 2nd edn. Sydney: MacLennan & Petty Pty Ltd, ©1991.)

FIGURE 43.27

allopurinol and non-steroidal anti-inflammatory drugs (NSAIDs). It is rare for SJS or TEN to be triggered by an infectious agent.

Cellulitis and erysipelas

Cellulitis (see Fig. 43.28) is inflammation of the deep dermis and subcutaneous tissue causing a unilateral erythematous lower limb. There may be associated lymphangitis and tender inguinal lymphadenopathy. In severe cases purple patches develop and may blister. It is usually due to beta-haemolytic *Streptococcus* or *Staphylococcus aureus* infection. In intravenous drug users it affects the upper limb (the usual sites of drug injection).

Erysipelas is a superficial variant of cellulitis caused primarily by beta-haemolytic *Streptococcus* that affects the dermis (see Fig. 43.29). It can occur on the face or the legs and consists of sharply demarcated erythema and a characteristic raised edge as a result of dermal involvement. There may be an obvious entry point for the organism, such as soft-tissue injury, tinea pedis, a varicose ulcer or a predisposing condition such as diabetes mellitus.

[e] Albert Mason Stevens (1884–1945), a New York paediatrician, and Frank C Johnson (1894–1934), an American physician.

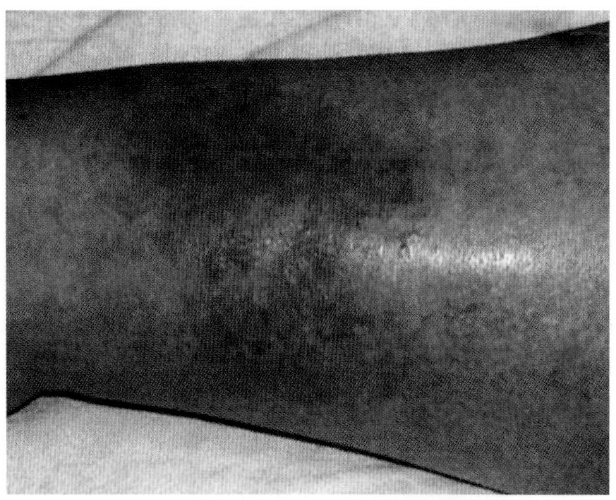

Cellulitis

(Courtesy of Dr A Watson, Infectious Diseases Department, The Canberra Hospital.)

FIGURE 43.28

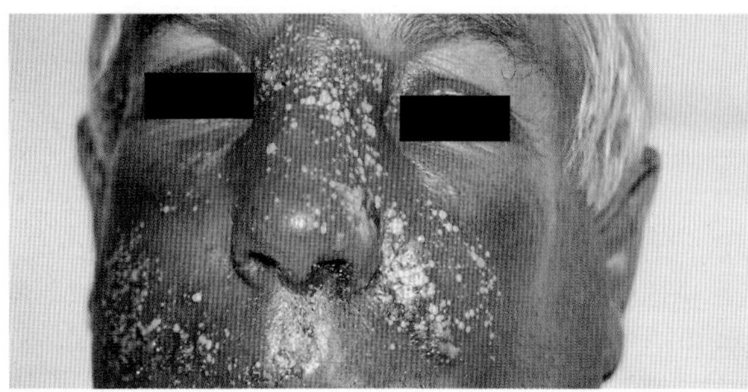

Erysipelas

(Courtesy of Dr A Watson, Infectious Diseases Department, The Canberra Hospital.)

FIGURE 43.29

Necrotising fasciitis is important to consider in the differential diagnosis. If there is severe pain, the skin is pale pink rather than floridly erythematous and the patient has signs of sepsis, consider necrotising fasciitis.

Folliculitis, furuncles and carbuncles

These conditions are all infections of hair follicles of varying severity.

Folliculitis is a very common disorder characterised by superficial inflammation of a hair follicle. Most cases are due to staphylococcal infection but they can be caused by other microorganisms (such as *Candida, Malassezia* or *Pseudomonas*) or topical medications, or be drug induced. If the infection becomes deeper, it becomes a *furuncle* (or boil) and if it spreads to involve a number of adjacent hair follicles it becomes a *carbuncle*. Lesions can occur anywhere on the skin but are commoner on the buttocks, neck and anogenital area. They are very painful and often associated with systemic symptoms. Staphylococcal organisms are usually responsible. The deep lesions heal by rupturing and exuding pus. They often leave a scar. Draining lymph nodes may be enlarged and tender.

The condition *hidradenitis suppurativa* is an inflammatory skin condition that is associated with nodules, cysts, abscesses and the sinus tract. It is more common in women and in overweight patients. The condition involves the apocrine glands in the axillae, the groin and the submammary areas and exhibits the pathognomonic double-ended comedone.

Other infections

Viral infections can lead to skin reactions. Measles is an example of an infection causing a *viral exanthem* (see Fig. 43.30). Many viruses including cytomegalovirus (CMV), Epstein–Barr virus (EBV), Coxsackie virus and the seroconversion illness after human immunodeficiency virus (HIV) infection can cause a similar rash. Patients with EBV infection treated with amoxicillin develop a characteristic rash (see Fig. 43.31). Meningococcal septicaemia causes a petechial rash, which can progress to purpura fulminans (see Fig. 43.32).

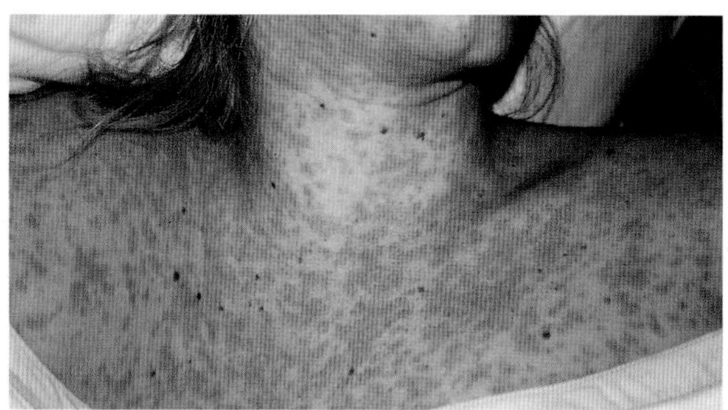

Viral exanthema

(Courtesy of Dr A Watson, Infectious Diseases Department, The Canberra Hospital.)

FIGURE 43.30

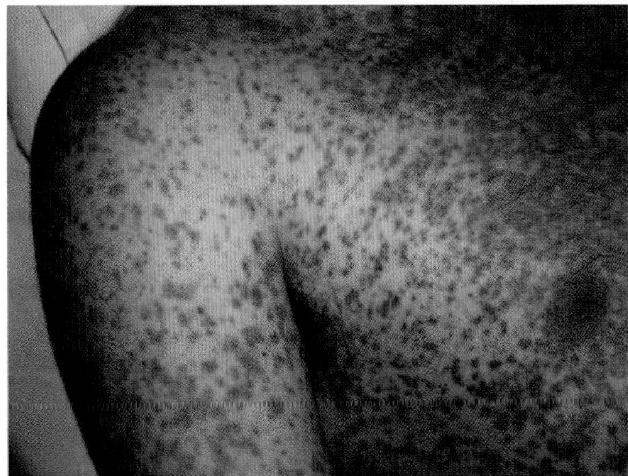

Epstein–Barr virus infection after amoxicillin

(Courtesy of Dr A Watson, Infectious Diseases Department, The Canberra Hospital.)

FIGURE 43.31

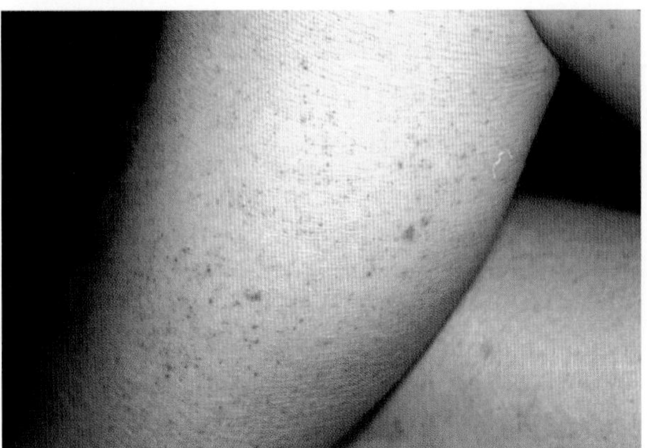

Petechial rash

(From Marks J, Miller J. *Lookingbill & Marks' principles of dermatology*, 4th edn. Philadelphia: Saunders, 2006.)

FIGURE 43.32

Keratoderma blennorrhagicum.

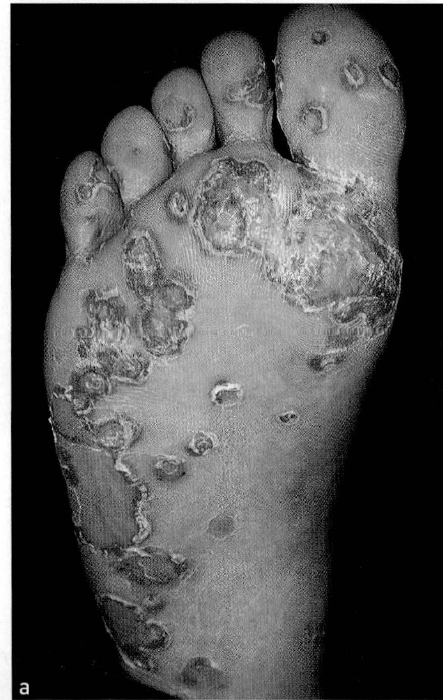

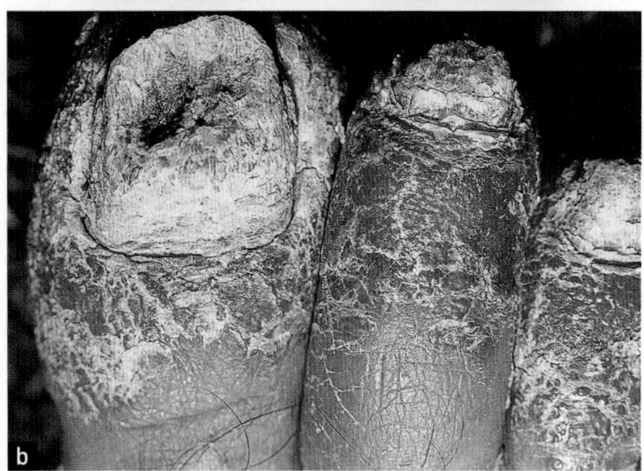

(a) Sole of foot; (b) toenails

(From Habif T. *Clinical dermatology*, 5th edn. St Louis MO: Mosby, 2009.)

FIGURE 43.33

Impetigo is the most common cutaneous bacterial infection, characterised by honey-coloured golden crusting, vesicles and pustules on an erythematous base. *S. aureus* and *Streptococcus pyogenes* are the most frequent agents. Reactive arthritis caused by genitourinary or gastrointestinal bacterial infection may be associated with *keratoderma blennorrhagicum*, in which tender hyperkeratotic nodules and plaques, sometimes with blisters or pustules, arise on the soles of the feet (see Fig. 43.33). Molluscum contagiosum is a common infectious viral disease of the skin characterised by discrete waxy dome-shaped papules, often with central umbilication (see Fig. 43.34).

Fungal skin infections include tinea, which often involves the foot (*tinea pedis*; see Fig. 43.35). It is caused by any of a number of dermatophyte species. Deep

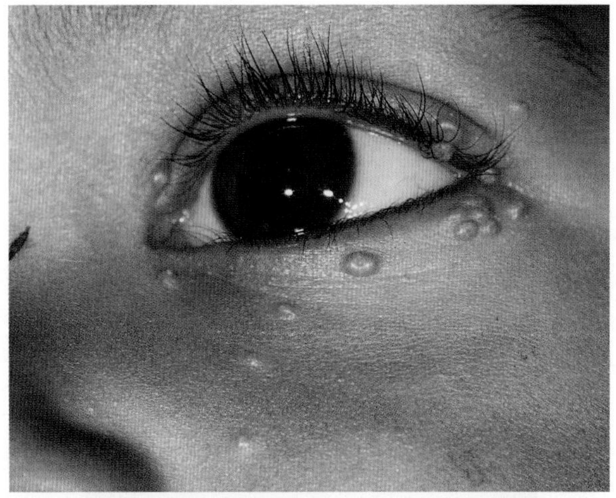

Molluscum contagiosum

(Black M. *Obstetric and gynecologic dermatology*, 3rd edn. St Louis MO: Mosby, 2008.)

FIGURE 43.34

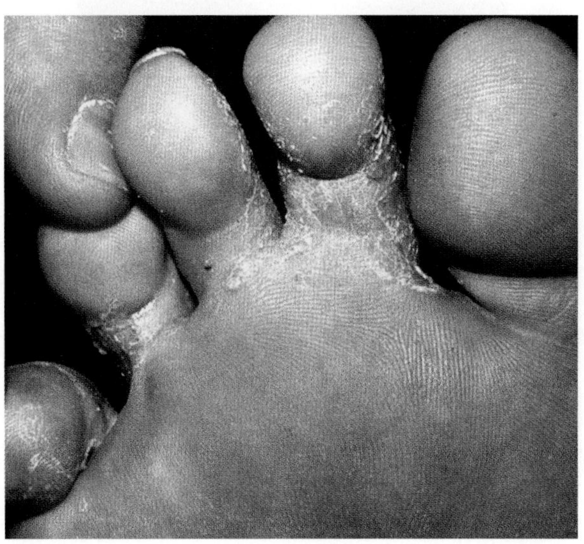

Tinea pedis

(From Busam Klaus J, ed. *Dermatopathology—a volume in the series foundations in diagnostic pathology*. Philadelphia: Saunders, 2010.)

FIGURE 43.35

cutaneous infections caused by organisms such as histoplasmosis, coccidioidomycosis and atypical mycobacterial species can present with ulceration, and are more common in immunosuppressed patients. Intertrigo is moist inflammation between skinfolds where skin rubs together; *Candida albicans* is often present (see Fig. 43.36).

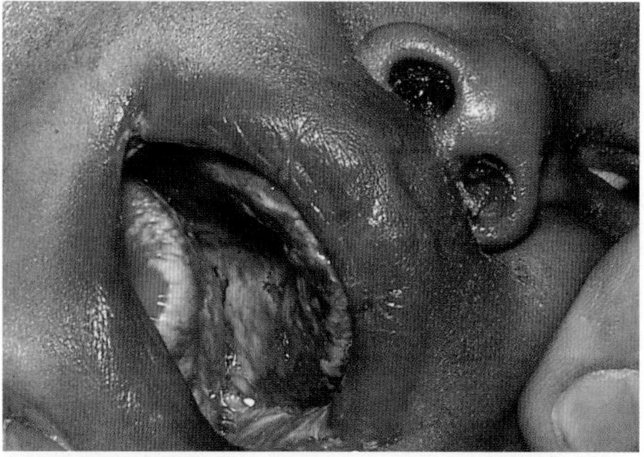

Candida albicans

(From Male D, Brostoff J, Roth D, Roitt I. *Immunology*, 8th edn. Philadelphia: Saunders, 2012.)

FIGURE 43.36

Hyperpigmentation, hypopigmentation and depigmentation

The presence of hyperpigmentation can be a clue to underlying systemic disease (see List 43.10) but commonly develops after inflammation in skin. This pattern is called postinflammatory hyperpigmentation. Hypopigmentation (decreased pigment) may also occur after inflammation, or with pityriasis versicolor where *Malassezia* yeast creates azaleic acid, which destroys melanin. Depigmentation (complete loss of pigment) may be caused by vitiligo, which is associated with other autoimmune diseases such as type I diabetes mellitus, Hashimoto thyroiditis and Addison disease.

Flushing and sweating

Flushing of the skin may sometimes be observed, especially on the face, by the examiner. Some of the causes of this phenomenon are presented in List 43.11.

Excessive sweating (hyperhidrosis) can be classified as primary or secondary. Primary hyperhidrosis is not associated with any systemic disorder and is the most common type. Secondary hyperhidrosis is associated with infection, tumours (e.g. phaeochromocytoma), hyperthyroidism, acromegaly, hypoglycaemia, menopause, autonomic dysfunction and drugs.

CAUSES OF DIFFUSE HYPERPIGMENTATION

Endocrine disease

Addison disease (excess ACTH)

Ectopic ACTH secretion (e.g. carcinoma)

The contraceptive pill or pregnancy

Thyrotoxicosis, acromegaly, phaeochromocytoma

Metabolic

Malabsorption or malnutrition

Liver diseases (e.g. haemochromatosis, primary biliary cirrhosis, Wilson disease)

Chronic kidney disease

Porphyria

Chronic infection (e.g. bacterial endocarditis)

Connective tissue disease (e.g. systemic lupus, scleroderma, dermatomyositis)

Racial or genetic

Other

Drugs (e.g. chlorpromazine, busulfan, arsenicals)

Radiation

ACTH=adrenocorticotrophic hormone.

LIST 43.10

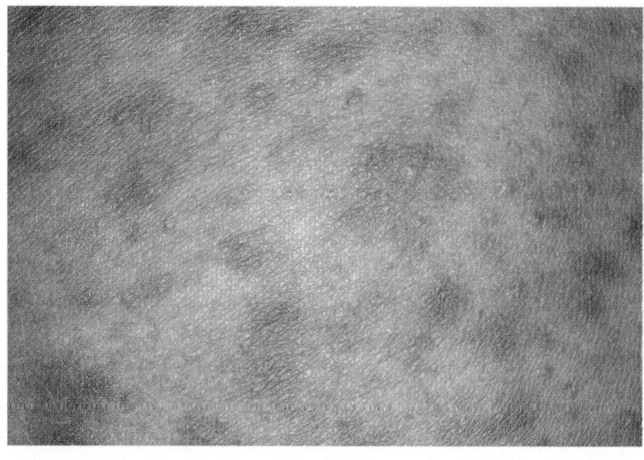

Adult patient with indolent systemic mastocytosis

FIGURE 43.37

CAUSES OF FACIAL FLUSHING

1. Menopause
2. Drugs and foods (e.g. nifedipine, sildenafil, monosodium glutamate [MSG])
3. Alcohol after taking the drug disulfiram (or alcohol alone in some people)
4. Systemic mastocytosis (see Fig. 43.37)
5. Rosacea
6. Carcinoid syndrome (secretion of serotonin and other mediators by a tumour may produce flushing, diarrhoea and valvular heart disease) (see Fig. 43.38)
7. Autonomic dysfunction
8. Medullary carcinoma of the thyroid

LIST 43.11

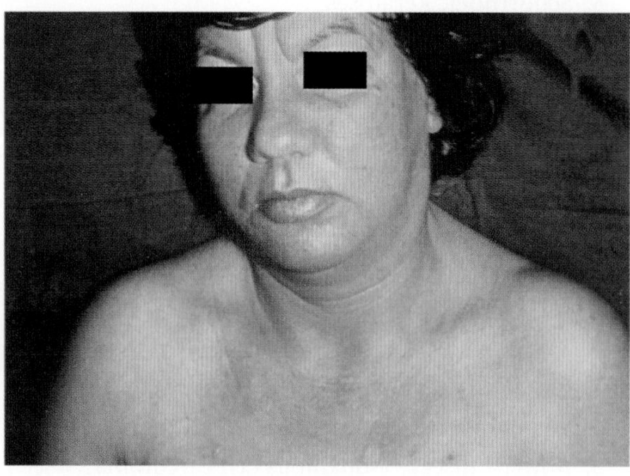

Patient with lung carcinoid and carcinoid syndrome with severe, long-standing flushing, lacrimation and a swollen face

FIGURE 43.38

Skin tumours

Skin tumours are very common and are usually benign (see List 43.12).[4] Most malignant skin tumours can be cured if they are detected early and treated appropriately (see List 43.13).

Skin cancer often occurs in those predisposed individuals (with the fair skin of Celtic or Northern European origin) who undergo chronic exposure to ultraviolet light. Skin cancers may present as flat scaly lesions or as raised scaly or smooth lesions. They may be large or small and they may eventually ulcerate. All non-healing ulcers should be considered to be skin cancer, until proven otherwise. Fifteen percent of melanoma patients present with little or no pigment (amelanotic subtype) and the lesion hence appears as a red patch or a nodule; these patients usually present late because their diagnosis is missed.

The earliest lesions are actinic (solar) keratoses, which are erythematous macules or papules surmounted by adherent scale (see Fig. 43.40), A small number of these may develop into Bowen disease (*squamous cell carcinoma* [SSC] in situ). This is typically an opaque papule or plaque that is often eroded or scaly (see Fig. 43.41). Metastasis can occur.

Basal cell carcinoma (BCC) is characteristically a translucent papule with a depressed centre and a rolled border with ectatic capillaries (see Fig. 43.42). Different subtypes include superficial, nodular, pigmented and sclerosing (morphoeic). These very rarely metastasise. Multiple BCCs may be associated with basal cell nevus syndrome (Gorlin syndrome) with other cardinal signs including jaw cysts, palmar pits and bony abnormalities.

Malignant melanomas are usually deeply pigmented lesions that are enlarging and have an irregular notched border (see Fig. 43.43). There is often variation of pigment within the lesion. Sometimes melanomas lack pigment altogether and are referred to as amelanotic melanomas. Consider malignant melanoma if the lesion follows the **ABCDE** checklist:[5,6]

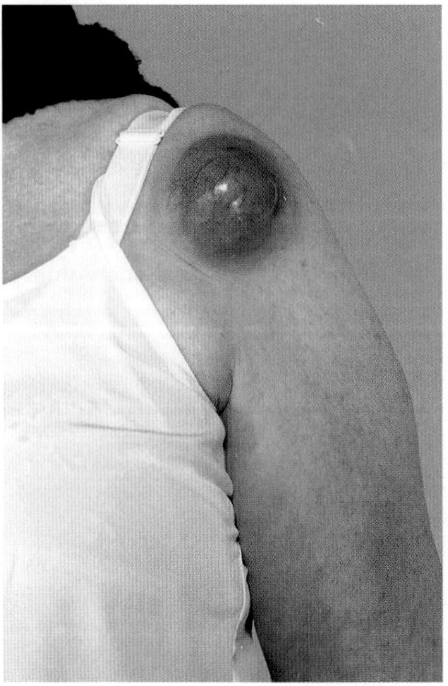

Metastatic melanoma

(From O'Neill JK, Khundar R, Knowles L et al. Melanoma with an unknown primary: a case series. *J Plast Reconstr Aesthet Surg* 2010; 63(12):2071–2080.)

FIGURE 43.39

BENIGN SKIN TUMOURS

1. Warts
2. Molluscum contagiosum
3. Seborrhoeic keratoses
4. Dermatofibroma
5. Neurofibroma
6. Angioma
7. Xanthoma

LIST 43.12

MALIGNANT SKIN TUMOURS

1. Basal cell carcinoma
2. Squamous cell carcinoma
3. Bowen* disease (squamous cell carcinoma confined to the epithelial layer of the skin—carcinoma in situ)
4. Malignant melanoma (which can be metastatic—see Fig. 43.39)
5. Metastatic deposits

*John Templeton Bowen (1857–1941), a Boston dermatologist.

LIST 43.13

Actinic keratosis, slightly eroded and scaly.

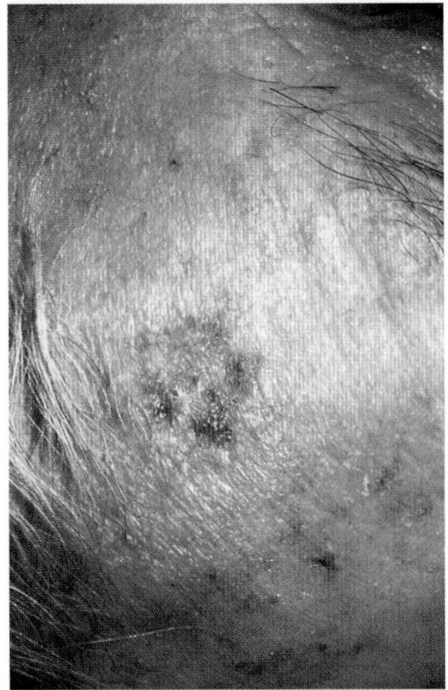

Higher on the forehead, additional granular keratosis could be easily palpated

(From Reeves JT, Maibach H. *Clinical dermatology illustrated: a regional approach*, 2nd edn. Sydney: MacLennan & Petty Pty Ltd, ©1991.)

FIGURE 43.40

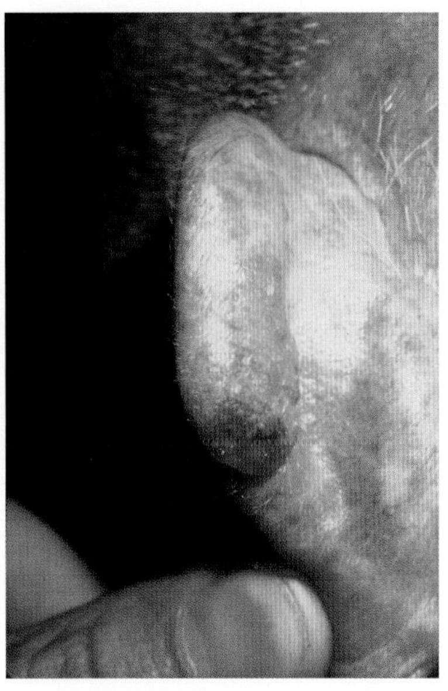

Squamous cell carcinoma

(From Reeves JT, Maibach H. *Clinical dermatology illustrated: a regional approach*, 2nd edn. Sydney: MacLennan & Petty Pty Ltd, ©1991.)

FIGURE 43.41

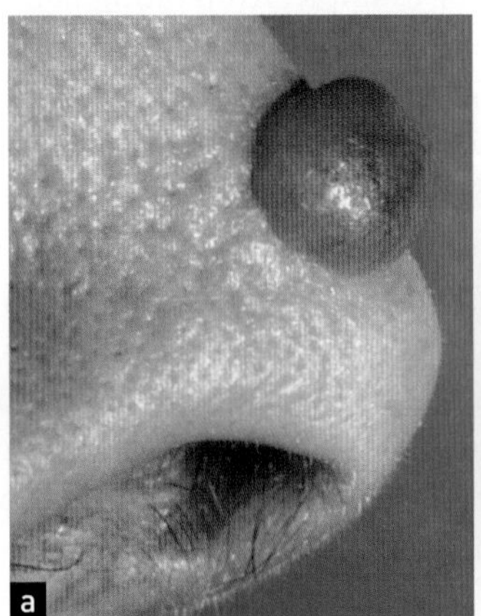

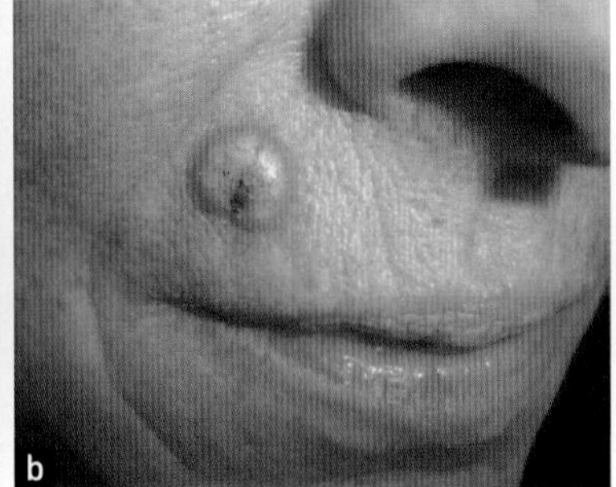

(a) Basal cell carcinoma: noted the rolled edges; (b) pigmented basal cell carcinoma, with pearly quality and depressed centre, in a patient with sun-damaged skin

(From Pfenninger J. *Pfenninger and Fowler's procedures for primary care*, 3rd edn. Maryland Heights, MO: Mosby, 2010.)

FIGURE 43.42

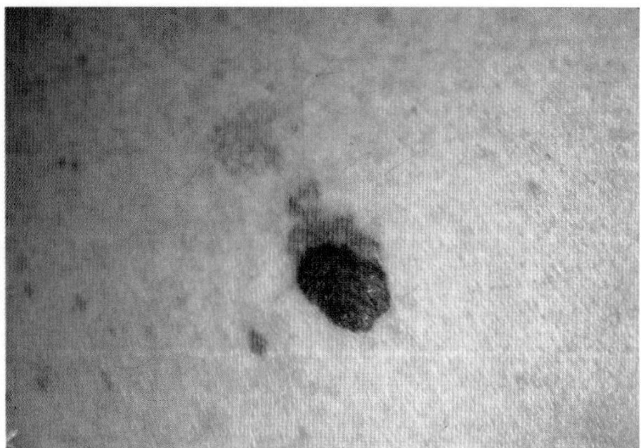

Superficial spreading melanoma, still confined to the upper dermis

(© Dr Loren Golitz.)

FIGURE 43.43

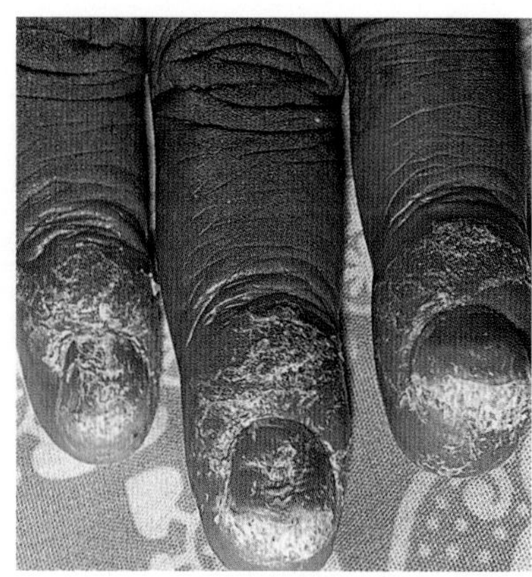

Onychomycosis: fungal infection of the nails

(From Reeves JT, Maibach H. *Clinical dermatology illustrated: a regional approach*, 2nd edn. Sydney: MacLennan & Petty Pty Ltd, ©1991.)

FIGURE 43.44

A symmetrical
B order irregularity
C olour variation
D iameter >6 millimetres
E volving (enlarging or changing) or **E** levated.

Patients with numerous large and unusual pigmented naevi (dysplastic naevus syndrome) are at an increased risk of developing malignant melanoma.[7]

THE NAILS

Systemic disease is commonly associated with changes in the patient's finger- and toenails and in the nail beds. The slow growth of the nails means that the temporal course of an illness may be seen in nail changes. Many of these findings have been described in other chapters, but important features of nail changes are dealt with here.

Fungal infection of the nails (**onychomycosis;** see Fig. 43.44) is the most common nail abnormality: it makes up 40% of all nail disorders and 30% of all cutaneous fungal infections. This infection is more common in people with diabetes, peripheral vascular disease and immunosuppression. The characteristic findings are thickened yellow nails, ridging, crumbling and deformity. The changes can be difficult to distinguish from psoriasis. A nail clipping should be taken to help confirm the diagnosis.

Acute paronychia is inflammation of the skin surrounding the nail; it can be acute or chronic. Acute paronychia is usually caused by *S. aureus* infection; other causes include ingrown nails, irritants, trauma (for example, from biting nails or sucking the thumb) or manicures. Chronic paronychia affects a number of fingers and causes red, swollen nail folds that have no cuticles. It leads to chronic ridging and dystrophy of the nail plate. The usual cause is chronic irritation from water or chemicals. Dermatophyes account for approximately 90% of fungal nail infections and *Candida* spp. make up the majority of the remainder. Candidal nail infection (diagnosed by microscopy and culture) suggests the possibility of chronic mucocutaneous candidiasis, which is a rare condition associated with polyendocrinopathies.

Nail involvement occurs in about 25% of patients with psoriasis (see Fig. 43.45). The characteristic abnormality is pitting. This can also occur in fungal infections, chronic paronychia, lichen planus, alopecia areata and atopic dermatitis. Psoriasis is also the most common cause of onycholysis. Rarer changes in psoriatic nails include longitudinal ridging (onychorrhexis), proximal transverse ridging, subungual hyperkeratosis and yellow-brown discoloration (the 'oil drop' sign).

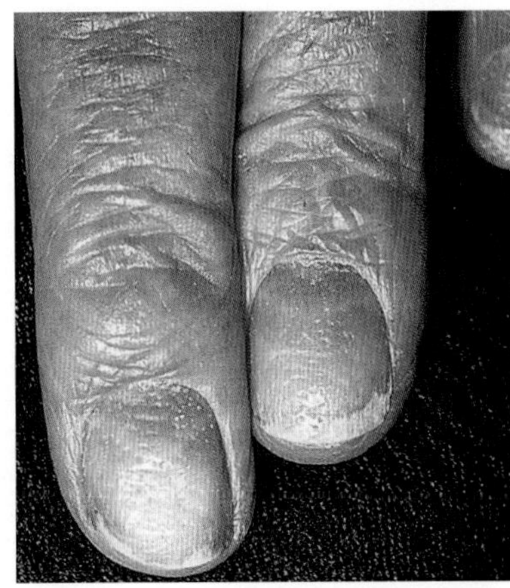

Nail involvement occurs in about 25% of patients with psoriasis

(From Reeves JT, Maibach H. *Clinical dermatology illustrated: a regional approach*, 2nd edn. Sydney: MacLennan & Petty Pty Ltd, ©1991.)

FIGURE 43.45

The presence of nailfold telangiectasias is an important sign in a number of systemic disorders, including systemic lupus erythematosus, scleroderma and Raynaud phenomenon. These changes are not very specific and considerable variation in nailfold capillary shape is present in healthy people. In patients with dermatomyositis, nailfold telangiectasiae are associated with hypertrophy of the cuticle and small haemorrhagic infarcts. Raynaud phenomenon is also associated with nail changes caused by the inadequate blood supply. These include brittleness, longitudinal ridging, splitting, flattening, onycholysis, koilonychia and a nail bed that is more erythematous than normal.

Clubbing is an important nail abnormality. It has been described in patients with HIV infection, and its severity seems proportional to the degree of immunosuppression. HIV infection is also associated with onychomycosis and longitudinal melonychia (dark line in the nail), secondary to treatment with zidovudine.

T&O'C ESSENTIALS

1. *The time course of a skin condition may be a clue to the diagnosis.*
2. *A careful medical history may reveal a systemic illness that underlies the skin problem.*
3. *Questioning about contact with new soaps or deodorants may help explain a new rash.*
4. *Many rashes may be assumed to be the result of a new medication unless proven otherwise.*
5. *A thorough dermatological examination must include the whole surface of the skin, nails, hair and accessible mucosal surfaces.*
6. *Many common dermatological abnormalities can be diagnosed on inspection (as long as the student has enough experience to recognise them).*
7. *For any pigmented lesion consider the melanoma* ***ABCDE*** *checklist:*
   A *symmetrical (typically)*
   B *order irregular*
   C *olour irregular*
   D *iameter large*
   E *levated above the skin or Evolving*
8. *Melanoma can have no or little pigment (amelanotic) in up to 15% of cases, and present as a red nodule.*

OSCE EXAMPLE – **SKIN**

Mr Talbot has a pigmented lesion on his chest. Please assess him.

1. Ask about sun exposure in childhood and as an adult.
2. Ask about any family history of melanoma (10% of melanomas have such a history).
3. Ask 'When was the lesion first noticed? Is it new?'
4. Ask 'Has the lesion changed in appearance?'
5. Ask 'Any itching or bleeding?'
6. Ask 'Has this lesion or any other pigmented lesion been biopsied or excised?'
7. Inspect the lesion: note whether symmetrical or not, regular or irregular border, raised or not, pigmentation uniform or variable and any ulceration or inflammation. Measure its size.
8. Inspect the skin all over the body including in the hair for other pigmented lesions. Inspect the draining lymph nodes if melanoma is suspected.
9. Present the ABCDE checklist.

References

1. Marks R. Diagnosis in dermatology. Tricks of the trade. *Aus Fam Physician* 2001; 30(11):1028–1032. A useful guide on clinical clues.
2. Ashton RE. Teaching non-dermatologists to examine the skin: a review of the literature and some recommendations. *Brit J Derm* 1995; 132:221–225. Presents a good scheme that can be used to describe any skin lesion.
3. Schwarzenberger K. The essentials of the complete skin examination. *Med Clin Nth Am* 1998; 82:981–999. Guidance on a thorough examination approach.
4. Preston DS, Stern RS. Nonmelanoma cancers of the skin. *N Engl J Med* 1992; 327:649–662. Provides useful information on discriminating between worrying and non-worrying lesions, and includes colour photographs.
5. Whitehead JD, Gichnik JM. Does this patient have a mole or a melanoma? *JAMA* 1998; 279:696–701. The ABCD checklist (asymmetry, border irregularity, irregular colour, diameter >6 millimetres) has a sensitivity over 90% and a specificity over 95% for identifying malignant melanoma.
6. Abbasi NR, Shaw HM, Rigel DS et al. Early diagnosis of cutaneous melanoma: rewriting the ABC criteria. *JAMA* 2004; 292:2771–2776. Changes (evolving) of symptoms or signs (size, shape, pruritus, tenderness, bleeding or colour) are additional evidence for the presence of melanoma.
7. Shenenberger DW. Cutaneous malignant melanoma: a primary care perspective. *Am Fam Physician* 2012; 85(2):161–168. An update on the clinical approach and management.
8. Bolognia JL, Jorizzo JL, Schaffer JV. *Dermatology*, 3rd edn. Philadelphia: Saunders, 2012.

CHAPTER 44

The older person assessment

Old men forget. SHAKESPEARE (1564–1616), Henry V

Older patients make up an increasing proportion of people admitted to hospital, their length of stay is often long and they need special consideration because of their often varied and complicated multiple medical problems.[1]

There is lack of universal agreement on what constitutes the age cut-off that defines a geriatric patient. Only 140 years ago, old age was set above 50. Today in the Western world as people (and their doctors) age, the cut-off may be extended above 65[a] (what highly competent older doctor in practice would want to be classified as geriatric?). Arbitrary distinctions currently drawn between the young old (65–74), the middle old (75–84) and the oldest old (85+) do not necessarily reflect biological age. The number of oldest old is growing steadily; this change will increasingly challenge health systems and has major resource implications for the future.

Geriatric patients tend to report fewer symptoms but have more chronic diseases. Hence, disease presentation is more likely to be atypical, so spending time taking the history is critical. Emphasis must be placed on the big four matters of concern for older people:

- immobility
- instability
- impaired intellect or memory
- incontinence.

These can be assessed as part of an activities of daily living (ADL) index (see Lists 44.4 and 44.5).[2,3]

Any of these may be caused or worsened by polypharmacy, which is a very common problem in elderly patients.

[a] Ask any relatives who are over 65 whether they think that they are old: 70 is the new 50!

THE COMPREHENSIVE GERIATRIC ASSESSMENT:[1] ASSESSMENT COMPONENTS (THE ABCs)

1. Activities of daily living
2. Balance, frailty testing
3. Cognition
4. Depression, drugs (polypharmacy), dentition (including nutrition and weight change)
5. Environment: home situation, social support, financial issues, living will (advance care planning)
6. Falls risk (history of falls, 'get up and go' test, functional reach test)
7. Gait speed (faster walkers have better survival)
8. Hearing, vision
9. Incontinence (urine, stool), sexual function

LIST 44.1

You need to find out about the risk of falls, mobility problems, ability to cope and risks to safety among other problems (see List 44.1 and Questions box 44.1). Functional and cognitive impairment are very important health problems to identify in older patients. Hearing and visual impairment, as well as cognitive decline, can impair history taking (see List 44.2).

HISTORY TAKING IN OLDER PERSONS: SPECIAL CONSIDERATIONS

1. *Presenting complaint:* a single complaint is unusual.
2. *Past history:* record the patient's immunisation status, especially for *Pneumococcus*, influenza and tetanus.

SPECIFIC QUESTIONS TO ASK THE ELDERLY PATIENT

1. What do you think your main problems are at the moment?
2. What tablets are you taking? Do you have trouble remembering to take them? Have any of your medications changed recently? Do you think they have caused you any problems?
3. Are you able to walk without difficulty: (a) in the house; and (b) to the shops?
4. Do you exercise regularly?
5. Have you fallen over in the past year? What happened? Were you hurt? How many times have you fallen? Do you have arthritis or Parkinson's disease? (See List 44.3)
6. Have you had any fractures of your spine? Wrists? Hips?
7. Do you drive?
8. With whom do you live?
9. Do you have any trouble managing cooking, washing or banking?
10. Do you feel that you eat well? Do your teeth give you trouble? Do you take them out to eat? What sort of meals do you have at night? Who cooks them?
11. How is your vision? Have you had cataracts? Do you wear glasses?
12. How is your hearing? Have you got hearing aids? Do they work?
13. Do you worry that you will not be able to cope in the future? Have you thought how you will manage if your health gets worse?
14. During the past month have you been feeling down, depressed or hopeless? During the past month, have you been bothered by little interest or pleasure in doing things?[6]
15. Would you allow me to talk to any of your relatives or friends about your health issues?

QUESTIONS BOX 44.1

CHANGES TO STANDARD HISTORY-TAKING TECHNIQUE FOR OLDER PATIENTS

- Slow down the speed of the interview.
- Adjust your interview approach if the patient has hearing or visual impairment issues, or dementia.
- To maximise the interaction, when you talk to the patient make sure that he or she can see your face.
- Do not patronise the patient.
- With the patient's permission, involve a relative or friend (but not too many) to help with the interview.

LIST 44.2

3. *Medications:* many patients will be taking multiple medications for several diseases, not all of which they may really need (polypharmacy). A comprehensive list including reason for use is important in terms of planning management. Always ask about over-the-counter medications, laxatives and sleeping medications.

   Any new symptoms may be from polypharmacy.
4. *Social history:*
   - *Accommodation:* find out whether the patient lives in a house or flat or in some form of assisted or serviced accommodation and who else lives there. Ask about the health and mobility of other people in the house and the proximity of younger relatives and friends.
   - *Exercise:* exercise is safe in the elderly, in general, and improves flexibility, balance, endurance and strength, which can assist with

RISK FACTORS FOR FALLS

1. A history of multiple previous falls (number, injuries)
2. Age over 80 years
3. Difficulty in getting up from a chair
4. Use of a walking stick or frame
5. Arthritis
6. Poor vision
7. Cognitive decline or depression
8. Muscle weakness
9. Parkinson's disease
10. Gait or balance problems (e.g. stroke)
11. Mechanical problems in the house (e.g. loose rugs, steep stairs)
12. Drug treatment (polypharmacy; particularly note sedatives, antidepressants, antihypertensives, anticholinergics)

LIST 44.3

INSTRUMENTAL ACTIVITIES OF DAILY LIVING (IADL) SCALE[3]

1. Ability to use the telephone
2. Shopping
3. Food preparation
4. Housekeeping
5. Laundry
6. Transport
7. Medication management
8. Ability to handle finances

Score 1 for each.

0=total dependence, 8=total independence for IADLs.

(Lawton MP, Brody EM. Assessment of older people; self maintaining and instrumental activities of daily living. *Gerontologist* 1969; 9:179 © Oxford University Press.)

LIST 44.4

maintenance of independent function as well as improving quality of life. It also reduces the risk of falls.

- *Smoking:* the details should be acquired as usual. Stopping smoking improves lung function even in people over the age of 60. Furthermore, advice to stop smoking is as successful in older patients as in younger ones.
- *Alcohol use:* alcohol intake is common and the details should always be recorded in the notes.
- *Abuse and neglect:* these can be problems in this age group. Careful questioning, often over a number of interviews, may help uncover such problems.[4]

5. *Review of systems:* concentrate especially on vision, hearing, chewing and dentition, weight changes, faecal and urinary incontinence, recurrent falls (see List 44.3), a history of fractures and foot disease, and chronic pain.
   - Falls are an important cause of mortality in the elderly and are usually multifactorial: postural dizziness, poor vision, cognitive impairment, foot problems, impaired bone mineral density and gait problems can all contribute to or exacerbate the problem. A patient is more likely to have further falls if he or she has a history of three or more falls, or if during the past year a fall resulted in injury or if he or she currently has arthritis or Parkinson's disease.[5]
   - Ask about the layout of the patient's house, including the number of steps and the presence of railings, for example, in the bathroom.
   - Ask about depression, because this is a common problem in the elderly and needs to be recognised and treated.[6]
6. *Specific areas of enquiry:*
   - *Instrumental activities of daily living (IADLs):* ask about using the telephone, shopping, preparing food, housekeeping, doing the laundry, driving, taking medicine and ability to handle finances (see List 44.4).
   - *Physical activities of daily living (ADLs):* ask about bathing, dressing, toileting, transfer (i.e. getting in / out of bed or chair), continence and feeding (see List 44.5); these can be affected by many different chronic illnesses.
   - *Driving:* older drivers share an increased risk of accidents with those under 25. Ask whether the patient still drives or has 'retired from driving'—a tactful way of approaching the loss of mobility and standing that comes with giving up a driver's licence. If the patient is

KATZ INDEX OF ACTIVITIES OF DAILY LIVING (ADLs)[2]

Activity

1. Bathing
2. Dressing
3. Toileting
4. Transferring
5. Continence
6. Feeding

1 point for each that can be done without help or supervision.

Score:

6 = fully functional

4 = moderately impaired

2 = severely impaired

Katz S, Down TD, Cash HR, Grotz RC. Program in the development of the index of ADL. *Gerontologist* 1970; 10:20, by permission of Oxford University Press.

LIST 44.5

FACTORS SUGGESTING DRIVING ABILITY MAY BE IMPAIRED

1. Passenger reports concern
2. Cognitive decline
3. Recent accidents or traffic offences
4. Driving of short distances (<100 km / week) and self-limited driving, e.g. not at night
5. Impaired mobility
6. Poor vision
7. Impulsive or aggressive behaviour
8. Use of alcohol or sedative drugs
9. History of syncope

LIST 44.6

still driving ask about his or her confidence when driving and whether certain situations are now avoided, e.g. driving at peak hour or at night. The assessment of relatives who may have been terrified passengers is more accurate than self-assessment. Certain risk factors have been identified for impaired driving (see List 44.6).

- *Urinary incontinence:* up to 30% of older women and men are affected by urinary incontinence—risk factors are listed in List 44.7. Ask if it has been a problem and how it affects daily life. Consider the types:
  - urge incontinence—the feeling of an urgent need to urinate followed by incontinence
  - stress incontinence—loss of urine when straining, coughing or exercising
  - mixed urge and stress incontinence
  - overflow incontinence—constant dribbling of urine, which affects men with prostatic obstruction
  - functional incontinence, which occurs in people too immobile to reach a bathroom or who have cognitive problems.

  Ask about drugs that may exacerbate the problem (e.g. diuretics, alpha-blockers) and about previous surgery (e.g. radical prostatectomy), radiation treatment, prostate symptoms and urinary tract infections.

  Find out tactfully how the patient and those around them cope and what has been done to help the problem.

- *End-of-life and treatment decisions:* patients generally prefer this topic to be brought up actively by their doctor. It is worth encouraging the patient to place his or her preferences in writing about decisions such as 'do not resuscitate' orders and advance care planning.

RISK FACTORS FOR URINARY INCONTINENCE IN THE ELDERLY

1. Obesity
2. Parity
3. Gynaecological surgery
4. Diabetes mellitus
5. Smoking
6. Diuretic drugs, calcium channel blockers
7. Immobility
8. Recurrent urinary tract infections
9. Previous radical prostatectomy
10. Cognitive impairment
11. Immobility

LIST 44.7

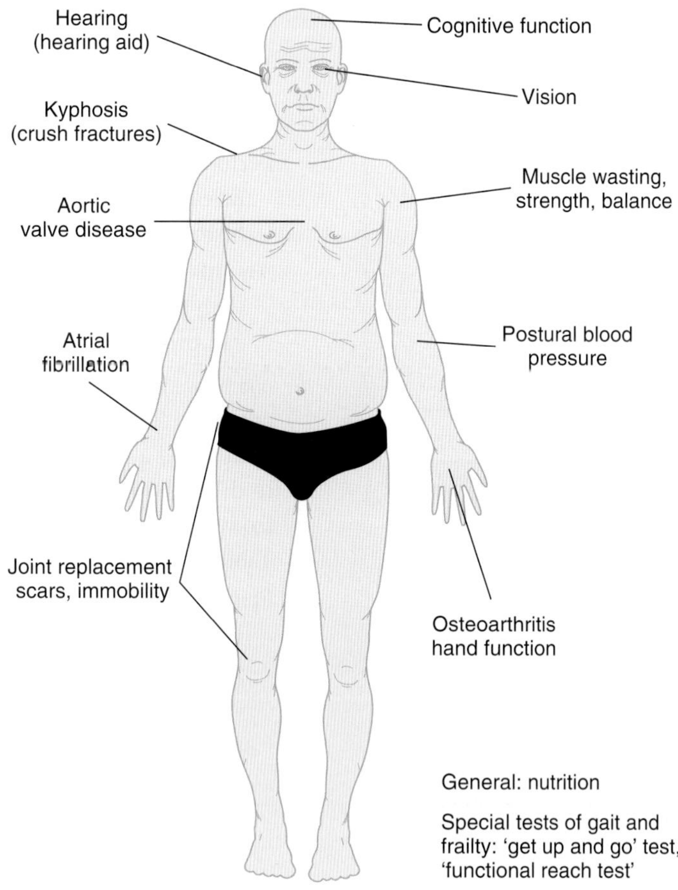

Examination of the geriatric patient: summary

FIGURE 44.1

PHYSICAL EXAMINATION IN OLDER PERSONS: SPECIAL CONSIDERATIONS

A complete examination is required as usual, but think about the following areas as you go about obtaining the data (see Fig. 44.1).

1. *General assessment:* check for postural blood pressure changes.

   Assess hydration, which may be impaired in older patients with cognitive dysfunction.

   Look at the patient's skin carefully for pressure sores. These are areas of injury to the skin or soft tissue and subcutaneous tissue as a result of localised pressure or shear injury and occur in immobile patients. Certain risk factors have been identified that increase the risk of a patient's developing pressure sores (List 44.8). Classify the severity and extent of the sores (Table 44.1).

   Look for evidence of bruises from falls or elder abuse. Look at the skin for any evidence of skin cancer.

   Measure the patient's weight and height to calculate the body mass index, as weight loss is common in the elderly.

2. *Heart:* if a systolic murmur is heard, consider whether this may be aortic stenosis, which, if severe, is likely to require evaluation.

   Ankle swelling may indicate venous insufficiency or antihypertensive drug use (e.g. calcium antagonists) rather than

RISK FACTORS FOR PRESSURE SORES

1. Cognitive impairment
2. Immobility
3. Advanced age
4. Sensory impairment
5. Low body weight
6. Oedema
7. Incontinence
8. Hypoalbuminaemia

LIST 44.8

Classification of bed sores

Stage	Description
I	Skin intact but non-blanching erythema
II	Partial thickness loss of skin. Shallow open ulcer, no slough or intact or burst blister
III	Full-thickness loss of tissue. Subcutaneous fat visible but not bone or muscle
IV	Full-thickness tissue loss and muscle or bone visible
Unstageable	Full-thickness but base covered in slough
Suspected deep tissue injury	Purple- or maroon-coloured area of intact skin or a blood-filled blister

TABLE 44.1

congestive cardiac failure. Ischaemic heart disease is common but often 'silent' in the elderly.

3. *Chest:* shortness of breath may be due to lung or cardiac disease, and these often coexist in the elderly.
4. *Gastrointestinal system:* look at the dentition and look for dry mouth, which may impair eating. Note signs of recent weight loss.

   A mass may be felt in the left lower quadrant in patients with constipation from hard stool; this will clear with treatment of the constipation.

   The aorta may be palpable in the thin elderly patient. This may be falsely interpreted as an aneurysm, but if the aorta seems significantly enlarged then an aortic aneurysm needs to be excluded. If the aneurysm is leaking, the classical presentation includes back pain, abdominal distension, shock and poor asymmetrical peripheral pulses in the legs.

   Perform a rectal examination and rule out faecal impaction, particularly if there is a history of faecal or urinary incontinence.

   An enlarged bladder may be felt in patients with acute urinary retention; this problem can present with delirium.
5. *Nervous system:* evaluation of mental status and cognitive function should be routine in older patients. If a patient is confused it is important to distinguish cognitive decline (dementia) from an acute confusional state (delirium; see Tables 46.5 and 46.6 on p 892).

   Primitive reflexes such as the glabellar tap (see Fig. 35.17 on p 619), palmomental reflex and grasp reflex are found in those of increasing age and may be evidence of dementia.

   Carefully assess gait (which may include gait speed over 8 metres with a stopwatch; normal gait speed in healthy elderly people ranges from 1.1 to 1.5 metres / second) and balance.[5]

   Further test gait with the 'get up and go' test (see Fig. 44.2): ask the patient to stand up out of a chair, walk 3 metres, turn around 180°, return to the chair and sit down. Assess the following:

   - Patient in the chair: does the patient have trouble getting out of a chair with or without arms?
   - Patient standing near the chair: is the patient unsteady?
   - Patient walking: is the gait abnormal—unsteady, Parkinsonian, hemiplegic, needs stick, frame, etc.?
   - Patient turning: is the patient slow or hesitant?
   - Patient sitting down: is the patient nervous or hesitant?

   Look for abnormalities in gait, balance and power. The test can be graded from 1 (normal) to 5 (severely impaired) but is usually timed (fixing the walking distance),

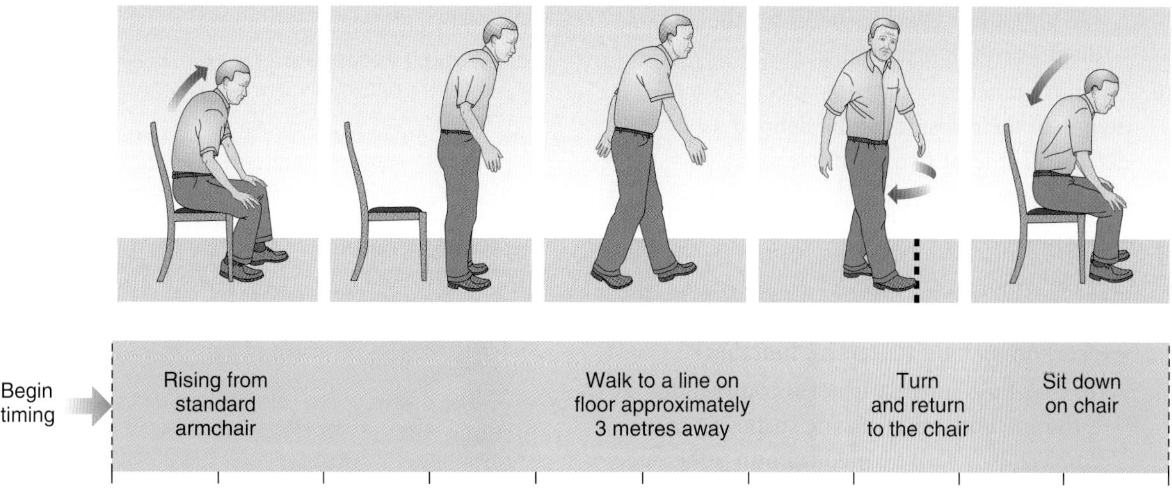

'Get up and go' test:
1. 'Stand up now for me and walk over to here.' 2. 'Now turn around and walk back.' 3. 'Now come and sit down again.' Difficulty in standing up from a chair indicates an increased falls risk

(From Douglas G, Nicol F, Robertson C. *Macleod's clinical examination*, 13th edn. Edinburgh: Churchill Livingstone, ©2013.)

FIGURE 44.2

comparing the time taken to age-adjusted normal values (however, these times appear to have limited diagnostic value).[7] Look carefully for lower leg weakness and test power if needed.[8,9]

Test for falls risk using the 'functional reach' test. Ask the patient to stand with his or her fist extended alongside a wall, then lean forwards as far as possible. The patient should be able to move the fist along the wall without taking a step or losing stability. Measure the length of movement. A distance of less than 15 centimetres suggests an increased falls risk.[10]

6. *Eyes and ears:* check the patient's vision and hearing as these may impair independent living. Does the patient have a hearing aid in place? (80% of 80 year olds have impaired hearing.) Hearing aids can be difficult to manage and patients need some enthusiasm to make them work, but there is some evidence that use of hearing aids reduces patients' sense of isolation. Hearing loss must not be confused with cognitive dysfunction. A whispered voice test may be useful for screening for hearing loss. Has the patient got cataracts interfering with vision?
7. *Rheumatological system:* examine for deformities and functional disabilities, including the feet.
8. *Breasts:* perform a breast examination in women, as the incidence of breast cancer greatly increases with age.
9. *Depression:* 5% of men and 7% of women over 60 have problems with depression. This can lead to lack of enthusiasm and engagement and must also not be confused with cognitive impairment.

   Ask: 'In the last month, have you been troubled by feeling little interest in doing things? Have you felt "low", "down" or depressed?' This simple questioning is very sensitive

(97%) but less specific (67%) for the diagnosis of depression.

10. *Cognitive function:* dementia affects 35% of people in their 90s. It can be defined as a decline in at least two cognitive areas:
    - memory
    - attention
    - language
    - visuospatial ability
    - decision making (executive function).

    Screening for dementia is not recommended as a routine but if there is any suspicion (e.g. concern by relatives, medical non-adherence, accidents or behavioural changes) then screening should be performed.[11]

Dementia screening

The mini-mental state examination (MMSE)[12] has a good evidence base but is protected by copyright; the Mini-Cog screening tool[13] is more readily available and is easy to use (see Ch 46, p 879).

OSCE REVISION TOPICS – **ASSESSMENT OF THE GERIATRIC PATIENT**

Use these topics, which commonly occur in the OSCE, to help with revision.

1. This 89-year-old man takes 11 regular medications. Take a drug history from him. (p 862)
2. This 77-year-old woman has some problems with her memory. Please take a history from her. (pp 565, 868, 888)
3. This 79-year-old man is having difficulty managing at home by himself. Please take a history from him. (p 863)
4. This elderly woman has had a number of falls recently and has fractured her wrist. Please take a history from her and perform an examination. (p 863)

References

1. Ellis G, Whitehead MA, O'Neill D et al. Comprehensive geriatric assessment for older patients admitted to hospital. *Cochrane Database Sys Rev* 2011; (7):CD006211.
2. Katz S, Down TD, Cash HR, Grotz RC. Progress in the development of the index of ADL. *Gerontologist* 1970; 10:20–30.
3. Lawton MP, Brody EM. Assessment of older people; self maintaining and instrumental activities of daily living. *Gerontologist* 1969; 9:179.
4. Lachs MS, Pillemer KA. Elder abuse. *N Engl J Med* 2015; 373(20):1947–1956. Like child abuse, clinicians should be alert to the possibility of elder abuse in patients who present with unexplained injuries.
5. Studenski S, Perera S, Patel K et al. Gait speed and survival in older adults. *JAMA* 2011; 305:50–58. Gait speed is a measure of frailty. Faster walkers have better survival.
6. Whooley MA, Avins AL, Miranda J, Browner WS. Case-finding instruments for depression: two questions are as good as many. *J Gen Intern Med* 1997; 12:439–445.
7. Schoene D, Wu SM, Mikolaizak AS et al. Discriminative ability and predictive validity of the timed up and go test in identifying older people who fall: systematic review and meta-analysis. *J Am Geriatr Soc* 2013; 61:202–208. 'Get up and go' test times have only poor-to-moderate diagnostic accuracy.
8. Nevitt MC, Cummings SR, Kidd S, Black D. Risk factors for recurrent nonsyncopal falls: a prospective study. *JAMA* 1989; 261:2663–2668. The history identifies those at higher risk of falls. Risk factors include three or more falls or a fall with injury in the previous year, arthritis, Parkinson's disease, difficulty in standing up from a chair or in performing a tandem walk.
9. Tinetti ME. Clinical practice. Preventing falls in elderly persons. *N Engl J Med* 2003; 348:42–49. Practical management advice.
10. Fleming KC, Evans JM, Weber DC, Chutka DS. Practical functional assessment of elderly persons: a primary-care approach. *Mayo Clin Proc* 1995; 70:890–910. Useful screening test advice is given. The 'functional reach' test is useful for predicting increased falls risk.
11. Lin JS, O'Connor E, Rossom RC et al. Screening for cognitive impairment in older adults: a systematic review for the U.S. Preventive Services Task Force. *Ann Intern Med* 2013; 159(9):601–612. Screening tests available for dementia include the Mini-Cog and the Clock Drawing Test.
12. Tangalos EG, Smith GE, Ivnik RJ et al. The mini-mental state examination in general medical practice: clinical utility and acceptance. *Mayo Clin Proc* 1996; 71:829.
13. Borson S, Scanlan JM, Chen P, Ganguli M. The Mini-Cog as a screen for dementia: validation in a population-based sample. *J Am Geriatr Soc* 2003; 51:1451.

CHAPTER 45

Approaching infectious diseases

The very first requirement in a hospital is that it should do the sick no harm. FLORENCE NIGHTINGALE (1820 – 1910)

We have selected two important presentations to be covered in this chapter to show how infectious diseases can be approached in a systematic manner.

PYREXIA OF UNKNOWN ORIGIN

Pyrexia of unknown origin (PUO) is defined as documented fever (>38°C) of more than 3 weeks' duration, where no cause is found despite basic investigations.[1] The most frequent causes to consider are tuberculosis, occult abscess (usually intra-abdominal), osteomyelitis, infective endocarditis, lymphoma or leukaemia, systemic-onset juvenile rheumatoid arthritis, giant cell arteritis and drug fever (drug fever is responsible for 10% of fevers leading to hospital admission[2]). In studies of fever of unknown origin,[3] infection is found to be the cause in 30%, neoplasia in 30%, connective tissue disease in 15% and miscellaneous causes in 15%; in 10% the aetiology remains unknown (see List 45.1). Remember: the longer the duration of the fever, the less likely there is to be

COMMON CAUSES OF PYREXIA OF UNKNOWN ORIGIN

Neoplasms

- Hodgkin's and non-Hodgkin's lymphoma, leukaemia, malignant histiocytosis
- Other tumours: hepatic, renal, lung, disseminated carcinoma, atrial myxoma

Infections

- *Bacterial:* e.g. tuberculosis, brucellosis and other bacteraemias, abscess formation (especially pelvic or abdominal), endocarditis, pericarditis, osteomyelitis, cholangitis, pyelonephritis, pelvic inflammatory disease, prostatitis, syphilis, Lyme disease, borreliosis, cat scratch disease, dental abscess
- *Viral:* e.g. infectious mononucleosis,* cytomegalovirus infection, hepatitis B or C, human immunodeficiency virus (HIV) infection, Ross River virus
- *Parasitic:* e.g. strongyloidiasis, schistosomiasis, malaria, Q fever, toxoplasmosis
- *Fungal:* e.g. histoplasmosis, cryptococcosis, blastomycosis

Connective tissue diseases

- Juvenile rheumatoid arthritis, adult Still's disease, systemic lupus erythematosus
- Vasculitis (e.g. giant cell arteritis, polyarteritis nodosa)
- Immunosuppressive drugs (occult infection)

Drug fever: e.g. anticonvulsants, antibiotics (e.g. minocycline), allopurinol, heparin

Miscellaneous

- Inflammatory bowel disease, acute alcoholic hepatitis, granulomatous disease (e.g. sarcoid), multiple pulmonary emboli, thyroiditis, adrenal insufficiency, phaeochromocytoma, familial Mediterranean fever and other hereditary periodic fever syndromes, haematoma, factitious fever

Uncertain

*Epstein–Barr virus is the cause of infectious mononucleosis.

LIST 45.1

an infectious aetiology. The majority of patients do not have a rare disease but rather a relatively common disease presenting in an unusual way.[4]

History

The history may give a number of clues in these puzzling cases. In some patients a careful history may give the diagnosis where expensive tests have failed. (See Questions box 45.1.)

The time course of the fever and any associated symptoms must be uncovered. Symptoms from the various body systems should be sought methodically. Examples include:

1. *gastrointestinal system*—diarrhoea, abdominal pain, recent abdominal surgery (inflammatory bowel disease, diverticular disease, cholangitis)
2. *cardiovascular system*—heart murmurs, dental procedures (infective endocarditis), chest pain (pericarditis)
3. *rheumatology*—joint symptoms, rashes, persistent back pain (spondylodiscitis may cause PUO and progress to quadriplegia)
4. *neurology*—headache (meningitis, cerebral abscess)
5. *genitourinary system*—history of renal disease or infection, dysuria
6. *respiratory system*—old tuberculosis (TB) or recent TB contact, chest symptoms.

Details of any recent overseas travel are important. Find out also about hobbies and exposure to pets. Occupational exposure may be important. Take a drug history. Find out whether the patient is involved in behaviour posing a risk of HIV infection. Patients who are already in hospital may have infected cannulas or old cannula sites. The new onset of fever in a hospitalised patient is an indication to remove a peripheral cannula (send the tip for culture).

Fever due to bacteraemia (the presence of viable bacteria in the bloodstream) is associated with a higher risk of mortality. Bacteraemia is present in up to 20% of hospital patients with acute fever.[5,6]

GENERAL QUESTIONS TO ASK THE PATIENT WITH A FEVER

! denotes symptoms for the possible diagnosis of an urgent or dangerous problem.

1. How long have you had high temperatures?
2. Have you taken your own temperature? How high has it been?
3. **!** Have you had shivers and shakes (rigors)? (Shaking chills suggest bacteraemia[4])
4. Has anyone you know had a similar illness?
5. What medications are you taking?
6. Have you had any recent illnesses?
7. Have you had any recent operations or medical procedures?
8. Have you travelled recently? Where to?
9. Did you take antimalarial prophylaxis and have the recommended vaccinations for your trip?
10. Have you any pets? Have they been sick lately?

QUESTIONS BOX 45.1

Examination

General

Look at the temperature chart to see whether there is a pattern of fever that is identifiable. Inspect the patient and decide how seriously ill he or she appears. Look for evidence of weight loss (indicating a chronic illness). Note any skin rash (see List 45.2). The details of the examination required will depend on the patient's history.[7]

DIFFERENTIAL DIAGNOSIS OF PROLONGED FEVER AND RASH

1. *Viral:* e.g. infectious mononucleosis, rubella, dengue fever
2. *Bacterial:* e.g. syphilis, Lyme disease
3. *Non-infective:* e.g. drugs, systemic lupus erythematosus, erythema multiforme (which may also be related to an underlying infection)

LIST 45.2

Hands

Look for the stigmata of infective endocarditis or vasculitic changes. Note whether there is clubbing. The presence of arthropathy or Raynaud phenomenon may point to a connective tissue disease.

Arms

Inspect for drug injection sites suggesting intravenous drug abuse (see Fig. 7.2 on p 127) as well as recent cannula sites. Peripheral cannulae are responsible for sepsis and death in hospitalised patients. The new onset of fever in a hospitalised patient is an indication to remove the peripheral cannula (send the tip for culture). Feel for the epitrochlear and axillary nodes (e.g. lymphoma, other malignancy, sarcoidosis, focal infections).

Head and neck

Feel the *temporal arteries* (over the temples for giant cell arteritis). In temporal arteritis these may be tender and thickened.

Examine the *eyes* for iritis or conjunctivitis (e.g. leptospirosis, measles, connective tissue disease e.g. reactive arthritis) or jaundice (e.g. ascending cholangitis, blackwater fever in malaria). Look in the fundi for choroidal tubercles in miliary tuberculosis, Roth's spots in infective endocarditis and retinal haemorrhages or the infiltrates of leukaemia or lymphoma.

Inspect the *face* for a butterfly rash (systemic lupus erythematosus, see Fig. 25.11 on p 434) or seborrhoeic dermatitis, which is common in patients with HIV infection.

Examine the *mouth* for ulcers, gum disease or candidiasis, and the teeth and tonsils for infection (e.g. abscess). Look in the *ears* for otitis media. Feel the *parotid glands* for evidence of infection.

Palpate the cervical lymph nodes. Examine for thyroid enlargement and tenderness (subacute thyroiditis).

Chest

Examine the chest. Palpate for bony tenderness. Carefully examine the respiratory system (e.g. for signs of pneumonia, tuberculosis, empyema, carcinoma) and the heart for murmurs (e.g. infective endocarditis, atrial myxoma) or rubs (e.g. pericarditis).

Abdomen

Examine the abdomen. Inspect for rashes, including rose-coloured spots (in typhoid fever—2- to 4-millimetre flat red spots, which blanch on pressure and occur on the upper abdomen and lower chest). Examine for evidence of hepatomegaly and ascites (e.g. spontaneous bacterial peritonitis, hepatic carcinoma, metastatic deposits), splenomegaly (e.g. haemopoietic malignancy, infective endocarditis, malaria), renal enlargement (e.g. renal cell carcinoma) or localised tenderness (e.g. collection of pus). Palpate for testicular enlargement (e.g. seminoma, tuberculosis). Feel for inguinal lymphadenopathy.

Perform a rectal examination, feeling for a mass or tenderness in the rectum or pelvis (e.g. abscess, carcinoma, prostatitis). Perform a vaginal examination to detect collections of pelvic pus or evidence of pelvic inflammatory disease. Look at the penis and scrotum for a discharge or rash.

Central nervous system

Examine the central nervous system for signs of meningism (e.g. chronic tuberculous meningitis, cryptococcal meningitis) or focal neurological signs (e.g. brain abscess, mononeuritis multiplex in polyarteritis nodosa).

Clinical scenarios for unexplained fever

Consider age, co-morbidities and the epidemiology, e.g. adult with a prosthetic heart valve (endocarditis), young female with a rash (systemic lupus), post neurosurgery on phenytoin (drug), middle-aged with easy bruising and fatigue (haematological malignancy), young migrant from Nepal (TB).

HIV INFECTION AND AIDS

The acquired immunodeficiency syndrome (AIDS), first described in 1981, is caused by the human immunodeficiency virus (HIV).[7-9] This is a T-cell lymphotrophic virus, which results in T4-cell destruction and therefore susceptibility to opportunistic infections and the development of tumours, notably Kaposi's[a] sarcoma and non-Hodgkin's lymphoma.

[a] Moritz Kohn Kaposi (1837–1902), a professor of dermatology in Vienna, described the sarcoma in 1892.

Features of the HIV seroconversion illness (acute retroviral illness) and their frequency

Feature	%
Fever	95
Lymphadenopathy	75
Pharyngitis	70
Rash	70
Arthralgia / myalgia	55
Diarrhoea	32
Headache	30
Nausea and vomiting	25
Hepatosplenomegaly	15
Loss of weight	13
Thrush	10
Neurological symptoms	10

TABLE 45.1

QUESTIONS TO ASK THE PATIENT WITH A RECENT DIAGNOSIS OF HIV INFECTION

1. Can you remember symptoms of a seroconversion illness?
2. Why was the diagnosis suspected?
3. How do you think you may have become infected?
4. Is your sexual partner(s) aware of your illness?
5. Are they taking precautions against infection?
6. Have you been tested for hepatitis?
7. Have you had a problem with chest or other infections?
8. Have you begun treatment?
9. What have you been told about your prognosis?

QUESTIONS BOX 45.2

History

HIV infection should be suspected particularly if the patient falls into a high-risk group (e.g. men who have sex with men, intravenous drug user, sexual tourist, sexual partner of HIV-infected person, haemophiliac, blood transfusion or blood product recipient, prostitute or someone having sexual contact with one of these).

The patient may have had a seroconversion illness (50% of cases) (Table 45.1). Ask about: fever, lymphadenopathy, maculopapular rash, arthralgia, pharyngitis, nausea and vomiting, headache, weight loss and oral candidiasis.

Careful questioning (see Questions box 45.2) about the mode of infection is important but should be left to a subsequent consultation if the patient seems reluctant to discuss this. Patients may be unwilling to inform their sexual partners that they are infected. This puts the latter at risk of infection and there is a duty on the treating clinician's part to ensure that these people are informed, tested and protected (e.g. by condom use).

HIV infection is often present in combination with other sexually transmitted infections, such as syphilis and gonorrhoea, and with the hepatic viruses B and C. The incidence varies in different countries, but hepatitis C is uncommon in Australian HIV patients.

HIV should be strongly suspected in patients who present with TB, and TB should be suspected in HIV patients with a chronic respiratory illness. HIV infection has replaced TB as the great imitator of other illnesses. HIV testing should be routine in any unexplained infectious illness.

Ask about features of chronic HIV infection including:

- fever, night sweats
- enlarged lymph nodes
- fatigue
- weight loss
- chronic diarrhoea
- seborrhoeic dermatitis
- psoriasis
- fungal infections, e.g. tinea, onychomycosis
- apthous ulcers, gingivitis
- peripheral neuropathy
- anaemia, leucopenia, thrombocytopenia ('Have you got reduced red or white cells or platelets in your blood?')
- nephropathy ('Have you had kidney problems?').

Patients treated for HIV infection have an increased risk of cardiovascular disease. This is partly because of their chronic inflammatory condition and partly because of the development of metabolic risk factors as a side effect of their antiviral treatment. Cardiovascular disease has become the most common cause of death for treated HIV patients. Ask about cardiovascular risk factors: smoking, diabetes, hypertension etc. Has the patient had any diagnosis of heart disease?

Examination

Examine the patient as follows.

General inspection

Take the patient's temperature. The patient may appear ill and wasted owing to chronic ill-health or chronic opportunistic infection. *Mycobacterium avium* complex (MAC) presents with fever and weight loss.

Look at the skin for rashes:

- The maculopapular rash of acute HIV infection (5- to 10-millimetre maculopapular lesions on the face and trunk and rarely on the palms and soles).
- Herpes zoster (shingles, which may involve more than one dermatome in this disease and is more commonly seen in early rather than advanced HIV infection).
- Oral herpes simplex (cold sores) or genital herpes.
- Oral and flexural candidiasis (once the CD4 level is below 200 / mm^3).
- Molluscum contagiosum, impetigo, seborrhoea or other non-specific exanthems.
- Kaposi's sarcoma: red-purple vascular non-tender tumours. These present typically on the skin but can occur anywhere.
- Skin lesions resembling Kaposi's sarcoma may also be seen. These are called bacillary angiomatosis and are caused by *Bartonella henselae* and *Bartonella quintana* (see Figs 45.1 and 45.2).
- Severe psoriasis is common in HIV patients.

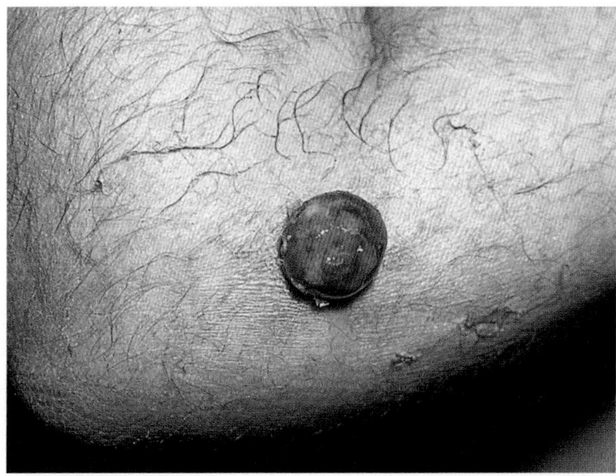

Angry red nodule of bacillary angiomatosis

(Reeves JT, Maibach H. *Clinical dermatology illustrated: a regional approach*, 2nd edn. Sydney: MacLennan & Petty Pty Ltd, ©1991.)

FIGURE 45.1

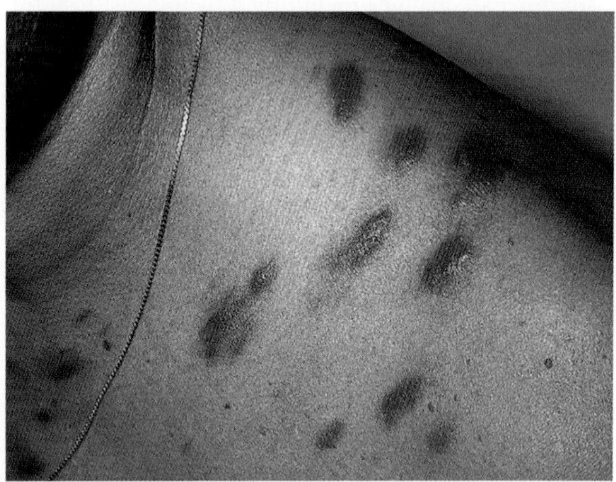

Late nodules of Kaposi's sarcoma

(Reeves JT, Maibach H. *Clinical dermatology illustrated: a regional approach*, 2nd edn. Sydney: MacLennan & Petty Pty Ltd, ©1991.)

FIGURE 45.2

Adverse drug reactions are more common in patients with HIV infection and may be the cause of a rash. Look for hyperpigmentation. Patients taking the drug clofazimine for MAC infection usually become deeply pigmented. Areas of peripheral fat atrophy—lipodystrophy—on limbs, cheeks and buttocks may be seen in patients treated with protease inhibitor drugs. Some of these patients have fat redistribution with central obesity.

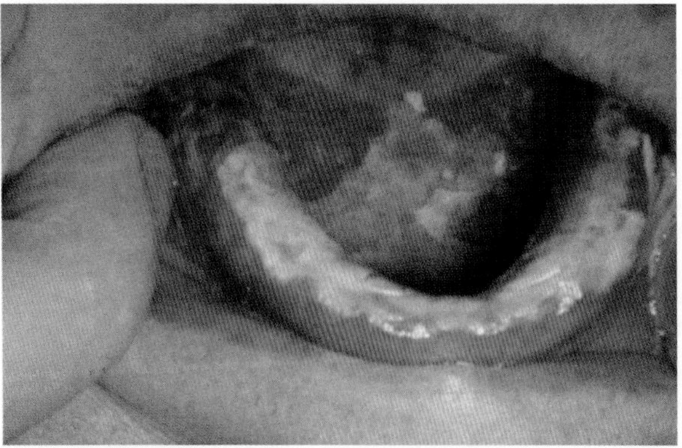

Oral candidiasis

(From McDonald FS, ed. *Mayo Clinic images in internal medicine*, with permission. © Mayo Clinic Scientific Press and CRC Press. Reproduced by permission of Taylor and Francis Group, LLC, a division of Informa plc.)

FIGURE 45.3

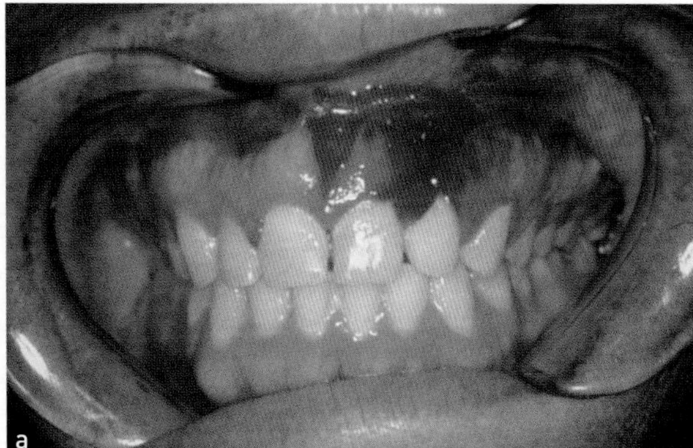

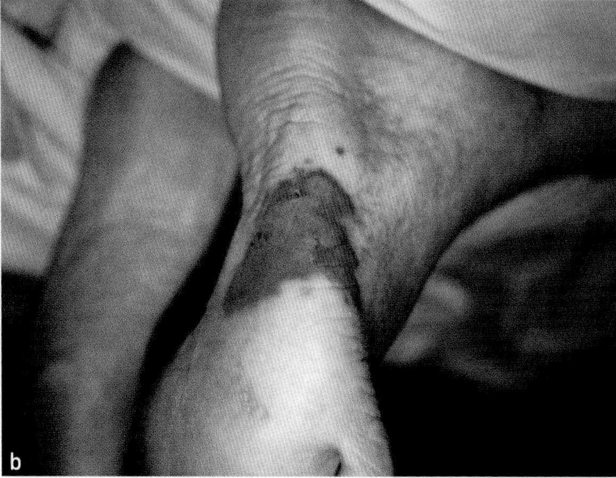

(a) Kaposi's sarcoma in the mouth.
(b) Kaposi's sarcoma on the foot

((a) From McDonald FS, ed. *Mayo Clinic images in internal medicine*, with permission. © Mayo Clinic Scientific Press and CRC Press. Reproduced by permission of Taylor and Francis Group, LLC, a division of Informa plc. (b) Courtesy of Dr A Watson, Infectious Diseases Department, The Canberra Hospital.)

FIGURE 45.4

Hands and arms

Look for nail changes including onycholysis. Feel for the epitrochlear nodes; a node 0.5 centimetres or larger may be characteristic.[10] Note any injection marks.

Face

Inspect the mouth for:

- candidal plaques (see Fig. 45.3)
- angular stomatitis
- aphthous ulcers
- tongue ulceration (e.g. herpes simplex, cytomegalovirus or candidal infections) or gingivitis[11]
- periodontal disease.

Kaposi's sarcoma (see Fig. 45.4) may also occur on the hard or soft palate (in which case associated lesions are almost always present elsewhere in the gastrointestinal tract). Oral squamous cell carcinoma and non-Hodgkin's lymphoma are more common in AIDS.

Parotidomegaly is sometimes seen as a result of HIV-associated Sjögren syndrome. These patients may have dry eyes and mouth for this reason.

Hairy leucoplakia is a unique raised or flat white, painless and often hairy-looking lesion typically present on the lateral surface of the tongue; it is caused by Epstein–Barr virus (EBV) infection in HIV-infected people and is almost diagnostic of HIV infection.

Palpate over the sinuses for tenderness (sinusitis). Examine the cervical and axillary nodes. There may be generalised lymphadenopathy, and all lymph node groups should be examined.

Chest

Note any tachypnoea or dry cough. Note chronic cough, either dry or productive of purulent sputum. On auscultation, crackles may be present at the bases owing to bronchiolitis obliterans. There are often, however, no chest signs despite the presence of pulmonary infiltrates on chest X-ray, due to *Pneumocystis jiroveci* (formerly *carinii*) or other opportunistic infections.

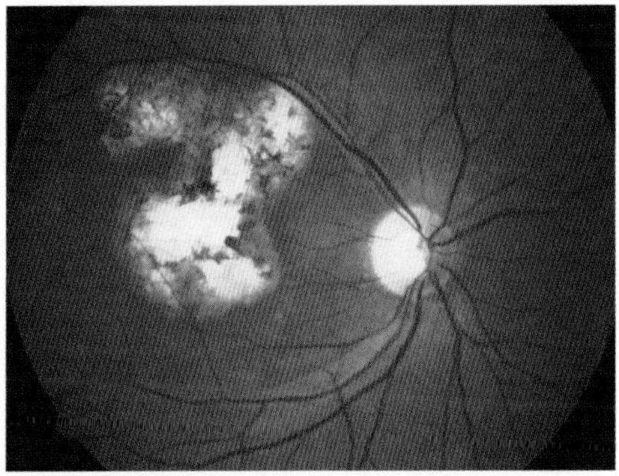

Retinal toxoplasmosis—old chorioretinal scar

(Courtesy of Dr Chris Kennedy & Professor Ian Constable, Lions Eye Institute.)

FIGURE 45.5

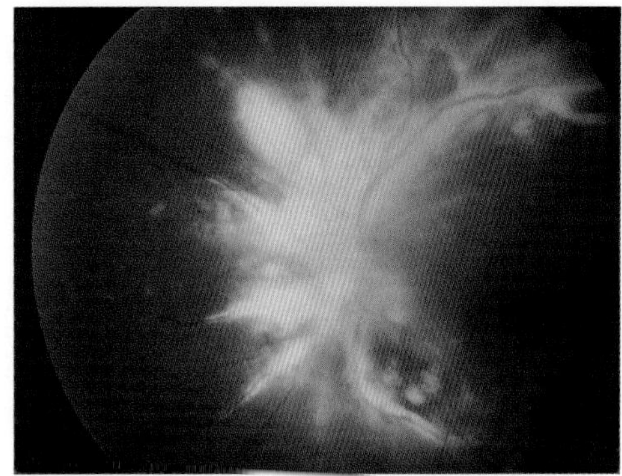

Cytomegalovirus retinitis

(Courtesy of Dr Chris Kennedy & Professor Ian Constable, Lions Eye Institute.)

FIGURE 45.6

Abdomen

Examine for hepatosplenomegaly (e.g. infection, lymphoma). Perform a rectal examination (e.g. perianal ulceration from herpes simplex) and a sigmoidoscopy looking for Kaposi's sarcoma or proctitis (e.g. cytomegalovirus, herpes simplex, amoebic dysentery or pseudomembranous colitis from antibiotic use). Examine the genitals for herpes simplex, warts, discharge or chancre.

Nervous system

Look for signs of meningism (e.g. cryptococcal meningitis). There may be focal signs due to a space-occupying intracranial lesion (e.g. toxoplasmosis, non-Hodgkin's lymphoma).

A syndrome similar to Guillain–Barré and a pure sensory neuropathy can occur. HIV infection itself, opportunistic infection or the drugs used in treatment can be responsible for peripheral sensorimotor neuropathy, polymyositis, radiculopathy, mononeuritis multiplex or a myelopathy.

Look in the fundi for soft exudates (common in AIDS patients), scars (e.g. toxoplasmosis—see Fig. 45.5) or retinitis (e.g. cytomegalovirus-induced retinitis with perivascular haemorrhages and fluffy exudates, which can cause blindness of rapid onset—see Fig. 45.6).[12] There may be signs of dementia (AIDS encephalopathy).

T&O'C ESSENTIALS

1. *Persisting fever may be due to a common illness that has presented in an unusual way.*
2. *Careful history taking and examination will help direct the investigations in a febrile or possibly septic patient.*
3. *Recent travel or contact with other sick people or animals may suggest a specific line of investigation.*
4. *Systemic inflammatory response syndrome (SIRS) refers to two or more of the following four features: fever >38.3°C (or temperature <36°C), tachycardia (>90 beats/minute), tachypnoea (>20 breaths/minute) and an elevated white cell count. This may be due to acute infection (you must rule out sepsis), but can occur after burns or surgery or with other inflammatory diseases (e.g. thromboembolism, pancreatitis).*
5. *HIV infection should be suspected in a patient with tuberculosis or any unexplained infectious illness.*
6. *Questioning a patient with newly diagnosed HIV about the possible mode of infection and contacts is important from a public health point of view.*

OSCE REVISION TOPICS – **INFECTIOUS DISEASES**

1. This woman has a prosthetic heart valve and has been unwell for 2 months. Please take a history from her and explain what examination you would perform. (p 870)
2. This man has recently been diagnosed with HIV infection. Please take a history from him. (p 872)

References

1. Hayakawa K, Ramasamy B, Chandrasekar PH. Fever of unknown origin: an evidence-based review. *Am J Med Sci* 2012; 344(4):307–316. The modern approach to diagnosis still relies on the history and physical examination initially.
2. Arbo M, Fine MJ, Hanusa BH et al. Fever of nosocomial origin: etiology, risk factors and outcomes. *Am J Med* 1993; 95:505–515.
3. Cunha BA, Lortholary O, Cunha CB. Fever of unknown origin: a clinical approach. *Am J Med* 2015; 128(10):1138.
4. Mourad O, Palda V, Detsky AS. A comprehensive evidence-based approach to fever of unknown origin. *Arch Intern Med* 2003; 163:545.
5. Coburn B, Morris AM, Tomlinson G, Detsky AS. Does this adult patient with suspected bacteremia require blood cultures? *JAMA* 2012; 308(5):502–511. Shaking chills but not fever alone suggests bacteraemia.
6. Bates DW, Cook EF, Goldman L et al. Predicting bacteremia in hospitalized patients: a prospectively validated model. *Ann Intern Med* 1990; 113:495–500.
7. Wood E, Kerr T, Rowell G et al. The rational clinical examination systematic review. Does this adult patient have early HIV infection? *JAMA* 2014; 312(3):278–285.
8. American College of Physicians and Infectious Diseases Society of America. Human immunodeficiency virus (HIV) infection. *Ann Intern Med* 1994; 120:310–319.
9. Nandwani R. Human immunodeficiency virus medicine for the MRCP short cases. *Br J Hosp Med* 1994; 51:353–356.
10. Malin A, Ternouth I, Sarbah S. Epitrochlear nodes as marker of HIV disease in sub-Saharan Africa. *BMJ* 1994; 309:1550–1551.
11. Weinert ML, Grimes RM, Lynch DP. Oral manifestations of HIV infection. *Ann Intern Med* 1996; 125:485–496. Details the 16 leading oral complications, based on an extensive literature review.
12. De Smet MD, Nessenbatt RB. Ocular manifestations of AIDS. *JAMA* 1991; 266:3019–3022. Provides a very good review of eye changes.

SECTION 13

Mental health history and examination

CHAPTER 46

The mental health history and mental state examination

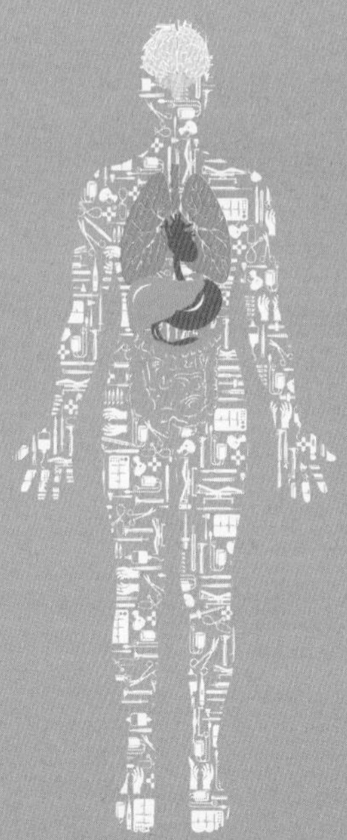

CHAPTER 46

The mental health history and mental state examination

Law number four: the patient is the one with the disease. SAMUEL SHEM (1944–), The House of God

This chapter deals with mental health, mental illness and the mental state examination. The practising clinician must have an understanding of psychiatric illness and know how to perform a psychiatric interview and a mental state examination. This is because there is considerable overlap between psychiatric and physical illness.

Psychiatric disorders (especially anxiety and depression) are common (one person in four will experience a mental illness in his or her lifetime) but most will fully recover. People suffering from these conditions often have medical problems or problems with drugs and alcohol. Appropriate management of these patients requires an understanding of the intercurrent psychiatric disorder and the effect of that disorder on the primary medical problem. A medical illness may, in some instances, present as a psychiatric illness. For example, some endocrine disorders, such as hypothroidism, may present with depression. On the other hand, some psychiatric disorders may present medically. Panic disorder (or acute anxiety) may be mistaken for an acute myocardial infarction. Furthermore, a patient's psychological state may interfere with the course of a medical illness; it may lead in some cases to exaggeration of the symptoms and in others to denial of the severity of physical symptoms. Medical illnesses, particularly chronic and / or life-threatening illnesses, have major psychological impacts and can be complicated by psychiatric symptoms (such as anxiety or depression) that can induce disability and affect recovery from illness.

THE HISTORY

The psychiatric history generally follows the same format as the standard medical history, and the principles described apply just as much here as in any history taking.[1] One should enquire about the history of the present illness, the past psychiatric and medical history, and the family and social history. However, the psychiatric history aims to elicit more detail about the patient's illness from a broad perspective, focusing not only on symptoms but also on the patient's social background, psychological functioning and life circumstances (a biopsychosocial approach). Within the psychiatric history, particular attention is paid to the developmental, personal and social history, although these factors are usually also relevant in the general medical history.

Every medical interview should aim to be therapeutic as well as diagnostic. The method of psychiatric history taking is somewhat different from the standard medical interview. In the course of the interview it is hoped that the patient will be able to talk about his or her concerns in detail, and their context. In doing so, patients should gain some relief from their distress by airing their problems. For this to take place, the clinician's attitude needs to be unhurried, patient and understanding. The psychiatric history also aims to gain an understanding of how the patient's problem arose from a biological, interpersonal, social and psychological perspective, so that the best management plan can be worked out. In this way, the psychiatric interview is similar to the general medical interview. These factors are also important in relation to any illness, especially if it is a chronic or life-threatening problem. Psychiatric and physical problems often coexist and each affects the other. A comprehensive medical interview should therefore encompass both physical and psychological concerns.

OBTAINING THE HISTORY

The clinician taking a psychiatric history wants the patient to tell his or her story in his or her own words. In this way the patient will be more likely to report the most important aspects of the illness. Of course, this technique also applies to the general medical interview. It is best achieved using a non-directive approach with open-ended questions. **Open-ended questions** are those to which the patient responds with a narrative (or a description about what has been happening) rather than a simple factual response. They give patients an opportunity to talk about their problems in their own words. **Closed questions**, on the other hand, are more likely to elicit 'yes' or 'no' responses. For example, in the assessment of a patient with depression, a closed question would be: 'Have you been depressed?' An open-ended question would be: 'Tell me about how you have been feeling.' At first glance it might appear that the open-ended question is less efficient, as it could take longer to find out about a range of symptoms. However, with a careful and judicious approach, open-ended questioning—by permitting the patient to tell the story—will enable the clinician to get a comprehensive history efficiently. This is not to say that targeted, more-closed questions must not be used—they are necessary to elicit information on certain symptoms.

It takes experience and practice to feel confident and unembarrassed when interviewing patients who have difficult psychiatric problems that may be associated with a certain stigma or where the questioning is about sexual or intimate problems. This is certainly not the place to make judgements about or appear shocked by what a patient is saying. Of course, appearing to be sympathetic about the patient's difficulties is necessary here, as it is with any medical interview.

While the patient is telling his or her story, you should begin to formulate hypotheses about the problem or diagnosis. These hypotheses are tested by asking more-focused questions later in the interview, at which point a diagnostic hypothesis can be rejected or pursued further. For example, a patient may describe tiredness and lethargy, an inability to concentrate and loss of appetite. These symptoms will suggest a diagnosis of depression. Follow-up questions should focus on this possibility. You should ask questions about other symptoms of depression such as: 'How have you been feeling in yourself?', 'What has your mood been like?' and 'How have you been sleeping?'

Introductory questions

The assessment of psychiatric symptoms should start with non-threatening questions. After introducing yourself, it can be useful to begin by asking about basic demographic information (age, marital status, occupation, whom the patient lives with) and then make the patient feel at ease by discussing some neutral topic. In some cases the presenting problem will be an obvious psychiatric or psychological one. For example, a patient may say, 'I've come to see you because I've been feeling very depressed.' However, even such an apparently definite psychiatric problem may have a medical cause, such as hypothyroidism or a recent serious medical illness. More often, the presenting problem will be a more general one, such as 'I have no energy and feel tired all the time.' This may be due to a depressive illness or it could have a medical cause such as anaemia. Remember that psychiatric and medical problems are intimately entwined. It is rare for an interview to focus purely on psychiatric problems.

History of the presenting illness

In assessing the history of the presenting illness, you need to cover a number of areas.

The problem

Find out the nature of the patient's problem, and the patient's perception of his or her difficulties. This can, of course, be difficult if the patient is psychotic and does not believe that a psychiatric problem exists at all. In these cases a corroborative history must be taken. For example, a manic patient may consider that there is nothing wrong and that his or her behaviour is reasonable, whereas the patient's partner is able to recognise that ordering an expensive new sports car when the family is impoverished is a problem.

A range of symptoms commonly found in psychiatric disorders needs to be reviewed in the course of assessing the history of the present illness. These include mood change, anxiety, worry, sleep patterns, appetite, hallucinations and delusions. A set of simple screening questions for each of the major diagnoses is listed within Table 46.1.

It is especially important to ask about symptoms of anxiety and depression (the most common psychiatric

Text continued on p 851

The common psychiatric disorders* and their screening questions

Disorder	Screening questions
Mood (affective) disorders	
Mood disorders have a pathological disturbance in mood (depression or mania) as the predominant feature. They are distinguished from 'normal' mood changes by their persistence, duration and severity, together with the presence of other symptoms and impairment of functioning.	
Manic–depressive illness—bipolar disorder	
Bipolar disorder is a broad term to describe a recurrent illness characterised by episodes of either mania or depression, with a return to normal functioning between episodes of illness.	
(a) Mania A disorder demonstrated by change in mood (*elation*), thought form (*grandiosity*) and behaviour disturbance (*increased energy and disinhibition*). Frequently associated symptoms and signs: increased talkativeness, irritability, distractibility, decreased need for sleep, loss of inhibition (e.g. engaging in reckless behaviour such as spending sprees, sexual indiscretion or social overfamiliarity).	**Questions box 46.1** Questions to ask the patient with possible mania 1. Have you felt especially good about yourself? 2. Have you been needing less sleep than usual? 3. Do you feel that you are special or that you have special powers? 4. Have you been spending more than usual?
(b) Depression A disorder characterised by depressed mood (or loss of pleasure) and the presence of somatic (*sleep disturbance, change in appetite, fatigue and weight*), psychological (*low self-esteem, worry–anxiety, guilt, suicidal ideation*), affective (*sadness, irritability, loss of pleasure and interest in activities*) and psychomotor (*retardation or agitation*) symptoms.	**Questions box 46.2** Questions to ask the patient with possible depression 1. How have you been feeling in yourself? 2. What has your mood been like? 3. Have you been feeling sad, blue, down or depressed? 4. Have you lost interest in things you usually enjoy? 5. How have you been sleeping?
Anxiety disorders	
Anxiety disorders are those in which the person experiences excessive levels of anxiety. Anxiety may be somatic (palpitations, difficulty breathing, dry mouth, nausea, frequency of micturition, dizziness, muscular tension, sweating, abdominal churning, tremor, cold skin) or psychological (feelings of dread and threat, irritability, panic, anxious anticipation, inner [psychic] tension, worrying over trivia, difficulty in concentrating, initial insomnia, inability to relax).	
1. Generalised anxiety disorder (GAD) A chronic disorder characterised by a tendency to worry excessively about everyday things. It is accompanied by: symptoms of anxiety or tension; mental tension (*feeling tense or nervous, poor concentration, on edge*); physical tension.	**Questions box 46.3** Questions to ask the patient with possible anxiety 1. Have you been feeling nervy or tense? 2. Do you worry a lot about things? Find it hard to relax / switch off? 3. Do you worry about things most other people would not worry about?
2. Panic disorder A disorder characterised by episodes of panic occurring spontaneously in situations where most people would not be afraid. A panic attack is characterised by the presence of physical symptoms (*palpitations, chest pain, a choking feeling, a churning stomach, dizziness, feelings of unreality*) or fear of some disaster (*losing control or going mad, heart attack, sudden death*). They begin suddenly, build up rapidly and may last only a few minutes.	**Questions box 46.4** Questions to ask the patient with possible panic disorder 1. Have you ever had an attack of acute anxiety or panic (suddenly feeling very anxious and frightened, feeling something terrible could happen)? 2. Did this occur in a situation in which most people would not feel afraid? 3. Can these attacks happen at any time?
3. Agoraphobia (phobic anxiety) A disorder in which an individual avoids places (such as supermarkets or trains) in which they fear they may have a panic attack and cannot escape.	**Questions box 46.5** Questions to ask the patient with possible phobic anxiety 1. Do you avoid going out? 2. Do you avoid going to places or situations because you fear you may have an anxiety attack?

TABLE 46.1

Continued

The common psychiatric disorders* and their screening questions *continued*

4. Obsessive–compulsive disorder A disorder in which the person has either obsessions or compulsions that interfere with everyday life.	**Questions box 46.6** Questions to ask the patient with possible obsessive–compulsive disorder 1. Are there any rituals or habits that you have to carry out every day? 2. Do they cause you problems or make you anxious? 3. Do you find yourself having to do things even though they seem unnecessary, to stop yourself feeling anxious (compulsions)? 4. Do you ever have a thought going round in your head that you cannot get rid of?
Stress-related disorders	
1. Acute stress disorder Individuals may present shortly after a traumatic event with a range of symptoms, such as *anxiety, depression, disturbed sleep, problems with memory or concentration.* Images, dreams or flashbacks of the traumatic event may also occur.	**Questions box 46.7** Questions to ask the patient with possible acute stress disorder 1. Have you been having any problems following … ? 2. Have you been feeling especially anxious or worried? Or depressed? Finding you cannot get the events out of your mind? 3. Have you had trouble sleeping? 4. Do you have bad memories?
2. Post-traumatic stress disorder (PTSD) Onset of persistent problems within 6 months of a traumatic event of exceptional severity. The individual experiences *repetitive and intrusive re-enactments* of the trauma in images, dreams or flashbacks. *Sleep, concentration, memory, mood and attention may be disturbed.* Individuals may feel emotionally detached and avoid things that act as reminders of the traumatic event.	**Questions box 46.8** Questions to ask the patient with possible PTSD 1. Since … happened, have you been troubled by bad memories of it? 2. Have you been having nightmares? 3. Have you had trouble with sleep? 4. Have you had trouble with your memory? 5. Do you try to avoid any reminders of the event or situation? 6. Are you jumpy?
Schizophrenia and delusional disorders	
A condition characterised by disorders of content (presence of delusions), thought form (shown by difficulty in understanding the connections between the patient's thoughts), perception (hallucinations—predominantly auditory), behaviour (erratic or bizarre) and / or volition (apathy and withdrawal).	**Questions box 46.9** Questions to ask the patient with possible schizophrenia or delusions 1. Have you ever heard people speaking when there is no one around? 2. Do you ever hear voices speaking as if someone is there? 3. Have you heard your thoughts spoken out loud, as if by someone else? 4. Do you have any thoughts or beliefs that others might find unusual or strange? 5. Have you felt people may be against you? 6. Have you felt that the TV or radio sends you messages? 7. Do you ever feel as if someone is spying on you or plotting to hurt you? 8. Do you have any ideas that you don't like to talk about because you are afraid other people will not believe you or will think there is something wrong with you?
Organic brain disorders	
These are disorders in which there is brain dysfunction manifested by cognitive disturbances such as memory loss or disorientation; there may be behavioural disturbance as well.	

TABLE 46.1

The common psychiatric disorders* and their screening questions *continued*

1. Delirium (acute brain syndrome) A disorder characterised by the acute onset of disturbed consciousness plus changes in cognition that are not due to a pre-existing dementia. It is a direct physiological consequence of a general medical condition (*substance intoxication or withdrawal, use of a medication, exposure to a toxin, or a combination of these factors*). Delirium is characterised by fluctuating confusion and clouding of consciousness. This may be accompanied by *poor concentration, poor memory, disorientation, inattention, agitation, emotional upset, hallucinations, visions or illusions, suspiciousness and disturbed sleep* (*reversal of sleep pattern*). **Hypoactive delirium** is characterised by withdrawal, slowing of thinking and behaviour, and a depression-like presentation.	**Questions box 46.10** Questions to ask the patient with possible delirium 1. What day is it today? 2. How long have you been here? 3. What is the name of the place we are in? 4. Do you remember my name? 5. Are you having trouble staying awake? Questions to ask the patient's attendant 6. Does …'s ability to concentrate vary from moment to moment? 7. Did these problems begin suddenly? Mental state examination (see Table 46.4)
2. Dementia (chronic brain syndrome) A generalised impairment of intellect, memory and personality with no impairment of consciousness. Characterised by *loss of memory* (especially short-term memory), *loss of orientation and deterioration in social functioning and behaviour and emotional control* (may be easily upset—tearful or irritable).	**Questions box 46.11** Questions to ask the patient with possible dementia 1. What day is it today? 2. How long have you been here? 3. What is the name of the place we are in? 4. Do you remember my name? Mental state examination (see Table 46.4)
Other disorders	
There are a number of other psychiatric disorders that may present with physical problems, or that may be seen in an emergency department with some complication (particularly after attempted suicide).	
A. Eating disorders (anorexia nervosa and bulimia nervosa)	
Here the sufferer (generally female) has a disturbed body image with an unreasonable fear of being fat, and makes extensive efforts to lose weight (strict dieting, vomiting, use of purgatives, excessive exercise). The patient may deny that weight or eating habits are a problem. *Bulimia nervosa* is characterised by binge eating followed by vomiting or purging. *Anorexia nervosa* is characterised by excessive dieting, but there may also be binges followed by vomiting or purging. Anorexic patients will be grossly underweight and may show signs of malnutrition. Amenorrhoea is generally present. *Binge-eating disorder (BED)* is characterised by 3 months or more of eating more food, more rapidly than normally, often secretly. Patients feel lack of control of their eating, and guilt, self-disgust, and physical discomfort after overeating.	**Questions box 46.12** Questions to ask the patient with a possible eating disorder 1. Do you worry about your weight? 2. Do you think that you are fat? *or* What are your feelings about your weight? 3. Do you diet? *or* What other things have you tried to control your weight? 4. Have you ever made yourself sick after a meal?
B. Somatoform disorders	
1. Somatisation disorder A disorder characterised by multiple physical complaints that cannot be satisfactorily explained by physical disease. An individual with this disorder will have unexplained complaints in several bodily systems (e.g. gastrointestinal, cardiac, respiratory, musculoskeletal, menstrual). Usually commences in teens or early adult life and there is a risk of iatrogenic complications.	**Questions box 46.13** Questions to ask the patient with possible somatoform disorder 1. Do you have any other medical problems? 2. Have you had symptoms that your doctor has not been able to find a cause for? 3. Are you often sick?

TABLE 46.1

Continued

The common psychiatric disorders* and their screening questions *continued*

2. Somatic symptom disorder (hypochondriacal disorder) These patients fear they have a serious illness despite repeated medical reassurance and are preoccupied with physical symptoms. They often seek repeated medical opinions. In some cases the disorder becomes delusional (e.g. of parasitic skin infection).	**Questions box 46.14** Questions to ask the patient with possible somatic symptom disorder (hypochondriacal disorder[†]) 1. Have you been very worried about your health? 2. What do you think might be wrong? 3. What have your doctors told you?
3. Medically unexplained symptoms (MUS) (conversion disorder, hysteria) These patients usually present with a neurological abnormality that is not fully explained medically. Common symptoms include: blindness, gait disturbances, sensory loss, limb paralysis and loss of speech. There is usually a precipitating psychological stress event, and often a past history of similar episodes.	**Questions box 46.15** Questions to ask the patient with possible MUS disorder 1. What have you noticed has been wrong? 2. What tests have you had? 3. What have you been told about your illness?
Substance misuse	
This category includes the misuse of alcohol, illegal drugs and prescription medications.	
Personality disorders	
In these disorders the individual, while not having specific symptoms, has behavioural disturbances and problems with impulse control, interpersonal relationships and mood. Typically there are problems involving many areas of personality. Individuals who have repeatedly and deliberately made self-harm attempts often have a personality disorder.[‡] They may also have unpredictable behaviour while in hospital, which may cause problems for staff.	**Questions box 46.16** Questions to ask the patient with a possible borderline personality disorder 1. Have you ever tried to harm yourself? 2. Have you ever had problems with relationships?
Neurasthenia (chronic fatigue syndrome)	
This is a somewhat controversial inclusion in the current WHO classification of psychiatric disorders.	
Puerperal mental disorders	
This category includes peripartum depression and psychosis. Early recognition of this disorder is important for the mother and the baby. It needs to be distinguished from the more common 'postpartum blues'. Mothers may present with quite specific symptoms, such as excessive anxiety about the baby or feelings of failure as a mother and of inability to cope. There may be loss of ability to enjoy the baby and women often become isolated from others. In postpartum psychosis, the baby may be included in the mother's psychotic symptoms.	**Questions box 46.17** Questions to ask the patient with a possible puerperal mental disorder 1. Have you ever been worried that you might want to hurt your baby? 2. Have you ever thought of hurting yourself?

**Based on the* WHO International Classification of Disease, *10th edn (ICD-10). ICD-11 was published in 2018.*

[†]Alfons Jakob (1884–1931), a professor of neurology in Hamburg from 1924, had more than 200 cases of neurosyphilis on his ward at a time; he died of osteomyelitis. Jakob described this cerebral atrophy in 1920 and before Hans Creutzeld (1885–1933).

[‡]Depression can be a cause of attempted self-harm but in this case it is not usually deliberate.

TABLE 46.1

disorders). A simple screening approach to determine whether the patient has depression is to ask him or her:[2]

- 'In the past month, have you felt down, depressed or hopeless?'
- 'Have you felt little interest or pleasure in doing things?'

If the patient answers 'yes' to either question, you need to explore the possibility of depression in detail (LR+, 2.9; LR–, 0.05).[2]

Screening is encouraged to reduce the high rate of undetected depression. Use of such screening questions in all patients (where there will be a low prevalence—i.e. a low pretest probability of depression) will lead to some false-positive responses so detailed follow-up questions are required to help confirm the results.[3]

The definitions of other symptoms are given in Table 46.2. It is important to ask about drug usage (legal and illegal) as well as alcohol and caffeine intake (which may be associated with anxiety disorders).

Assessment of suicide risk

Suicide may be the tragic outcome of psychiatric illness. Assessing the risk of suicide is an essential part of the psychiatric interview. Asking about this does *not* increase the risk or put the idea into the patient's head; it may reduce the risk, as the patient may feel relief in talking about his or her fears. The risk of suicide is assessed by asking directly whether the person has ever contemplated it.

1. Have you thought that life was not worth living?

   Or

2. Have you ever felt so bad that you have considered ending it all?

   If 'yes'

- Have you thought of killing yourself?
- Have you thought how you might do this?
- Have you made any plans for doing this?

TEXT BOX 46.1

Precipitating events

Psychiatric illness can occur for no reason (e.g. bipolar disease episodes) but there is often an event that has precipitated the illness, even though this may not be obvious at the beginning. Such events include a range of experiences that may have affected the patient or a member of the patient's social network. Events such as physical illness, drug treatment or treatment non-adherence may be implicated as precipitants. Patients with psychiatric illnesses have a possibly undeserved reputation for non-adherence to treatment. It may be no more common than in non-psychiatric patients but when it occurs it can be a major contribution to relapse.

Risk

An assessment of the patient's risk of harm, either to others or to him- or herself, is essential: this will indicate any urgent steps that need to be taken to ensure safety and whether the patient needs to be treated involuntarily. Patients with psychotic illness may, in some circumstances, need to be treated involuntarily under the relevant legislation (e.g. *Mental Health Act*). Although the exact details for involuntary treatment are different under individual mental health laws, the essential features are generally that: (1) a person has a mental illness, and (2) the person is a danger to self or others. Assessment of danger to others is difficult, with the best predictor being a history of past threat or harm to others. It is best to err on the side of caution in such cases and seek advice from psychiatry colleagues and mental health services. Assessment of suicide risk needs to be made with sensitivity and using a direct approach, as shown in Text box 46.1.

Past history and treatment history

Both the past psychiatric history and the medical history should be assessed. The past medical history should be evaluated in the same way as the general medical history. An assessment should be made of stresses that may have contributed to past episodes of illness and that may have led to relapse. For the past psychiatric history, it is important to obtain not only the diagnosis but also the treatment the patient has had, and its outcome.

Ask about previous non-drug treatment including counselling, psychotherapy and electroconvulsive therapy (ECT), and whether the patient thought the treatment was effective. Was the patient ever admitted to a psychiatric unit, and for how long?

Symptoms of psychiatric illness	
Affect	The observable behaviour by which a person's internal emotional state is judged.
Agitation (psychomotor agitation)	Excessive motor activity associated with a feeling of inner tension. The activity is usually non-productive and repetitious and consists of such behaviour as pacing, fidgeting, wringing the hands, pulling the clothes and inability to sit still.
Anxiety	The apprehensive anticipation of future danger or misfortune. It is associated with feelings of tension and symptoms of autonomic arousal.
Conversion symptom (hysteria)	A loss of, or alteration in, motor or sensory function. Psychological factors are judged to be associated with the development of the symptom, which is not fully explained by anatomical or pathological conditions. The symptom is the result of unconscious conflict and is not feigned.
Delusion	A false unshakable idea or belief that is out of keeping with the patient's educational, cultural and social background.
Depersonalisation	An alteration in the awareness of the self—the individual feels as if he or she is unreal.
Derealisation	An alteration in the perception or experience of the external world so that it seems unreal.
Disorientation	Confusion about the time of day, date or season (time), where one is (place) or who one is (person).
Flight of ideas	A nearly continuous flow of accelerated speech with abrupt changes from topic to topic that are usually based on understandable associations, distracting stimuli or plays on words. When severe, speech may be disorganised or incoherent.
Grandiosity	An inflated appraisal of one's worth, power, knowledge, importance or identity. When extreme, grandiosity may be of delusional proportions.
Hallucination	A sensory perception that seems real, but occurs without external stimulation of the relevant sensory organ. The term *hallucination* is not ordinarily applied to the false perceptions that occur during dreaming, while falling asleep (hypnagogic) or when awakening (hypnopompic).
Ideas of reference	The feeling that casual incidents and external events have a particular significance and unusual meaning that is specific to the person.
Illusion	A misperception or misinterpretation of a real external stimulus.
Mood	A pervasive and sustained emotion that colours the perception of the world.
Overvalued idea	An unreasonable belief that is held, but not as strongly as a delusion (i.e. the person is able to acknowledge the possibility that the belief may not be true). The belief is not one that is ordinarily accepted by other members of the person's culture or subculture.
Personality	Enduring patterns of perceiving, relating to and thinking about the environment and oneself.
Phobia	A persistent irrational fear of a specific object, activity or situation (the phobic stimulus) that results in a compelling desire to avoid it.
Pressured speech	Speech that is increased in amount, accelerated and difficult or impossible to interrupt. Usually it is also loud and emphatic. Frequently the person talks without any social stimulation and may continue to talk even though no one is listening.
Psychomotor retardation	Visible generalised slowing of movements and speech.
Psychotic	Psychotic can be used to mean a loss of contact with reality, but is generally used to imply the presence of delusions or hallucinations.

(Based on American Psychiatric Association. *Diagnostic and statistical manual of mental disorders*, 5th edn. Washington, DC: APA, 2013.)

TABLE 46.2

Classes of psychiatric drugs and their major indications	
Antianxiety (e.g. benzodiazepines, beta-blockers [control somatic symptoms])	For anxiety disorders, insomnia, alcohol withdrawal
Antipsychotic (e.g. atypical antipsychotics, phenothiazines, butyrophenones, major tranquillisers)	For schizophrenia, mania, delirium
Antidepressants (e.g. tricyclics, selective serotonin reuptake inhibitors [SSRIs] and serotonin–noradrenaline reuptake inhibitors [SNRIs])	For depression, anxiety disorders, obsessive–compulsive disorder
Mood-stabilising (e.g. lithium, anticonvulsants—carbamazepine, sodium valproate)	For prevention of manic depression or treatment of mania

TABLE 46.3

COMMON SIDE EFFECTS OF THE ANTIPSYCHOTIC DRUGS

1. *Anticholinergic*—dry mouth, blurred vision, urinary retention, erectile dysfunction, sedation, metabolic syndrome (weight gain, insulin resistance and hyperlipidaemia)
2. *Hypersensitivity reactions*—photosensitivity dermatitis, cholestatic jaundice, agranulocytosis (clozapine)
3. *Effects due to dopamine blockade*—Parkinsonianism, motor restlessness (akathisia), tardive dyskinesia, dystonia, gynaecomastia, malignant neuroleptic syndrome

LIST 46.1

Find out what drug treatment has been tried, the class (see Table 46.3) of psychiatric medication, its effectiveness and any side effects. The antipsychotic drugs in particular have common long-term side effects (see List 46.1).

Family history

Some mental illnesses have a genetic association and in other family situations behaviours are learned.

First, ask the patient tactfully whether anyone in the family has had any psychiatric or mental illness or has committed suicide. Also ask whether anyone in the family has had any treatment for psychological problems, such as anxiety, depression, agoraphobia,[a] eating disorders or drug and alcohol problems (these last few areas are often not considered by patients to be psychiatric or mental illnesses).

Second, try to gain an understanding of the patient's family origin. Drawing up a family tree is a useful way of finding this out. Factual details about each family member can be included in this family tree (age, mental state, health). In the psychiatric history one also needs to know what type of person each family member is, about any important family events (such as bereavements, separations) and how family members get on with each other. It is worth exploring the quality of care the patient received from each parent, and how controlling or protective each was. These two factors have been shown to be important in contributing to psychiatric illness. Ask about the quality of the parental relationship and the general family atmosphere.

Childhood abuse (emotional, physical or sexual)[4] may be an important predisposing event for many illnesses, and should be enquired about. This can be elicited by saying something like, 'Sometimes children can have had some unpleasant experiences—I wonder if you had any? Did anyone ever harm you? Or hit you? How about interfering with you sexually? Could you tell me more about that and what happened?'

Taking a detailed family history in this way sets the scene for the patient's developmental history, which should be taken next.

Social and personal history

Open-ended questions are again the best way to initiate discussion of personal and social history. Ask the patient something like, 'Could you tell me a bit about your background, your development, what sort of childhood you had, what are the important things you remember from your childhood?', and then allow the patient to tell his or her own story. During the course of this narrative, the patient may require some prompting to add information about important issues such as the birth history (schizophrenia is known to be associated with perinatal morbidity) and early development, and whether there were significant problems in early

[a] From the Greek, meaning 'fear of the market place'.

childhood, such as head injuries or serious infections. How did the patient cope with early separations, particularly when starting primary school and going on to secondary school (difficulty in separation may be a risk factor for panic disorder or abnormal illness behaviour)? The patient should be asked about peer relationships, friendships, school, academic ability, adolescence and teenage relationships. The adult history should focus predominantly on the quality of intimate relationships and the social support network, especially whether there are people in whom the patient can confide, and about significant events that may have occurred and about the patient's ability to cope with such events.

The patient's living circumstances should be asked about in the same way as for a medical history. There should also be a focus on the patient's occupation: not only on the type of job but also on how he or she copes with work or, if he or she does not work, how that is coped with.

Premorbid personality

An assessment should be made of the patient's premorbid personality. Ask the patient to describe him- or herself (e.g. 'How would your friends or family describe you?'). The personality can be described using the predominant trait, such as obsessional, nervy or highly strung; it is not necessary to use official systems to describe a patient's personality. In the assessment of premorbid personality it is important to evaluate both positive and negative aspects of the person, how he or she copes or responds to the strains of life, what type of interests he or she has, and what other strengths and weaknesses are present.

THE MENTAL STATE EXAMINATION

While assessing the patient, carefully make observations about appearance, behaviour, patterns of speech, predominant concerns, attitude to the examiner and ways of interacting. These observations are brought together in a systematic fashion in the mental state examination. This is not something that is 'done' at the conclusion of taking a history; it is an essential part of the total process of assessing the patient.[5]

However, there are a number of tests or specific tasks that need to be conducted in a formalised way as part of the mental state examination. These include assessing the patient's cognitive state (orientation, memory, attention, registration) and enquiring about perceptual disturbances and, in some cases, disorders of thought. The mental state examination provides valuable diagnostic information; with some disorders, it is this examination that gives most of the diagnostic clues.

The headings under which the mental state is recorded are shown in Table 46.4, together with some simple bedside tests for assessing cognitive function. Also shown in Table 46.4 are some abnormal features of the mental state examination that are commonly found in psychiatric disorders.

When cognitive dysfunction is suspected, as in patients with delirium or dementia,[6] a more detailed examination of cognitive function should be carried out. A widely used screening tool for doing this has been the mini-mental state examination (MMSE),[6] which assesses aspects of orientation, memory and concentration. The MMSE is copyright protected. Another useful screening tool is the simple three-step (3-minute) Mini-Cog test.[7] For this test, ask the patient to remember three words (repeat them up to three times to make sure that he or she has captured the words correctly). Next, ask the patient to draw a clock face with numbers and then draw the hands at a specified time (e.g. 11.10). Then ask the patient to repeat the original three words. Scoring is out of 5: 1 point for each word remembered and 2 for a correct clock face drawing (0 if not fully correct). A total score of 0–2 supports a diagnosis of dementia.

Some of the common causes of delirium and dementia are listed in Tables 46.5 and 46.6 respectively.

THE DIAGNOSIS

At the conclusion of the psychiatric history, which should include a general physical examination, a provisional diagnosis and formulation should be made. Essentially, the diagnostic formulation is a means of summarising, in a succinct yet comprehensive manner, your understanding of the patient's problem.

Psychiatric disorders generally arise through a combination of biological, psychological and psychosocial factors, and each of these needs to be considered when a patient's problem is being assessed (a biopsychosocial approach). The patient's problem

The mental state examination

	What is assessed, described or observed	Common findings indicating psychopathology	Types of illness
General description			
Appearance	A general description of the patient's appearance, including body build, posture, clothing (appropriateness), grooming (e.g. make-up) and hygiene. Note any physical stigmata (e.g. tattoos) and facial expression (depression, apprehension, worry, etc.).	Bizarre appearance	Psychotic disorders (schizophrenia, mania), personality disorder
		Unkempt, poorly groomed	Schizophrenia, depression, dementia or delirium
		Apprehensive, anxious	Anxiety disorders
		Over-bright clothing / disinhibited	Mania
		Scarred wrists, non-professional tattoos	Personality disorder
Behaviour	All aspects of the patient's behaviour. Note the appropriateness of the patient's behaviour within the interview context. Abnormal motor behaviour: mannerisms, stereotyped movements, tics. Variants of normal motor behaviour: restlessness, psychomotor change (agitation, retardation).	Uncooperative behaviour	Psychotic disorder, personality disorder, delirium, substance intoxication
		Manneristic behaviour	Psychotic disorder
		Stereotypical behaviour	Psychotic disorders, developmental disability, organic syndromes
		Bizarre behaviour	Psychotic disorders, substance intoxication, delirium
		Assaultive, threatening	Personality disorders, intoxication, neurological disorders, mania, delirium
		Restlessness	Akathisia from antipsychotic medication
		Psychomotor change (withdrawn)	Depression, delirium
Attitude towards examiner	The way the patient responds to the interviewer, the level of cooperation, willingness to disclose information. A range of attitudes and deviation from appropriateness may occur, ranging from hostility to seductiveness.	Uncooperative attitude, belligerence	Psychotic disorder, personality disorder, delirium, substance intoxication
		Seductiveness	Mania or hypomania, personality disorder
Mood and affect			
Mood	A relatively persistent emotional state: describe the depth, intensity, duration and fluctuations of mood. Mood may be neutral, euphoric, depressed, anxious or irritable.	Depressed	Depression
		Anxious / irritable	Depression / anxiety disorders
Affect	The way a patient conveys his or her emotional state. Affect may be full, blunted, restricted or inappropriate.	Depressed	Depression
		Blunted, restricted	Schizophrenia
Appropriateness	Are the patient's responses appropriate to the matter being discussed?	Inappropriate	Schizophrenia

TABLE 46.4

Continued

The mental state examination *continued*

	What is assessed, described or observed	Common findings indicating psychopathology	Types of illness
Speech	The tempo, modulation and quality of the patient's speech should be described here. Note should be made of dysphasia or dysarthria.	Increased tempo Slowed	Mania, acute schizophrenia Depression
Perceptual disturbances	The presence of hallucinations (auditory, visual, gustatory or tactile) should be noted. It is important to check whether they occurred with a clear sensorium. Hypnagogic or hypnopompic hallucinations are normal experiences. Other perceptual disturbances (e.g. illusions, depersonalisation or derealisation) should be noted.	Visual hallucinations Auditory Tactile / gustatory	Acute brain syndrome (delirium), epilepsy, alcohol withdrawal, drug intoxication Schizophrenia, delirium, organic states (hallucinosis) Epilepsy, schizophrenia
Thought			
Thought form	The process of the patient's thinking. This involves the quantity of ideas (pressured thought, poverty of ideas) and the way in which the ideas (thoughts) are produced. Are they logical and relevant, or are they fragmented and irrelevant? The link between ideas should be assessed—do they flow logically or are they disconnected and 'fragmented'? Are ideas connected by spurious concepts (rhyming, the way they sound—'clang' associations)?	Disorder of thought form Flight of ideas Poverty of ideas	Schizophrenia, mania, delirium Mania, schizophrenia Schizophrenia, depression, dementia
Thought content	The content of the patient's thoughts. Abnormalities range from preoccupation, obsessions and overvalued ideas to delusions. Themes should also be assessed: suicidal or homicidal thoughts or paranoid ideas. In the medical setting, preoccupation with illness (hypochondriacal thoughts) should be assessed, as well as thoughts of omnipotence—denying illness when it is present.	Delusions	Schizophrenia, mania, depression, delirium and other organic states
Sensorium and cognition			
Listed below are bedside tests for a basic assessment of cognitive function.			
Alertness and level of consciousness	The level of consciousness should be assessed. Clouding or fluctuating levels of consciousness should be noted.	Clouding	Delirium
Orientation	Orientation to time, place and person. Ask the day, date, month and year. Ask where he or she is. Ask for the names of his or her close family members.	Disorientation	Dementia, delirium

TABLE 46.4

The mental state examination *continued*

	What is assessed, described or observed	Common findings indicating psychopathology	Types of illness
Short-term memory	Short-term memory refers to the ability to retain information over a period of 3–5 minutes. Less than this refers to immediate recall. Ask the patient to recall a list of three objects after 3–5 minutes.	Loss of short-term memory Loss of immediate recall in delirium due to poor concentration	Dementia, delirium
Long-term memory	This refers to memory of remote events. Ask the patient to recall events of the previous few days, as well as events of a year ago.	Loss of long-term memory	Dementia
Concentration	Ask the patient to subtract 7 from 100 and keep subtracting 7, or spell 'world' backwards.	Poor concentration	Dementia, delirium
General knowledge and intelligence	Ask about some recent events. Intelligence can be gauged from the language used. Ask the patient to do some simple arithmetical tasks. Literacy should be assessed.	Poor general knowledge	Delirium, acute psychosis, dementia
Judgement and insight			
Judgement	The capacity to behave appropriately. Describe a hypothetical situation and ask how the patient would behave in it (e.g. 'What would you do if you smelt smoke while sitting in a cinema?').	Impaired judgement	Psychoses, dementia, personality disorders, delirium
Insight	Determine whether the patient is aware that he or she has a problem, and the level of understanding of this.	Lack of insight	Psychoses, dementia, delirium

TABLE 46.4

needs to be understood longitudinally, by defining biophysical factors that may have predisposed to the illness and, more immediately, may have precipitated the illness, and factors that may be contributing to the person remaining ill (perpetuating factors). A simple grid can be used for assessing the patient in this manner (see Table 46.7). Here biological, psychological or psychosocial factors that predispose to, precipitate or perpetuate the psychiatric illness are identified. Perpetuating factors are very important, particularly among medically ill patients, as it may be the medical or physical illness that maintains the patient's psychiatric problem. By the same token, psychological factors may perpetuate a patient's medical illness.

An example of such a formulation grid is shown in Table 46.8 for a 53-year-old man who becomes depressed after a myocardial infarction. He has a family history of depression (a genetic predisposing factor) and chronic low self-esteem (a psychological predisposing factor), which he coped with by succeeding in business. He has few friends and his marriage is unsatisfactory (a psychosocial factor). He had his infarct 1 week after he heard that he would not be promoted at work (a psychological factor) and his job was at risk (a psychosocial precipitant). His insecurity about work and his failing marriage, together with his low self-esteem, are maintaining his illness, as are the biological changes to the neurotransmitter system.

Common causes of delirium

Drug intoxication	Alcohol Anxiolytics Digoxin L-dopa 'Street drugs'
Withdrawal states	Alcohol (delirium tremens) Anxiolytic sedatives
Metabolic disturbance	Chronic kidney disease Liver failure Anoxia Cardiac failure Electrolyte imbalance Postoperative states
Endocrine disturbance	Diabetic ketosis Hypoglycaemia
Systemic infections	Pneumonia Urinary tract infection Septicaemia Viral infections
Intracranial infection	Encephalitis Meningitis
Other intracranial causes	Space-occupying lesions Raised intracranial pressure
Head injury	Subdural haemorrhage Cerebral contusion Concussion
Nutritional and vitamin deficiency	Thiamine (Wernicke's encephalopathy) Vitamin B_{12} Nicotinic acid
Epilepsy	Status epilepticus Postictal states

TABLE 46.5

Common causes of dementia

Hereditable Alzheimer's	Mutation of presenilin-1
Degenerative type	Senile dementia of Alzheimer's Dementia with Lewy bodies Parkinson disease Frontotemporal dementia* Huntington's chorea
Vascular	Multi-infarct dementia Chronic kidney disease
Intracranial space-occupying lesions	Tumour Subdural haematomas
Traumatic	Head injuries Boxing encephalopathy
Infections and related conditions	Encephalitis Neurosyphilis HIV (AIDS dementia) Jacob–Creutzfeldt disease
Metabolic	Chronic kidney disease Hepatic failure
Toxic	Alcoholic dementia Heavy-metal poisoning
Anoxia	Carbon monoxide poisoning Cardiac arrest Chronic respiratory failure
Vitamin deficiency	Vitamin B_{12} Folic acid Thiamine (Wernicke–Korsakoff syndrome)
Endocrine	Myxoedema, Addison disease

AIDS=acquired immunodeficiency syndrome; HIV=human immunodeficiency virus.
**Motor neurone disease may precede or follow onset.*

TABLE 46.6

A formulation grid

	Predisposing	**Precipitating**	**Perpetuating**
Biological			
Psychological			
Psychosocial			

TABLE 46.7

Understanding the patient in this manner helps you to plan an effective management approach that will focus on all the relevant factors, so that, for the patient in this example, a combination of antidepressants, marital counselling and assertiveness training (to build self-esteem) can be organised.

A good psychiatric history will provide a comprehensive understanding of the patient and will permit appropriate management to be planned. This is immensely rewarding for the clinician, and will also be of considerable benefit to the patient.

A completed formulation grid (see text)

	Predisposing	Precipitating	Perpetuating
Biological	Genetic predisposition	Acute myocardial infarct	Neurotransmitter changes
Psychological	Low self-esteem	Not promoted	Low self-esteem and insecurity
Psychosocial	Poor social support Dysfunctional marriage		Dysfunctional marriage

TABLE 46.8

PERSONALITY DISORDERS

A. Eccentric thinking or behaviour

1. **Paranoid**: pervasive and unjustified suspicion of others, hostile reactions to perceived insults
2. **Schizoid**: seemingly indifferent, cold in manner, not good at responding to social clues, prefer to be alone
3. **Schizotypal**: odd thinking, e.g. ability to influence others with powerful or magical thoughts, believe ordinary events have hidden meanings, may behave and dress eccentrically

B. Unpredictable thinking and behaviours, emotional problems

1. **Antisocial**: behaviour may include lying, stealing and aggression and violence. Little regard for the feelings or safety of others. Not remorseful. Often in legal difficulties.
2. **Borderline**: fragile self-image. Chaotic relationships with others, labile and intense emotions and mood, risky behaviour e.g. sexual activity and gambling. They may injure themselves and are at risk of suicide.
3. **Histrionic:** attention seeking and emotional behaviour, melodramatic. They can be sexually provocative.
4. **Narcissistic:*** inflated self-regard and need for attention.

C. Anxious and fearful thinking and behaviours

1. **Avoidant:** shy, sensitive to criticism, avoids encounters with others, particularly with strangers.
2. **Dependent:** fears being alone, excessively dependent on others, lacks self-confidence.
3. **Obsessive compulsive:** preoccupied with orderliness and rules. Controlling of self, situations and others; rigid values. This is a different condition from obsessive–compulsive disorder, which is an anxiety problem.

*Narkissos in Greek legend fell in love with his own reflection and pined away.

LIST 46.2

EXAMPLES OF IMPORTANT PSYCHIATRIC ILLNESSES

Some mental or possible mental disorders present as possible medical illnesses (see Table 46.1).

Patients with personality disorders have patterns of behaviour and thought that differ from that person's cultural norm. These characteristics are deeply entrenched and stable over long periods. They cause the patient considerable distress and usually begin in adolescence. The diagnosis requires evidence of problems across most areas of a person's life over many years. In some instances they may not be aware of the nature of their behaviour or interactions. List 46.2 sets out the current classification of these disorders.

Disorders that lead to physical illness

Eating disorders put patients at risk of physical illness and can be associated with a high mortality. There are three main types: binge eating and purging (bulimia nervosa), restricting without binge eating (anorexia nervosa), and binge-eating disorder (BED).

MEDICAL COMPLICATIONS OF BULIMIA NERVOSA

- Electrolyte changes and arrhythmias—a result of underweight and use of diuretics and purgatives
- Oesophagitis
- Mallory–Weiss oesophageal tears
- Oesophageal rupture
- Depression, anxiety, suicide risk

LIST 46.3

1. **Bulimia nervosa** is a condition in which frequent (more than once a week) episodes of binge eating are followed by compensating behaviours that are promoted by fear of weight gain. These include induced vomiting, and use of laxatives, enemas or diuretics. Patients are at risk of the medical complications summarised in List 46.3.

   Examination findings include erosion of dental enamel from vomiting, parotid gland enlargement, xerosis (dryness of the mouth, eyes and skin) and scarring on the dorsum or knuckles of the hand used to induce vomiting (Russell's sign).[b,8] The sign is not present if an object such as a pencil or toothbrush is used to induce vomiting.
2. **Anorexia nervosa** is associated with a considerable mortality risk. It occurs predominantly in women. They aggressively restrict food intake because of a distorted body image and fear of gaining weight. Adolescent girls and young women are most commonly affected. The severe medical complications are slightly different from those of bulimia nervosa (List 46.4).

   Amenorrhoea is common but no longer required for the diagnosis. The examination findings include: emaciation, xerosis, brittle hair and nails, bradycardia, hypothermia, oedema and lanugo.[c]

MEDICAL COMPLICATIONS AND ASSOCIATIONS OF ANOREXIA NERVOSA

- Loss of bone density (more than 30% of patients)
- Sinus bradycardia
- Hypotension
- Hypothermia
- Electrolyte changes—hypokalaemia, hypomagnesaemia, hypophosphataemia
- Cardiac arrhythmias including ventricular tachycardia associated with the long QT interval caused by electrolyte changes
- Depression, anxiety, suicide risk

LIST 46.4

3. **Binge-eating disorder** is defined as more-than-weekly episodes over 3 months or more of eating more food and eating more rapidly than normally. Patients feel lack of control of their eating. Unlike people who are merely greedy, these patients feel guilt and self-disgust after eating, often eat secretly to avoid embarrassment and feel physically uncomfortable after eating too much.

Schizophrenia

This psychotic illness is associated with an increased risk of death (2–3 times), of suicide (13 times) and of cardiovascular disease (twice). Patients have increased rates of cardiovascular risk factors including: hypertension, smoking, hyperlipidaemia, obesity and diabetes. They need medical assessment and help with these problems, some of which are exacerbated by their medication.

The condition begins usually in adolescence. At least two of the following symptoms are required for the diagnosis:

- hallucinations
- delusions
- disorganised or catatonic behaviour
- disorganised speech
- negative symptoms—a flattened affect, alogia, avolition.[d]

[b] Gerald Russell, b. 1928, a British psychiatrist who published the first description of bulimia nervosa in 1979.

[c] This is short, colourless, downy hair like that which covers unborn babies from the fourth month of gestation. It can also grow on people with malignancies. Lana means wool in Latin and lanugo means the downy hair that covers some plants and the cheeks of young people.

[d] Not talking, not doing anything spontaneously.

MEDICAL CONDITIONS THAT MAY RESEMBLE DEPRESSION

- Hypothyroidism
- Androgen deficiency
- Menopause
- Parkinson disease
- Multiple sclerosis
- Chronic illness—HIV infection, heart failure
- Drug treatment—interferons, chemotherapeutic agents

HIV=human immunodeficiency virus.

LIST 46.5

The symptoms must interfere with work, study, relations with other people or self-care, and have been present for 6 months. (See Questions box 46.9.)

Depression

About a fifth of women and 10% of men experience depression during their lives. The peak age of onset is 40 for women and 55 for men. Depression is both more common in people with medical illnesses and adversely affects their recovery. Depression is a common reason for presentation to a doctor and a few simple questions can help the clinician decide whether depression is a major problem.

A number of medical conditions can resemble depression (see List 46.5).

Major depressive disorder

The current diagnosis of this requires that the patient has five of the following symptoms within a 2-week period including at least symptom 1 or 2:

1. Mood is depressed most of the time—reported either by the patient or by others—with feelings of hopelessness and sadness.
2. Greatly reduced interest in life, activities or pleasure most of the time.
3. Unintended loss or gain in weight or appetite.
4. Sleeping poorly or too much.
5. Agitation or psychomotor retardation every day.
6. Loss of energy and fatigue.
7. Inability to concentrate.
8. Feelings of worthlessness or guilt.
9. Recurrent thoughts of death and of suicide.

Persistent depressive disorder (dysthymia)

This is a less severe illness than major depressive illness. The criteria are similar but symptoms occur on most days rather than on nearly every day and over an extended period, often years. Thoughts of suicide are less prominent. Periods of more severe major depression are common.

Seasonal affective disorder

These patients have 3 successive years of major symptoms of depression beginning in the autumn or winter and resolving in spring. More women than men are affected.

Peripartum depression

This condition is no longer called postpartum depression as 50% of women develop their symptoms during pregnancy. Up to 15% of women are affected within 6 months of giving birth. It is considered a major depressive disorder.

Bipolar disorder

People affected by this relatively common mood disorder (1% of people) have periods of mania or hypomania (see Table 46.1), usually with a history of major depressive disorder. The onset is usually in early adult life. Most patients also have periods of depression. The features of an episode of mania include:

- abnormally euphoric or irritable mood
- pressured speech
- flight of ideas
- grandiosity (inflated self-importance)
- agitation
- disinhibited behaviour (spending sprees, sexual promiscuity)
- little need for sleep
- severe disruption of normal life.

Bipolar I disorder is diagnosed after one or more manic episodes lasting at least a week. Bipolar II disorder is diagnosed when patients have less severe symptoms of mania (hypomania) that last at least 4 days. These patients have episodes of major depression.

Anxiety disorders

Panic disorder

Up to 30% of people have a panic attack during their lives but panic disorder is much less common. Patients with panic disorder have recurrent and unexpected periods of extreme anxiety that builds up in minutes. The features include at least four of the following:

- sweating
- trembling
- a choking sensation
- breathlessness
- chest pain
- abdominal pain
- nausea
- dizziness
- feeling hot or cold
- paraesthesias
- a feeling of being separated from self
- fear of dying
- fear of losing control of oneself.

For the diagnosis to be made, attacks must be followed by a least a month of anxiety that another attack will occur. Because there are so many physical symptoms the condition may be diagnosed as a medical condition. Certain other medical conditions may need to be excluded including:

- hyperthyroidism
- phaeochromocytoma
- drug use
- myocardial infarction
- acute abdomen.

Generalised anxiety disorder (GAD)

Women are affected more than men. Some of the symptoms are like those of panic attacks but less dramatic in onset (see Table 46.1). They include:

- sweats
- abdominal pain
- palpitations and tachycardia
- chest pain
- breathlessness
- fatigue
- diarrhoea
- inability to sleep
- a feeling of muscle tension
- headache
- tremor.

Many patients have multiple unexplained physical symptoms.

A number of criteria are required for the diagnosis of GAD. These include:

- Anxiety that seems excessive about activities or events (e.g. work, school, social events) occurring on more days than not and for 6 months or more.
- Acknowledgment from the patient that the worry is difficult to control.
- The worry itself is associated with three or more of the following: restlessness, fatigue, irritability, insomnia, tiredness, difficulty in concentrating or muscle tension.
- The symptoms interfere with life—work or school.
- There is no other medical or drug cause for the symptoms.

Social anxiety disorder

This used to be called social phobia. The lifetime occurrence is about 2.5% of people. Patients with this condition have a persisting exaggerated fear of public performances (e.g. public speaking) or of unfamiliar social situations (e.g. meeting new people). The symptoms last for 6 months or longer. The anxiety is accompanied by physical symptoms such as breathlessness, flushing and palpitations. Patients realise their anxiety is excessive but may go to great lengths to avoid situations that bring them on. Their normal lives (work, etc.) are affected by their symptoms.

Post-traumatic stress disorder (PTSD)

PTSD occurs to people in response to seeing or directly experiencing traumatic events such as violence, threatened death, sexual assault or finding out about such an event happening to someone close. The diagnosis requires at least 1 month of symptoms that include upsetting memories of the events, nightmares or flashbacks. Patients avoid reminders and have a persisting change in mood and thoughts. There are changes in arousal: sleep disturbances, hypervigilance, startle reactions and sometimes risky behaviours.[9]

Risk factors for PTSD include: severe traumatic events, other stressors (loss of job, marriage failure), parental neglect, and history within the family or for the patient of another psychiatric illness. Many patients have other psychiatric problems including depression, anxiety and alcohol or drug problems. They are at increased risk of suicide, marriage failure and loss of employment.

Obsessive–compulsive disorder (OCD)

Obsession is defined as the occurrence of intrusive and persistent thoughts, impulses or images that cause distress (see Table 46.1). Compulsions are repetitive behaviours such as counting, inspecting, hand washing or saying ritualised phrases in order to offset the anxiety the obsession causes. These thoughts and actions cause difficulty with normal daily activities, waste time and cause distress. About 2% of women and men are affected.

T&O'C ESSENTIALS

1. *The psychiatric interview can be therapeutic as well as diagnostic.*
2. *The mental state examination is a routine part of the assessment of a patient with suspected cognitive impairment.*
3. *It may take a number of interviews with a patient to gain his or her confidence.*
4. *Open-ended questions are more likely to produce accurate responses.*
5. *Depression is often overlooked. Ask the patient about current symptoms of depression in the setting of any chronic physical illness or alcohol abuse, or whether he or she has a past history of depression.*
6. *An acute decline in cognition suggests delirium, which usually has a medical cause.*

OSCE REVISION TOPICS – THE PSYCHIATRIC HISTORY AND THE MENTAL STATE EXAMINATION

Use these topics, which commonly occur in the OSCE, to help with revision.

1. Please perform a mini-mental examination on this patient who has had recent memory problems. (p 889)
2. This woman has had recent problems with anxiety. Please take a history from her. (p 880)
3. This thin woman has been very concerned about being overweight. Please take a history from her. (p 883)
4. This man has been troubled by disturbing thoughts. Please take a history from him. (p 882)

References

1. Kopelman MD. Structured psychiatric interview: psychiatric history and assessment of the mental state. *Br J Hosp Med* 1994; 52:93–98. Know how to take a psychiatric history.
2. Arroll B, Khin N, Kerse N. Screening for depression in primary care with two verbally asked questions: cross sectional study. *BMJ* 2003; 327:1144–1146. Two questions help identify depression: one positive answer should be followed up.
3. Gilbody S, Sheldon T, Wessely S. Should we screen for depression? *BMJ* 2006; 332:1027–1030. Routinely screening for depression in practice is questioned because of the low pre-test probability.
4. Drossman DA, Talley NJ, Lesserman J et al. Sexual and physical abuse and gastrointestinal illness. *Ann Intern Med* 1995; 123:782–794. An excellent clinical summary of abuse in the genesis of illness and how to screen for abuse.
5. Johnson J, Sims R, Gottlieb G. Differential diagnosis of dementia, delirium and depression. Implications for drug therapy. *Drugs and Aging* 1994; 5:431–445. The differential diagnosis hinges on a careful clinical evaluation. Dementia is defined as a chronic loss of intellectual or cognitive function of sufficient severity to interfere with social or occupational function. Delirium is an acute disturbance of consciousness marked by an attention deficit and a change in cognitive ability.
6. Folstein MF, Folstein SE, McHugh PR. Mini Mental State. A practical method for grading the cognitive state of patients for the clinician. *J Psychiatr Res* 1975; 12:189–198. This is a useful instrument but is now copyright protected (see Wikipedia for details).
7. Borson S, Scanlan J, Brush M et al. The Mini-Cog: a cognitive 'vital signs' measure for dementia screening in multi-lingual elderly. *Int J Geriatr Psychiatry* 2000; 15(11):1021–1027. A useful and quick screening test for dementia.
8. Russell G. Bulimia nervosa: an ominous variant of anorexia nervosa. *Psychol Med* 1979; 9(3):429–448.
9. Spoont MR, Williams JW Jr, Kehle-Forbes S et al. Does this patient have posttraumatic stress disorder?: Rational clinical examination systematic review. *JAMA* 2015; 314(5):501–510.

SECTION 14

Acute care and end of life

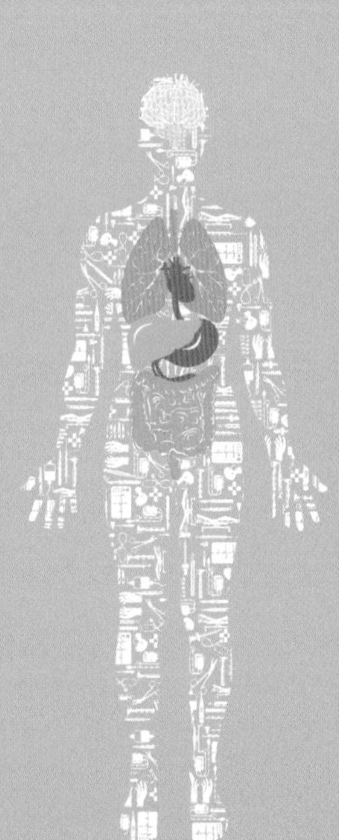

CHAPTER 47

The acutely ill patient

To be or not to be? That is the question. WILLIAM SHAKESPEARE (1564 – 1616), Hamlet

INITIAL ASSESSMENT

During your training, you will be expected to become expert in advanced life support and this training must be refreshed regularly. If you come across an obviously very ill patient, the first step is to ask, 'Are you okay?' If the patient is unresponsive on gentle shaking, quickly check whether the airway is patent and if he or she is breathing, then rapidly assess the circulation. This should all take no more than 10 seconds. Start cardiopulmonary resuscitation (CPR; see Fig. 47.1) if the patient is not breathing (or is just gasping) or has no pulse, and try to send someone else to call for help. Current guidelines emphasise the importance of adequate chest compressions during CPR (at least 100 / minute, compressing the centre of the chest 5 centimetres with each downward compression, and no interruptions—remember to push hard and fast).[1]

If the patient is clearly responding appropriately to questions, and the skin is normal in colour as well as warm and dry, the patient is much less likely to need urgent intervention before appropriate history taking and a full examination are completed. If the patient's level of consciousness becomes impaired, recheck the **a**irway, **b**reathing and **c**irculation (**ABCs**), check the serum glucose (you must not miss hypoglycaemia) and obtain intravenous access immediately.

An acutely ill patient who presents to hospital may be able to give some history. Ask:

- What is wrong?
- What has happened?'
- Have you been injured? Are you in pain anywhere?

If possible, while beginning your physical assessment (see Fig. 47.2) ask about previous medical problems such as heart disease, diabetes, asthma or depression. If the patient is accompanied by others, ask these people if they have any more information. Look for an alert bracelet and for a list of medications in the patient's pockets or wallet.

LEVEL OF CONSCIOUSNESS

Assess the patient's **level of consciousness** using the **AVPU** system:

A lert (normal)
V erbal stimulus responsive
P ainful stimulus responsive
U nresponsive patient.

If the patient only responds to a painful stimulus or is unresponsive, assess him or her using the Glasgow Coma Scale (see Table 35.4, p 623).[2]

Gather key data, as summarised by the mnemonic **AMPLE**:

A llergies
M edication currently being taken and most recent medications taken
P ast medical history
L ast meal
E vents preceding the current incident.

If the patient is tachypnoeic, check pulse oximetry and start oxygen therapy unless there is a known contraindication.

If the patient is bradycardic or tachycardic, obtain an ECG.

DELIRIUM

Delirium is an acute change in cognitive function that occurs over hours or a few days. It is often associated with acute medical conditions and therefore is often seen in hospital patients. It is important that it be recognised and the cause removed or treated. Risk factors include:

Resuscitation.

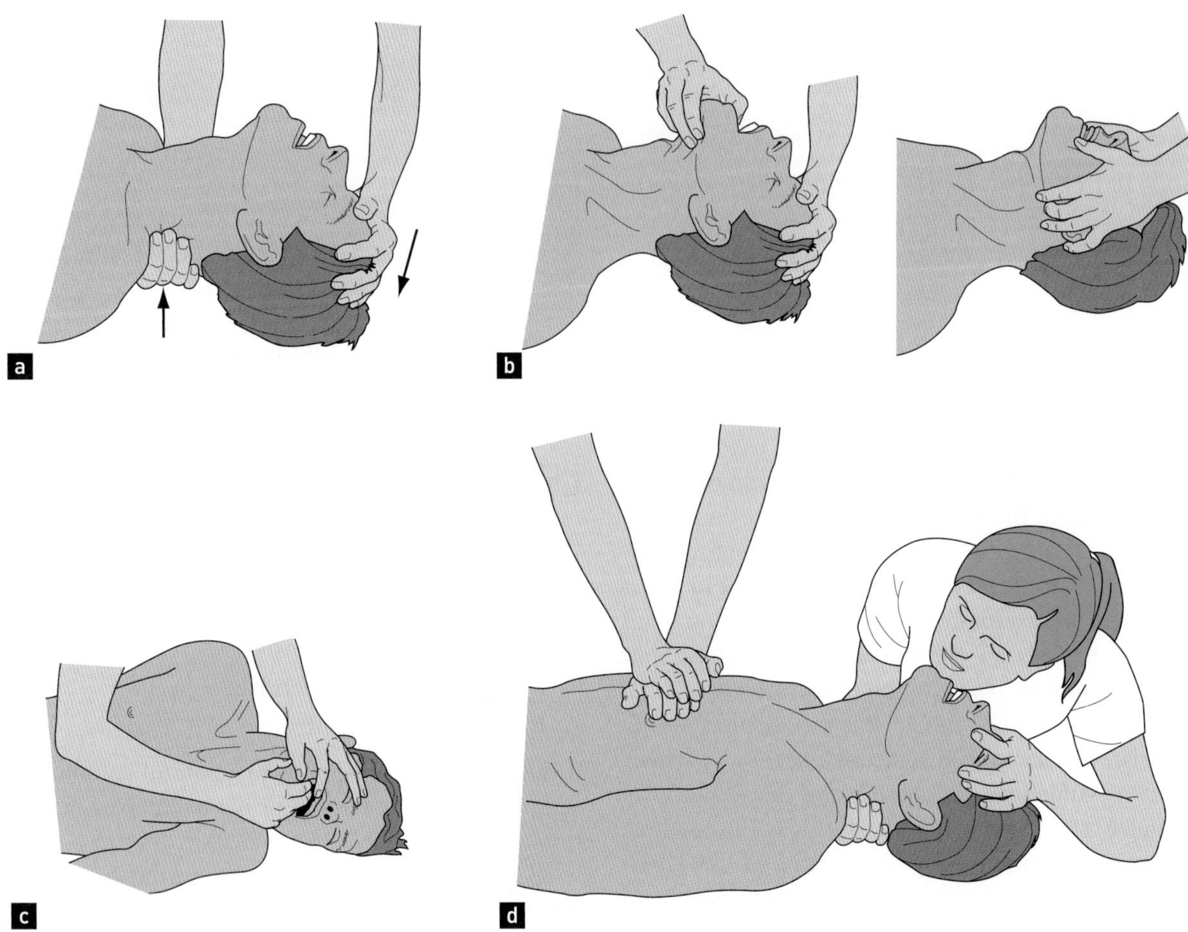

(a) Head-tilt; (b) jaw-thrust and jaw-tilt manoeuvres to open the airway; (c) clearing the airway; (d) cardiopulmonary resuscitation

(Baker T, Nikolic G, O'Connor S. *Practical cardiology*, 2nd edn. Sydney: Elsevier, 2008.)

FIGURE 47.1

- pre-existing dementia or other neurological disease, e.g. Parkinson's disease
- severe illness, e.g. mechanical ventilation
- age over 65
- alcoholism.

The diagnosis should be considered in all patients with risk factors. Relatives or nursing staff may be concerned about the patient's being confused. Ask the staff or relatives about typical features (Questions box 47.1).

A diagnosis of delirium is confirmed if the answers to questions 1 and 2 are 'yes' and that to either or both 3 and 4 is also 'yes'.

If delirium seems confirmed, look into possible causes (List 47.1)

FURTHER EXAMINATION

(See List 47.2.)

Check the patient's blood pressure and other vital signs. Assess fluid status (see Ch 18). If the patient is hypotensive, consider an intravenous fluid challenge, and organise to regularly measure the heart rate, blood pressure, respiratory rate and hourly urinary output (if necessary by inserting a urinary catheter).

Assess the capillary refill time by depressing the finger- or toenail until it blanches and recording the

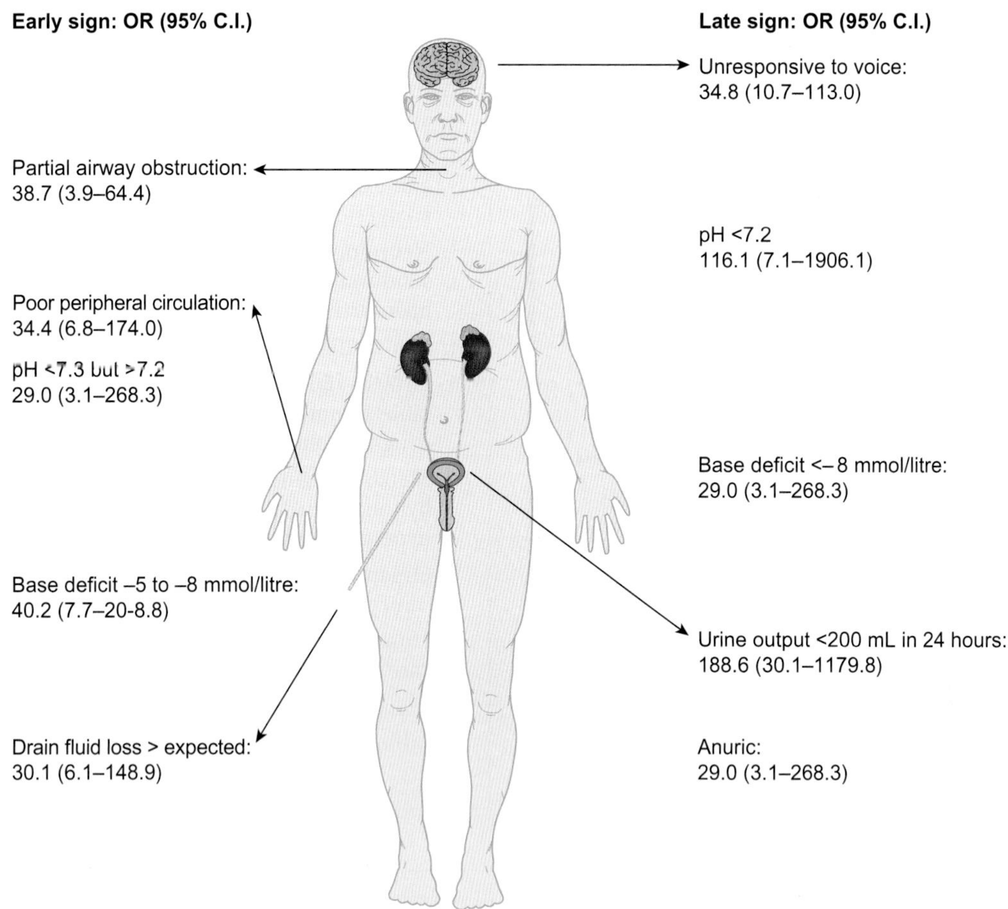

Assessment of the acutely ill patient: 'Top five' early and late signs of physiological deterioration with the odds ratio (OR) for death (95% confidence interval)

A=Airway

Obstructed? Look for injury

B=Breathing

1. Inspect chest for trauma
2. Look for chest wall movement
3. Is the patient using the accessory muscle of respiration?
4. Auscultate lungs for equal breath sounds

C=Circulation

1. Pulse: radial or femoral; rate and rhythm
2. Blood pressure
3. Perfusion: colour, temperature

D=Disability

1. Conscious state: Glasgow Coma Scale (see Table 35.4, p 623)
2. Pupillary responses
3. Abnormal movements: epileptiform
4. Localising signs (e.g. hyperreflexia)

Other

1. Signs of injury
2. Medical alert bracelet
3. Medication list in pocket

(Robertson LC. Recognizing the critically ill patient. *Anaesthesia and Intensive Care Medicine*, 2013; 14(1):11–14.)

FIGURE 47.2

QUESTIONS TO ASK RELATIVES OR STAFF ABOUT A PATIENT WHO MAY HAVE DELIRIUM

1. Has there been a recent change in the patient's mental state and has this been coming and going during the day or been worse at night?
2. Does the patient have difficulty in concentrating or following things said to him or her? Is he or she easily distracted?
3. Does he or she seem to have incoherent thinking with rambling conversation? Is there odd switching from one idea to another?
4. Does the patient seem alert, drowsy or comatose, or to have increased alertness (vigilance or agitation)?

QUESTIONS BOX 47.1

IMPORTANT CAUSES OF DELIRIUM

1. Infections—especially urinary tract infections and pneumonia
2. Surgery—postoperative delirium is common and exacerbated by anaesthetic drugs and analgesics
3. Neurological illnesses—stroke, seizures, subdural haematoma, intracranial haemorrhage
4. Myocardial infarction
5. Drugs—opioids, sedatives (including sleeping tablets), anticonvulsants, anti-Parkinsonian drugs, alcohol or drug withdrawal
6. Metabolic abnormalities—hypoxia, hyponatraemia, hypoglycaemia or hyperglycaemia, hypercarbia
7. Organ failure—heart failure, acute kidney injury
8. Hospital ward—sensory deprivation (intensive care ward), lack of sleep
9. Urinary retention

Combinations of these causes are common.

LIST 47.1

SIGNS OF A CRITICALLY ILL PATIENT

1. Respiratory signs
   - Stridor and intercostal recession
   - Threatened or obstructed airway (e.g. from injury or swelling; angio-oedema—see Fig. 47.4)
   - Abnormal respiratory rate >35 breaths / minute or <8 breaths / minute
   - No spontaneous respiratory effort
   - Respiratory distress: use of accessory muscles, unable to speak in sentences (e.g. severe asthma)
   - Abnormal oximetry: S_pO_2 <90% even with supplementary oxygen
   - Increasing P_aCO_2: blood gas measurements (indicates reduced respiratory effort)
2. Cardiovascular signs
   - Absent pulse
   - Heart rate <40 or >180 b.p.m.
   - Systolic blood pressure <100 mmHg (where blood pressure previously normal)
   - Poor peripheral perfusion (suggests tissue hypoxia)
   - Low urine output: <0.5 mL / kg / h (urinary catheter in situ)
   - ECG—asystole (no cardiac rhythm), ventricular fibrillation, fast ventricular tachycardia, complete heart block
3. Neurological signs
   - Airway threatened by absent gag reflex
   - Not obeying commands
   - Not responding to painful stimuli
   - Moving only one side in response to stimuli (stroke, cerebral haemorrhage)
   - Reduced respiratory rate
   - Sudden reduction in level of consciousness
   - Pupil size and reaction to light (pinpoint pupils suggest a pontine haemorrhage)
   - Recurrent seizures (tonic–clonic movements)
   - Glasgow Coma Scale score <10 (see Table 35.4, p 623)

LIST 47.2

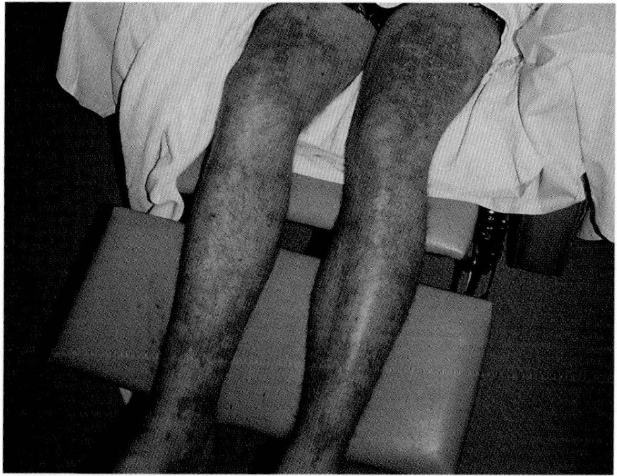

Meningococcal rash

(Courtesy of Dr A Watson, Infectious Diseases Department, The Canberra Hospital.)

FIGURE 47.3

time it takes for the colour to become normal again, which is usually less than 2 seconds. A delayed capillary refill time occurs in hypovolaemic or cardiogenic shock.

Examine the patient's chest for any obvious evidence of tension pneumothorax—features include unilateral pleuritic chest pain, respiratory distress, decreased breath sounds and increased percussion over the affected side, tachycardia and hypotension, tracheal deviation (away from affected side), palpable subcutaneous emphysema and greatly distended neck veins.

Assess the patient for possible cardiac tamponade (features include dypspnoea, tachycardia, hypotension, distended neck veins, difficult-to-hear heart sounds, and pulsus paradoxus).

Examine the body for any evidence of obvious bleeding or other trauma.[3]

Look at the skin for a meningococcal rash (see Fig. 47.3). Angio-oedema (see Fig. 47.4) can occur in anaphylaxis.

Measure the patient's temperature. If it is elevated, consider taking blood and urine cultures.

The **systemic inflammatory response syndrome (SIRS)** refers to two or more of the following four features: fever >38.3°C (or temperature <36°C), tachycardia (>90 beats / min), tachypnoea (>20 breaths / min) and an elevated white cell count (although it may be suppressed).

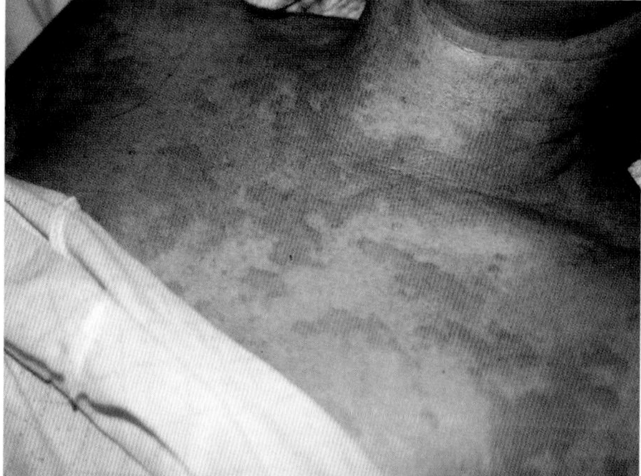

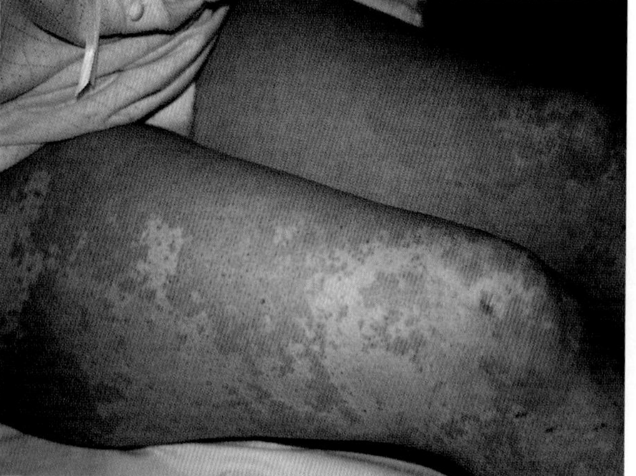

Angio-oedema

(Courtesy of Dr A Watson, Infectious Diseases Department, The Canberra Hospital.)

FIGURE 47.4

SIRS may be due to acute infection but can also occur after burns or surgery or with other inflammatory diseases (e.g. thromboembolism, pancreatitis, vasculitis, autoimmune disease). Sepsis refers to the presence of infection in the setting of SIRS, so SIRS is sensitive but not specific for bacteraemia. Early identification of sepsis remains a clinical diagnosis, and immediate treatment with antibiotics saves lives.[4]

A useful prognostic score in sepsis is the quick sequential organ failure assessment (SOFA) score (1 point each for: a high respiratory rate—22 or higher per minute, low systolic blood pressure—100 mmHg or lower, and altered mentation; 2 or more indicates a poor outcome).[4]

OSCE EXAMPLE – EMERGENCY CARE

Mr Sherlock has had episodes of sudden loss of consciousness. Please examine him.

1. Assess the patient's level of consciousness, and test orientation in time, place and person.
2. Neurological examination: examine the patient's gait, then limbs and cranial nerves, looking for focal neurological signs (stroke, intracranial tumour).
3. Note whether there are tongue lacerations (seizures).
4. Auscultate for carotid bruits (carotid stenosis).
5. Take the patient's pulse (arrhythmias including atrial fibrillation or heart block) and blood pressure lying and sitting (postural hypotension).
6. Examine the praecordium (signs of new murmurs, tamponade).
7. Take the patient's temperature and assess for neck stiffness (sepsis, meningism).

References

1. Berg RA, Hemphill R, Abella BS et al. Part 5: adult basic life support: 2010 American Heart Association Guidelines for Cardiopulmonary Resuscitation and Emergency Cardiovascular Care. *Circulation* 2010; 122:S685–S705. Know how to do basic and advanced cardiac life support—and remain competent.
2. Easter JS, Haukoos JS, Meehan WP et al. Will neuroimaging reveal a severe intracranial injury in this adult with minor head trauma?: The Rational Clinical Examination Systematic Review. *JAMA* 2015; 314(24):2672–2681. Following head trauma, a patient may initially appear fine (Glasgow Coma Scale [GCS] scores ≥13) yet still have severe intracranial injury as documented by head CT scan. A history of being struck by a car (LR up to 4.3) or two or more vomiting episodes (LR 3.6) is worrying. Examine for physical signs of a skull fracture (LR 16). Watch for a decline of GCS score.
3. Joshi N, Lira A, Mehta N et al. Diagnostic accuracy of history, physical examination, and bedside ultrasound for diagnosis of extremity fractures in the emergency department: a systematic review. *Acad Emerg Med* 2013; 20(1):1–15. Physical examination is not sufficient to diagnose a limb fracture: an X-ray remains the gold standard.
4. Singer M, Deutschman CS, Seymour CW et al. The Third International Consensus Definitions for Sepsis and Septic Shock (Sepsis-3). *JAMA* 2016; 315(8):801–810.

CHAPTER 48

The pre-anaesthetic medical evaluation (PAME)

Whenever ideas fail, men invent words. MARTIN H FISHER (1879–1962)

An appropriate medical evaluation of the patient who has been admitted for elective surgery is always required. It includes a history and examination that is sufficient to uncover any likely major problems with anaesthesia or the procedure itself.

THE HISTORY

The first thing to find out, of course, is the presenting problem, what operation is intended and whether the surgery is expected to be performed under general or local anaesthesia. Clearly the assessment of a patient having a small lesion removed under local anaesthesia can be briefer than the assessment of a patient undergoing extensive bowel resection under general anaesthesia. As a rule, before any patient undergoes surgery under general anaesthesia or spinal anaesthesia, careful attention must be given to identifying whether he or she is at higher risk.

Cardiovascular history

The most important questions here relate to a history of ischaemic heart disease. Patients who have had a myocardial infarct in the preceding 3 months should not usually undergo elective surgery; the risks of further infarction or malignant arrhythmia and death are high during this period. A patient who has symptoms of angina that have recently become unstable is also at greater risk. A history of stable angina that has not changed for months or years is not a contraindication to most forms of surgery. The recent placement of a coronary stent may mean that cessation of antiplatelet drugs is not safe for 1 month after insertion of a bare metal stent and 6 months to 1 year after the insertion of a drug-eluting stent.

Symptoms of cardiac failure should be sought. Any patient with uncontrolled cardiac failure is at considerable risk of severe cardiac failure postoperatively. This is particularly true if large amounts of intravenous fluids are given during and after surgery while the patient's antifailure drugs (e.g. diuretics) are omitted.

Cardiac drugs should be asked about, particularly antianginal and antifailure drugs. It is important to attempt to ensure that the patient receives these drugs, particularly beta-blockers, on the day of the operation. The surgeon may require the patient to stop aspirin a week or more before surgery. This is usually a safe thing for the patient to do but may be a problem in the first month at least after a coronary angioplasty because of the risk of thrombosis of the stent in this early period. Previous coronary artery bypass grafting or angioplasty is not a contraindication to surgery.

A history of infective endocarditis or the presence of a prosthetic cardiac valve or complex congenital cardiac condition is an indication for antibiotic prophylaxis for any procedure that may result in bacteraemia—the circulation of bacteria in the bloodstream. These procedures include most types of dental work and surgery on the bowel or bladder and some gynaecological operations and vaginal delivery.

Patients who take oral anticoagulants such as warfarin or the new oral anticoagulants (dabigatran, apixaban or rivaroxaban) require special attention. When the drug is being used to protect the patient from embolic events associated with atrial fibrillation it may be reasonable, on the balance of risks, to have the drug stopped an appropriate period before surgery and resumed as soon as practical afterwards. If the patient takes the drug to protect a mechanical heart valve from clot, the drug should, in general, be replaced by intravenous unfractionated or subcutaneous fractionated heparin. The last dose of fractionated heparin can be given about 12 hours before surgery and the drug recommenced as soon as the surgeon feels it is safe. Many patients can administer the drug themselves at home. Patients with mechanical valves, especially in the mitral position, are at high risk of embolic events if their warfarin is stopped without replacement with some form of heparin.

The presence of a cardiac pacemaker or implanted defibrillator may be a problem if the surgeon intends to use a diathermy device.

The respiratory history

Enquire about a history of respiratory disease, particularly chronic obstructive pulmonary disease or severe asthma. Patients who have continued to smoke up to the time of their surgery have a much higher risk of postoperative chest infections than those who have not. Even stopping a few weeks before will reduce this risk. Severe respiratory disease is a relative contraindication to surgery. It may be difficult to reverse the anaesthetic and muscle relaxant drugs in such a patient, and he or she may require ventilation postoperatively. Doctors in charge of intensive care units are always happier to be warned that a patient may require ventilation postoperatively than to have it come as a surprise.

Drug therapy for respiratory disease must be asked about. Steroids may impair wound healing, and steroid doses may need to be increased during the operative period because of steroid-induced adrenal suppression.

Other

Enquire about any history of bleeding diathesis, diabetes mellitus, renal disease, hepatitis, jaundice or drug abuse. The control of blood sugar in diabetic patients can be difficult in the perioperative period, especially while normal diet is impossible. The fasting preoperative diabetic on insulin may need to be advised to have half the normal insulin dose on the morning of surgery. This may be important to avoid ketoacidosis.

Specific enquiries about *previous operations and anaesthetics*, particularly with reference to any complications, should be made. *Allergies* to anaesthetic agents or other drugs must be asked about. Attempt to distinguish a true allergy or anaphylaxis from an adverse effect such as vomiting after a morphine injection. Some operations involve the use of contrast media, and an allergy to iodine may be a contraindication to their use. This risk is now much less with the new non-ionic contrast media. There may occasionally be a *family history of anaesthetic complications* or deaths. This raises the possibility of malignant hyperthermia, which is an inherited disorder leading to fever and muscle destruction after administration of muscle relaxants.

Ask about exercise tolerance. How far can the patient walk? How many flights of stairs can the patient climb? Poor functional status is indicated by an inability to walk one or two blocks on the flat.

THE EXAMINATION

Examination according to the rapid screening method outlined in Chapter 51 represents the best approach. Record height, weight and vital signs (pulse rate, blood pressure, respiratory rate). The cardiovascular and respiratory systems must be fully examined. Patients with a short thick neck may be difficult to ventilate and intubate. It is better for the anaesthetist to be aware of this possible problem before the patient is given a muscle relaxant and is unable to breathe spontaneously. The presence of loose or fragile teeth must also be noted because of the risk of their dislodgement during attempted intubation.

If a previously undiagnosed symptom or sign of significance is uncovered, some further investigations may be required before surgery, and the operation may have to be deferred. For example, the discovery of a new and significant heart murmur, uncontrolled hypertension, respiratory failure, a bleeding diathesis, uncontrolled diabetes mellitus or renal failure should be brought to the attention of the surgeon and anaesthetist.

CHAPTER 49

Assessment of death

I'm not afraid of death; I just don't want to be there when it happens. WOODY ALLAN

We all die eventually, although most of us try not to ruminate on the subject. The certification of a patient's death is one of the legal responsibilities of a doctor. The experience can be distressing for the doctor as well as the patient's relatives. Students should be given the opportunity to observe senior colleagues performing these tasks and to learn what is required technically and emotionally. Clearly, the declaration that a patient has died must be correct, as well as sympathetically performed.

Death is not easy to define in absolute terms but generally means brain death—an irreversible loss of consciousness, usually but not always linked to an irreversible loss of spontaneous respiration.

ASSESSMENT

If you are called to assess an unresponsive patient, do *not* assume that the patient has died: start cardiopulmonary resuscitation (CPR) immediately (see p 868) and call for help, *unless* there is a confirmed and current advance care directive or resuscitation plan.

Do-not-resuscitate (DNR) orders

Most hospitals have specific policies in place about resuscitation. Patients have the right to make a *living will* or *advance directive* outlining their wishes concerning resuscitation; for example, a patient with a terminal condition can elect to refuse CPR or life support if cardiac arrest occurs. The directive, if known, should be honoured. Remember, however, that if the patient had changed his or her mind before collapsing and notified staff verbally, the current verbal decision rather than the written directive must be honoured (i.e. you should provide CPR or life support). Sometimes, directives may be more specific. For example, a directive may forbid intubation. It would be wrong in this case to deny the patient an attempt at cardioversion from ventricular fibrillation, but it may be reasonable not to proceed to more invasive resuscitation. If the patient is unknown to you, it is important to err on the side of caution and begin resuscitation.

Do not misdiagnose death

The dead patient is unresponsive, has no spontaneous respiratory movements, has no pulse or heart sounds, is very pale and usually the eyes are open and blankly staring. Red–purple discoloration in gravity-dependent areas occurs about half an hour after death, while rigor mortis (muscle stiffening) occurs hours later.

Note that death can be and has been diagnosed in error most often in patients on a ventilator. Important conditions to exclude before declaring a person is dead include:

- hypothermia
- near-drowning
- drug overdose (especially alcohol and tranquillisers)
- hypoglycaemia
- other causes of deep coma, or severe catatonia.

In these cases, some cardiac and respiratory activity will be present.

Examining a suspected death

List 49.1 summarises the physical examination to confirm death. After brain death there may still be spontaneous movements from the denervated spinal cord or peripheral nerves—examples include flexion of the neck, elbows and trunk (when dramatic, known as the 'Lazarus sign') or finger flexor movements.

Remember, certifying death has medicolegal consequences. As a doctor you will be required to examine the patient and record your findings in the medical record, including the date and time that life became extinct. Where possible, you should include the likely cause of death, and sign your name (legibly). You are required to notify the authorities of any unexpected or suspect death.

Brainstem death

Patients on a *mechanical ventilator* require additional testing to confirm that they are truly dead.

Potentially reversible causes must always be excluded (especially drugs; see above). There have been cases where brain death has been pronounced and the patient has later woken up.

Do not miss the rare **locked-in syndrome**. This can occur following an embolus blocking the basilar artery or some other local injury to the base of the pons. The unfortunate patient is not unconscious at all, but cannot move any face, limb or trunk muscles. You can identify the syndrome by asking the patient to blink once for 'yes' and twice for 'no'; voluntary blinking as well as vertical eye movements are not affected.

Testing protocols are based on the law, which vary by country and state (check the requirements in your state). Traditionally, testing is carried out by two different doctors on two separate occasions, typically 24 hours apart, to ensure that the state is irreversible (but the timing of repeat testing is dependent on the patient's age and likely cause of death). Testing typically includes a physical examination (as per List 49.1), an obvious lack of any response to suctioning the tracheal tube, plus an *ice-water (oculovestibular reflex) test:* no eye response to irrigation of ice-cold water into the ears. If the examination indicates brain death, a *medullary brainstem hypercapnia test* is performed, whereby the ventilator is ceased while giving 100% oxygen and the arterial CO_2 is permitted to rise above a preset threshold (>6.7 kPa). Seeing no respiratory effort after 8–10 minutes indicates that there is no medullary function.

CONFIRMING DEATH: THE PHYSICAL EXAMINATION

Look

- Inspect the chest wall for any movement (nil).
- Look for any spontaneous movements (nil).
- Check the reflexes (eyes) for pupillary response to bright light (fixed, dilated, non-reactive).
- Assess the corneal reflexes (absent response to cottonwool).
- Assess the gag reflex (absent).

Feel

- Palpate the carotid or femoral artery (nil pulse over 1 minute).
- Check for a motor response to pain (nil after supraorbital pressure).

Listen

- Auscultate for heart sounds (nil over 1 minute).
- Auscultate for breath sounds (nil over 3 minutes).

LIST 49.1

INFORMING RELATIVES

Informing relatives is always difficult but is the responsibility of the certifying doctor. It is one of the hardest things doctors have to do. Give the news in person—this will usually be deeply appreciated. Break the bad news professionally and compassionately. Seek a private and quiet environment, speak clearly and concisely, be supportive, respect cultural and religious beliefs and engage the help of the team (e.g. nurse, social worker, and cleric). Relatives often want to know what happened, particularly if the death is unexpected. If the patient is well known to you, you may be able to provide that explanation; if not, you should suggest the relatives arrange to meet the consultant responsible for the patient to discuss the issues.

COMPLETING THE DEATH CERTIFICATE

The death certificate is a legal document. If the death was expected (and not suspect), you should complete the certificate as soon as possible. The World Health Organization (WHO) provides a certificate format that is applied internationally. Certify the disease that led directly to death (in part I of the form), as well as any other diseases that contributed (in part II of the form).

POSTMORTEM

The relatives must agree to a postmortem (PM) before it can be undertaken unless mandated by law. There has been a major decline in the undertaking of postmortems in recent decades because of a reluctance to ask relatives and a community reluctance to agree. If the reasons for the request are communicated clearly and compassionately, many will sign the consent.

Remember, the information gleaned from a postmortem not uncommonly leads to significant surprises about the causes of death, and potentially can inform the profession, helping to prevent future diagnostic and treatment mistakes.

If the cause of death is uncertain, a postmortem becomes even more important, and certain events such as recent surgery or trauma mean the case should be referred to the coroner, who will usually insist on a postmortem examination.

ORGAN DONATION

In settings where there is brain death but mechanical ventilation can be continued, consent to organ donation should be explored and is ethical. The patient's wishes may be known (e.g. on the driver's licence or an organ donation register, or as a result of previous discussion between the patient and relatives). Organ donation may provide some comfort to grieving relatives.

SECTION 15

Adult history taking and examination in the wards and clinics

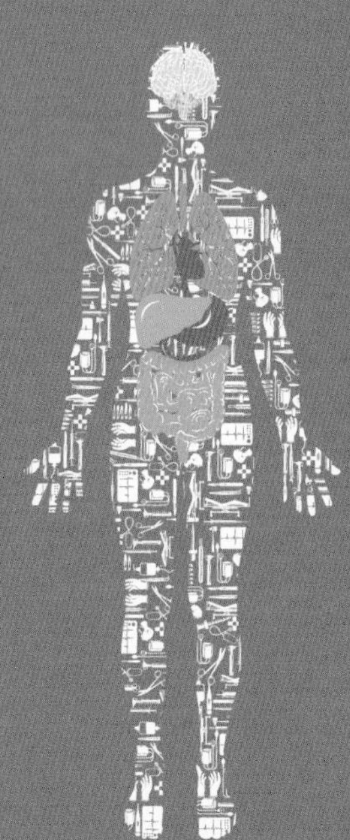

CHAPTER 50

Writing and presenting the adult history and physical examination

Medical education is not completed at the Medical School; it is only begun. WILLIAM H WELCH (1850–1934)

None of us can know what we are capable of until we are tested. ELIZABETH BLACKWELL (1821–1910, first woman in the United States to earn a medical degree)

It is important that the medical record be kept succinct and relevant. The following approach is the one recommended by the authors. The detail of the history and examination and its record varies of course, depending on whether this is a first visit and on the complexity of the presenting problem. It is not necessary to ask every patient every question.

HISTORY

Personal information

Record the name, sex, date of birth and address. Write down the date and time of the examination.

Presenting (principal) symptoms (PS)

A short sentence identifies the major symptoms and their duration; it is often useful to quote the patient's own words.

History of present illness (HPI)

Don't record every detail; rather, prepare short prose paragraphs telling the story of the illness in chronological order. Describe the characteristics of each symptom. Note why the patient presents at this time. Also, describe any past medical problems that are related to the current symptoms. Include the relevant positive and negative findings on the system review here. Note how the diagnosis was reached, side effects and response to treatment. If there are many seemingly unrelated problems, summarise these in an introductory paragraph and present the history of each problem in separate paragraphs.

List current medications and doses and the indications for their use, if they are known, and any side effects, or known or measured therapeutic effects. For example, if the patient takes antihypertensive drugs ask whether blood pressure control has been satisfactory as far as the patient knows, or haemoglobin A_{1c} (HbA_{1C}) if the patient has diabetes mellitus. Finally, record your impression of the reliability of the history and, if the patient was unable to give the history, describe the source of this information.

Past history (PH)

List, in chronological order, past medical or surgical problems (sometimes called inactive problems), past medication use, if relevant, and any history of allergy (particularly drug allergy) or of drug intolerance. Find out what the problem with the drug was. The patient may know the results of certain previous important investigations (e.g. 'The scan showed I had clots in my lung'). A history of blood transfusions should be noted.

Social history (SH)

This may include recording the patient's occupation, schooling, hobbies, marital status, family structure, personal support system, living conditions and recent travel. The number and gender of sexual partners may be relevant. Smoking, alcohol and other recreational drug use should also be described. Ask about ability to perform the activities of daily living (ADL) if elderly. If a patient has a chronic illness, ask about the effect of this on his or life. If it is appropriate, ask about advance care planning.

Family history (FH)

Describe causes of mortality in the first-degree relatives and, if indicated, draw a family tree.

Systems review (SR)

All directly relevant information should be incorporated in the HPI or PH.

PHYSICAL EXAMINATION (PE)

Under each of the major systems, list the relevant positives and negatives using brief statements. (See Ch 51.)

PROVISIONAL DIAGNOSIS

Ask yourself the following questions when considering the differential diagnosis of a patient's major symptoms.

1. What is the likely diagnosis based on the patient's age, sex and background?
2. Are there other conditions that resemble the likely diagnosis but can present in the same way?
3. Is there a serious disorder, even if rare, that must not be missed?
4. Could the patient have a specific condition that often masquerades as (or mimics) other conditions (e.g. depression, drugs, diabetes mellitus, thyroid dysfunction, anaemia, malignancy, spinal cord disease, urinary infection, renal failure, alcoholism, syphilis, tuberculosis, HIV infection, infective endocarditis or connective tissue disease)?
5. Is the patient trying to really tell me that there is an emotional or psychological problem?

An example of a patient history is presented in Box 50.1.

PROBLEM LIST AND PLANS

Using a sentence or two, summarise the most important findings and then give a provisional diagnosis (PD) and differential diagnosis (DD).

Remember Occam's razor: choose the simplest hypothesis to explain any new observations. Also remember Sutton's law: the famous bank robber said he robbed banks because 'That's where the money is'—that is, consider a common diagnosis before resorting to a rare one to explain the symptoms and signs. Older patients are more likely to have multiple co-morbidities.

It is often useful to ask yourself whether the patient's problem is a diagnostic or management one (or both). For example, a patient with the new onset of dyspnoea presents both a diagnostic problem—'What is the cause of the breathlessness?' and a management problem—'How should the condition be treated?' The patient who presents with a worsening of previously diagnosed angina presents only a management problem—'How should the symptoms be treated?'

List all the active problems that require management. Outline the diagnostic tests and therapy planned for each problem.

Sign your name and then print your name and position underneath.

CONTINUATION NOTES

Date (and time) each progress note in the record. The SOAP (**S**ubjective, **O**bjective, **A**ssessment and **P**lans) format can be useful.

Subjective data refer to what the patient tells you; list relevant current problems and note any new problems. Have the patient's previous symptoms improved on the current treatment?

Objective data are physical or laboratory findings; relevant data for each active problem are summarised.

Assessment refers to the interpretation of any relevant findings for each problem.

Plans describe any interventions that will be started for each problem.

Many patient records are now kept in a computer file. Parts of this can be used to provide referral information for the patient to take to a specialist or if he or she is travelling. It is important that such files be kept up to date and especially that lists of medications that are no longer used are deleted from the current list before it is given to the patient.

PRESENTATION[1]

In their formal examinations and less formally on the wards, students and resident medical officers will often be expected to present the history and physical examination of a patient to an examiner or senior colleague. This is excellent training for clinical practice, as the need to discuss patients with colleagues or

An example of an intern hospital admission note

Presenting symptom (PS)

Mr W Witheridge, age 75, a retired botanist, presents with progressive dyspnoea over the past 3 weeks.

History of present illness (HPI)

Progressively worsening dyspnoea over the past 3 weeks. Initially he noticed dyspnoea on exertion but it is now at rest on minimal exertion. Two-day history of orthopnoea, unable to sleep except while sitting in a chair, with associated paroxysmal nocturnal dyspnoea. Currently his exercise toleranceis approximately 10metres. Previously he has only had mild shortness of breath when walking over the last 5 years.

No associated chest tightness or pain on exertion or at rest.

No wheeze.

No cough or sputum.

No fever.

No recent change in medications.

No asthma or known lung disease.

No other relevant positive symptoms on systems review.

Past cardiac history

Previous myocardial infarction 5 years ago, treated with thrombolysis.
No known valvular heart disease or history of rheumatic fever.

Risk factors for heart disease

Hypertension on treatment for 15 years.
Hypercholesterolaemia: total cholesterol 6.7 mmol/L (patient report)but not on a statin because he developed muscle pain.

Smoked 25 cigarettes a day until the time of his infarct—30 pack-years.

Family history of ischaemic heart disease.
No history of diabetes mellitus.

Other symptoms

10 years of nocturia three times per night and urgency during the day. He denies other urinary tract symptoms. No history of known renal disease.

Family history of colon cancer but is not participating in colon cancer screening. No history of gastrointestinal bleeding, weight loss or other alarm symptoms.

Current medications

Aspirin, 100 mg daily; metoprolol (a beta-blocker), 100 mg twice a day,perindopril (ACE inhibitor) 2.5mg daily. Occasional paracetamol. No use of over-the-counter medications.

Past history (PH)

New onset epigastric pain 3 years ago-- peptic ulcer disease secondary H.pylori identified at upper endoscopy, successfully eradicated infection with triple therapy; no recurrence of symptoms.

Appendectomy aged 10.

Tonsillectomy aged 6.

No known drug allergies.

Unsure whether his vaccinations are all up to date.

Social history

Lives in his own home with his wife, who is well.Mobilises independently.

Interests: gardening, history of medicinal plants. No other hobbies.

No pets.

No recent overseas travel.

Family history

Father died of a myocardial infarct at age 64 years.

Mother died of colon cancer at age 54 years.

Both sons (42 and 39 years) are alive and well.

Brother has hypertension.

Physical examination

Breathless and using accessory muscles of respiration at rest.

BOX 50.1

Continued

An example of an intern hospital admission note *continued*

Respiratory rate—24 breaths per minute.

Temperature 37°C.

Oxygen saturation 93% on room air; improving to 98% with 2L oxygen delivered via nasal prongs.

Cardiovascular

No cyanosis. Not clubbed. No splinter haemorrhages.

Pulse rate 90 beats per minute and regular.

Blood pressure 180/110 mmHg lying, with no postural drop on sitting.

Jugular venous pressure (JVP) not elevated.

Apex beat 2 cm displaced, dyskinetic.

Heart sounds (HS): S1 and S2 present and normal; S3 present.

Pansystolic murmur grade 3/6 maximum at the apex consistent with mitral regurgitation.

Chest

Trachea in the midline.

Normal expansion bilaterally.

Normal percussion note bilaterally.

Bilateral medium basal midinspiratory crackles with occasional expiratory wheeze.

No areas of bronchial breathing.

No lymphadenopathy (cervical and axillary).

Abdomen

Well-healed appendix scar present.

Abdomen soft, no tenderness.

Liver, spleen and kidneys not palpable.

No ascites.

Normal bowel sounds.

Rectal examination deferred (the patient was too unwell at the time of admission).

Legs

No calf tenderness.

No peripheral oedema.

Peripheral pulses present and equal.

No visible varicose veins.

Central nervous system (CNS)

Alert and orientated (time, place, person).

No neck stiffness.

Cranial nerves (assessed after initial treatment)

II—acuity and fields normal; fundi normal.

III, IV and VI—pupils equal, circular and concentric—react normally to light and accommodation; eye movements normal; no nystagmus.

V—sensation and motor function normal.

VII—muscles of facial expression normal.

VIII—hearing normal.

IX, X—no uvular displacement.

XI—normal power.

XII—no fasciculation or displacement of tongue.

Upper and lower limbs

No wasting, fasciculations, tremor.

Tone normal.

Power normal.

Reflexes normal and symmetrical.[1]

	Right	Left
Biceps	++	++
Triceps	++	++
Brachioradialis	++	++
Knee	++	++
Ankle	++	++
Plantar response normal	↓	↓

Coordination normal.

Sensation—pain, proprioception normal.[2]

Provisional diagnosis

Left ventricular failure secondary to ischaemicheart disease.

BOX 50.1

Continued

An example of an intern hospital admission note *continued*

Differential diagnosis:

Left ventricular failure secondary to hypertension or mitral regurgitation.

Acute myocardial infarct, acute exacerbation of COPD, bilobar pneumonia and pulmonary embolus are all less likely given the history and clinical findings.

Impression

72-year-old male who presents with:

- *Left sided cardiac failure. This most likely secondary to ischaemic heart disease.*
- *Clinical signs of mitral regurgitation likely secondary to cardiac failure rather than the primary cause of left cardiac failure. This is in the context of no diagnosed history of chronic lung disease; however, he has a 30-pack-year history and may have underlying chronic obstructive pulmonary disease (COPD). The history and examination are not suggestive of pulmonary embolism, acute respiratory infection or acute myocardial ischaemia.*

Investigations and treatment plan

List all major health issues identified in a problem list (here these include left-sided cardiac failure as described above; need for age- and risk factor-appropriate colon cancer screening; urinary urgency and nocturia that may reflect overactive bladder syndrome or prostatic hyperplasia, or possibly urinary tract infection or renal disease; vaccination status uncertain).

Formulate a plan of management (investigations, treatment) under each problem (e.g. family history of colon cancer, no gastrointestinal symptoms-- plan follow-up screening after discharge; request general practitioner follow-up of vaccination status).

1. The reflexes may be recorded as:
   O (absent)
   + (reduced)
   ++ (normal)
   +++ (increased)
   ++++ (exaggerated with clonus)
   ↓ shorthand for downward (normal) Babinski sign (flexor plantar response)
2. In the absence of a history suggesting neurological disease, the normal CNS examination can be summarised in the notes briefly as follows:
   Alert, orientated
   Cranial nerves: grossly normal
   Upper and lower limbs: normal power
   Symmetrical normal reflexes, down-going plantar responses
   Coordination: normal
   Sensation (pain): normal

BOX 50.1

specialists arises frequently in both hospital and non-hospital practice.

A successful case presentation is both succinct and relevant. The examiner is most interested in what the patient's problems are now. One should aim to convey basic biographical information and an assessment of the patient's presenting problem in the first few sentences. It is often helpful to frame the presentation of the case as a diagnostic or management problem, or both.

The information will have been obtained from the patient by taking the history as set out above. The examination of the patient should be performed with particular attention to the areas most likely to be abnormal. This information must then be assembled into a form that can easily be conveyed to others. The following is a suggested method.

1. Begin with a sentence that tells your colleague about the essence of the patient and the clinical problem. For example, one might say 'Mr Jones

is a 72-year-old retired cabinet minister who presents with 2 hours of chest pain which is not typically ischaemic'. This gives an idea about the patient himself and indicates that the problem is likely to be a diagnostic one.

2. One should then go on to explain in what way the pain is atypical of ischaemia and whether it has features suggestive of any other diagnosis.
3. Once the presenting symptom or problem has been described, relevant past history should be discussed. In a patient with chest pain this would include any previous cardiac history or investigations, and a summary of the patient's risk factors for ischaemic heart disease.
4. Present a list of the patient's current medications.
5. Important previous health problems should be outlined briefly. This retired cabinet minister might also have a history of intermittent claudication and of chronic obstructive pulmonary disease. These facts will affect possible treatment for ischaemic heart disease, e.g. the use of beta-blockers.
6. Present the physical examination in two parts.
   a. Abnormal and important normal examination findings in the presenting system—in this patient's case this would mean giving the pulse rate and blood pressure but not details of normal heart sounds. If there was a history of claudication, the examination of the peripheral pulses should be presented even if it is normal.
   b. Abnormal findings in the rest of the examination.
7. Offer the most likely diagnosis and the differential diagnosis.
8. Suggest a plan for investigation and treatment.
9. Much more detail will have been obtained in the assessment of the patient than should be presented routinely, but further details may be asked for by your colleague. These may include information about the patient's living conditions and the availability of support from the family. This may determine how soon the patient can be sent home from hospital after treatment.

By the end of your presentation your colleague should know what you think is wrong with the patient and what you intend to do about it.

Reference

1. Kroenke K. The case presentation: stumbling blocks and stepping stones. *Am J Med* 1985; 79:605–608.

CHAPTER 51

A suggested method for a rapid screening adult physical examination

A good teacher knows the rules; a good pupil, the exceptions. MARTIN H FISHER (1879–1962)

To all students of medicine who listen, look, touch and reflect: may they hear, see, feel and comprehend. JOHN B BARLOW (1924–2008)

Begin by positioning the appropriately undressed patient in bed. Use this opportunity to make a spot diagnosis if this is possible. Look particularly for any of the diagnostic facies or body habits. Decide whether the patient looks ill or well. Note whether there is any dyspnoea or other distress. Take the blood pressure. Repeat the measurement a few minutes later if the first reading is abnormal.

KEY TO CHAPTER 51

CNS	central (and peripheral) nervous system
CVS	cardiovascular system
ENDO	endocrine system
GIT	gastrointestinal system
HAEM	haematological system
INF	infectious diseases
RENAL	renal system
RESP	respiratory system
RHEUM	rheumatological system

HANDS AND ARMS

Begin by picking up the patient's right hand and examine the nails for clubbing (RESP, CVS, GIT) and for the stigmata of infective endocarditis (CVS) or chronic liver disease (GIT). The nail changes suggesting chronic renal disease or iron deficiency must also be spotted (RENAL, HAEM). Note any evidence of arthropathy (RHEUM). Examine the other hand.

Take the patient's pulse, and note the rate and regularity or irregularity (CVS). While this is being done the arms can be inspected for bruising or scratch marks (GIT, HAEM, RENAL). Determine the state of hydration (GIT, RENAL, CVS). Go on and examine for axillary lymphadenopathy (HAEM). (see Table 51.1).

FACE

Look at the eyes for jaundice (GIT, HAEM) or exophthalmos (ENDO). Look at the face for evidence of a vasculitic rash (RHEUM). Inspect the mouth for mucosal ulcers (RHEUM, GIT, HAEM, INF) and the tongue for glossitis (nutritional deficiencies) or cyanosis (RESP, CVS) or macroglossia (ENDO).

FRONT OF THE NECK

Feel the carotid pulses (see Fig. 51.1) and at 45° pay careful attention to the state of the jugular venous pressure (CVS). Feel gently for the position of the trachea (RESP). Then palpate the supraclavicular lymph nodes (HAEM, GIT).

CHEST

Examine the front of the chest for scars and deformity. Note any spider naevi (GIT) or hair loss (GIT, ENDO). Palpate the chest wall and auscultate the heart (CVS). Then percuss and auscultate the chest (RESP) and examine the breasts.

BACK OF THE CHEST AND NECK

Sit the patient up and lean him or her forwards. After inspection, test chest expansion of the upper and lower lobes of the lungs. Percuss and auscultate the back of the chest (RESP). Feel for cervical lymphadenopathy (RESP,

Nail signs in systemic disease

Nail sign	Some causes	Example
Clubbing	Lung cancer, cyanotic congenital heart disease, endocarditis, inflammatory bowel disease, cirrhosis	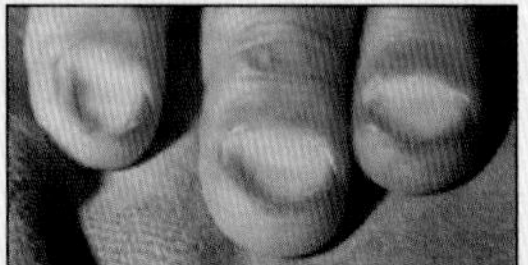
(From Zipes DP, Libby P, Bonow RO, et al. *Braunwald's heart disease: a textbook of cardiovascular medicine*, 7th edn. Philadelphia: WB Saunders, 2005.)		
Koilonychia (spoon-shaped nails)	Iron deficiency anaemia	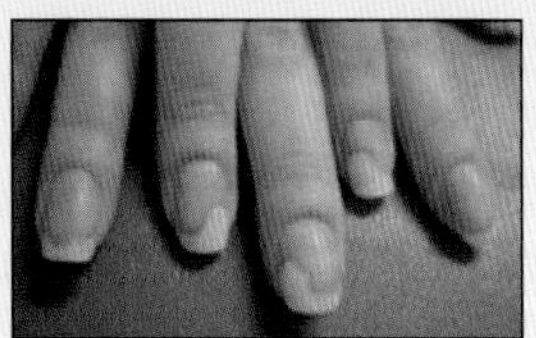
(From James DW. *Andrews' diseases of the skin*. Philadelphia: Elsevier, 2011, Figure 33.41.)		
Onycholysis (separation of nail from nail bed)	Psoriasis, infection, hyperthyroidism, trauma	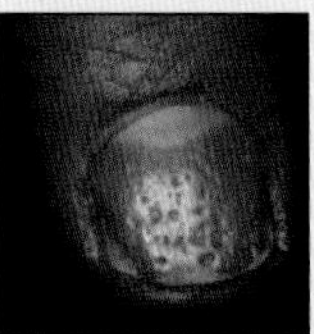
(From Bernard A, Cohen MD. *Pediatric dermatology*, 4th edn. © 2013, Elsevier Limited, Figure 8.67.)		
Pitting	Psoriasis, Reiter syndrome	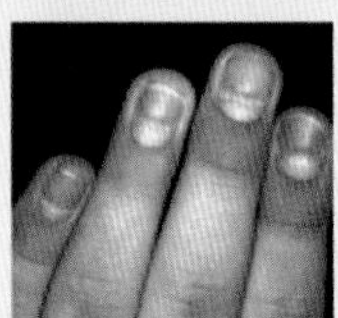
(From Bolognia J, Jorizzo JJ, Schaffer JV. *Dermatology*, 3rd edn. Philadelphia: Elsevier, 2012, Figure 71.4.)		
Beau's lines	Any severe systemic illness that disrupts nail growth, Raynaud disease, pemphigus, trauma	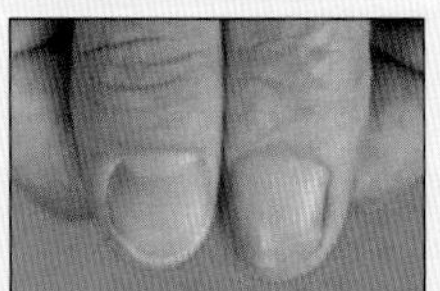
(From Habif TP. *Clinical dermatology: a color guide to diagnosis and therapy*. Philadelphia: Elsevier, 2010, Figure 14-13.)		
Yellow nails	Lymphoedema, pleural effusion, immunodeficiency, bronchiectasis, sinusitis, rheumatoid arthritis, nephrotic syndrome, thyroiditis, tuberculosis, Raynaud disease	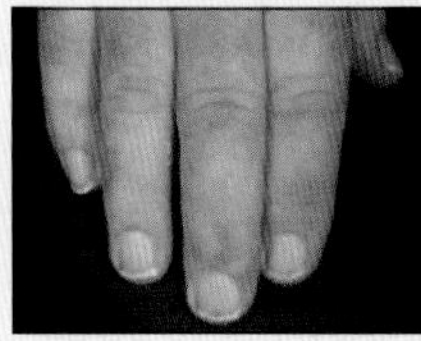
(From Simon RW, Bundi B. Yellow nails, chronic cough, and edema. *American Journal of Medicine* 2010; 123(2):125–126. Philadelphia: Elsevier, Figure 2.)		
Terry's (white) nails	Cirrhosis, malnutrition	
(Callen JP, Jorizzo JL, Bolognia JL, Piette WW, Zone JJ. *Dermatological signs of internal disease*. Elsevier, 2009, Figure 26-5.)		

TABLE 51.1

Nail signs in systemic disease—cont'd

Nail sign	Some causes	Example
Azure lunula (blue nails)	Hepatolenticular degeneration (Wilson's disease), silver poisoning	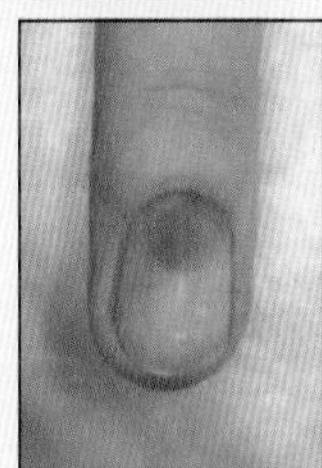
(Naylor EMT, Ruben ES, Robinson-Bostom L, Telang GH, Jellinek NJ. *Journal of the American Academy of Dermatology* 2008; 58(6):1021–1024. Copyright © 2008 American Academy of Dermatology, Inc., Figure 1.)		
Half-and-half nails	Chronic kidney disease	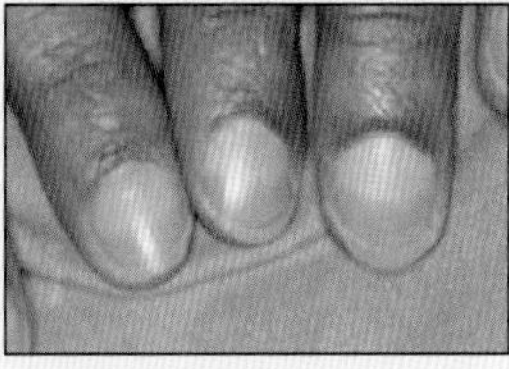
(Schwarzenberger K, Werchniak AE, Ko CJ. *General dermatology*. © 2009, Elsevier Limited, Figure 2-5.)		
Muehrcke's lines Hypoalbuminaemia (any cause)		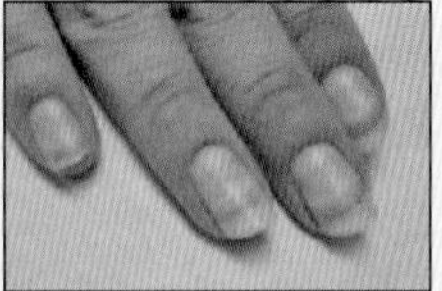
(Short N, Shah C. *American Journal of Medicine* 2010; 123(11):991–992. Copyright © 2010 Elsevier Inc.)		
Mees' lines	Arsenic poisoning, Hodgkin lymphoma, chemotherapy	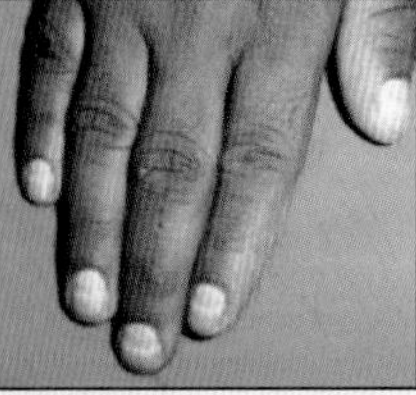
(Chauhan S, D'Cruz S, Singh R, Sachdev A. *The Lancet* 2008; 372(9647):1410–1410. Copyright © 2008 Elsevier.)		
Dark longitudinal streaks	Melanoma, benign naevus, chemical staining	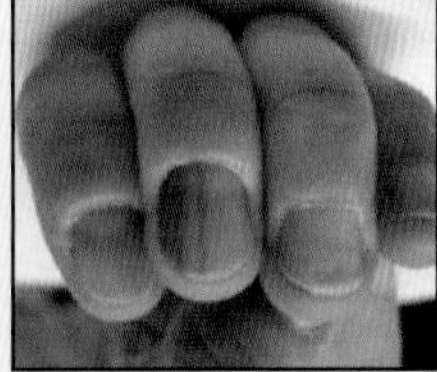
(Piraccini BM, Dika E, Fanti PA. Tips for diagnosis and treatment of nail pigmentation with practical algorithm. *Dermatologic clinics*. Copyright © 2015 Elsevier Inc., Figure 20.)		
Longitudinal striations	Alopecia areata, vitiligo, atopic dermatitis, psoriasis	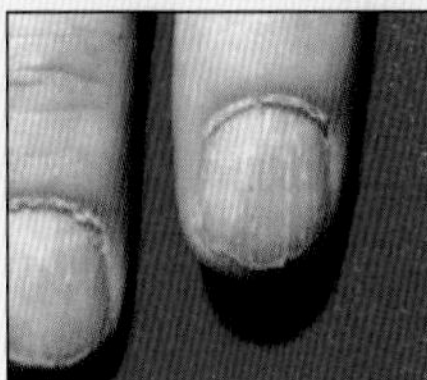
(Paller AS, Mancini AJ. *Hurwitz clinical pediatric dermatology*. Elsevier, Figure 7.54.)		

TABLE 51.1 (Continued)

Nail signs in systemic disease—cont'd

Nail sign	Some causes	Example
Splinter haemorrhages	Infective endocarditis, SLE, rheumatoid arthritis, antiphospholipid syndrome, trauma	
(Forbes & Jackson. *Color atlas and text of clinical medicine* 3rd edn. Elsevier; 2002.)		
Telangiectasia	Rheumatoid arthritis, SLE, dermatomyositis, scleroderma	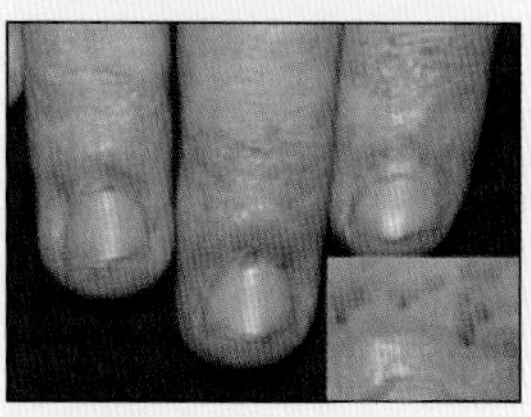
(Bolognia JL, Jorizzo JL, Schaffer JV, et al. *Dermatology*. Elsevier, Figure 42.1. Courtesy Julie V Schaffer, MD.)		

SLE, systemic lupus erythematosus.

TABLE 51.1 (Continued)

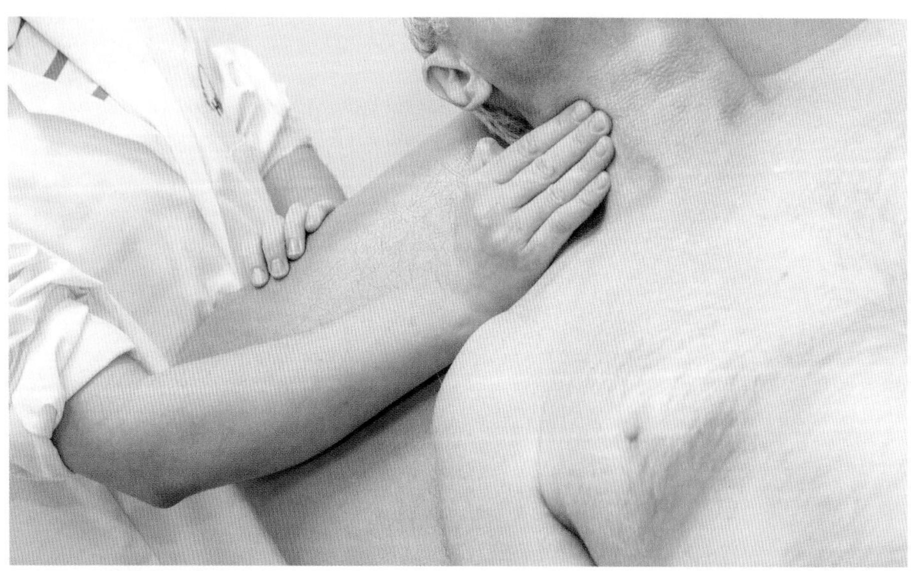

Feeling for the right carotid pulse

FIGURE 51.1

GIT, HAEM). Then examine formally for a goitre from behind (ENDO). Test for sacral oedema (CVS, RENAL).

ABDOMEN

Lay the patient flat on one pillow. Inspect the abdomen from the side and then palpate for organomegaly and other abdominal masses. Percuss for shifting dullness if this is appropriate and auscultate over the abdomen. Palpate for inguinal lymphadenopathy and hernias, and in men palpate the testes (GIT, RENAL).

LEGS

Look for peripheral oedema (CVS, RENAL) and leg ulcers (HAEM, RHEUM, CVS, CNS). Feel all the peripheral pulses (CVS).

NEUROLOGICAL EXAMINATION

Find out whether the patient is right- or left-handed.

Begin with examination of the higher centres and cranial nerves. Test orientation and note any speech defect. Ask about any noticed problem with the sense of smell (I). Then examine the visual acuity, visual fields, the fundi (II), the pupils and eye movements (III, IV, VI). Screen for the other cranial nerves by testing pain sensation over the face (V), the strength of upper and lower facial muscles (VII), whispered voice hearing (VIII), the palatal movement ('Ah') (IX, X), poking out the tongue (XII) and rotation of the head (XI).

Next look for wasting and fasciculation in the upper limbs. Test tone, power (shoulders, elbows, wrists and fingers) and the biceps, triceps and brachioradialis reflexes. Assess finger–nose movements. Then test pinprick sensation on the tip of the shoulder, outer and inner forearms and on the median, ulnar and radial areas of the hands.

Go to the lower limbs. Test gait: ask the patient to walk several paces, turn around rapidly and walk back. Then test heel–toe walking (cerebellum), ability to stand on the toes (S1) and heels (L4, L5) and squatting (proximal muscles). Finally look for Romberg's sign (posterior columns). Next, test hip and knee flexion and extension, and dorsiflexion and plantar flexion of the feet in bed. Then do knee, ankle and plantar reflexes and heel–shin tests. Test pinprick sensation on the middle third of the thighs, both sides of the tibia, the dorsum of the feet, the little toes, on the buttocks and three levels on the trunk on both sides.

COMPLETING THE EXAMINATION

Thorough physical examination may include a rectal or pelvic examination, analysis of the patient's urine, a temperature reading and measurement of height and weight and calculation of the BMI.

Particular details of the examination will be altered depending on what is found. An important guide to the areas where examination should be particularly directed, apart from the history, is the general inspection. A minute spent standing back to inspect the patient before the detailed examination begins is never wasted.

Occam's razor as applied in medicine is as follows: the simplest explanation is the most likely, so consider if a single diagnosis can explain all of the symptoms and signs, and if so according to Occam's razor it's most likely (so keep it simple!).

WILLIAM OF OCKHAM.
Ockham was a brilliant theologian, philosopher and logician in the medieval period.

Hickam's dictum is the antithesis: A man [and refers to all, not just men] can have as many diseases as he damn well pleases.

JOHN HICKAM, MD,
US physician in the mid 20th century.

Index

Page numbers followed by "f" indicate figures, "t" indicate tables, and "b" indicate boxes.

C

D

E

F

I

J

K

L

M

N

O

P

Q

R

S

T

U

Y

Z